HOSPITAL-ACQUIRED INFECTIONS

HOSPITAL-ACQUIRED INFECTIONS

JULIA B. WILCOX
EDITOR

Nova Science Publishers, Inc.
New York

WX
161
H8278
2009

Copyright © 2009 by Nova Science Publishers, Inc.

All rights reserved. No part of this book may be reproduced, stored in a retrieval system or transmitted in any form or by any means: electronic, electrostatic, magnetic, tape, mechanical photocopying, recording or otherwise without the written permission of the Publisher.

For permission to use material from this book please contact us:
Telephone 631-231-7269; Fax 631-231-8175
Web Site: http://www.novapublishers.com

NOTICE TO THE READER
The Publisher has taken reasonable care in the preparation of this book, but makes no expressed or implied warranty of any kind and assumes no responsibility for any errors or omissions. No liability is assumed for incidental or consequential damages in connection with or arising out of information contained in this book. The Publisher shall not be liable for any special, consequential, or exemplary damages resulting, in whole or in part, from the readers' use of, or reliance upon, this material.

Independent verification should be sought for any data, advice or recommendations contained in this book. In addition, no responsibility is assumed by the publisher for any injury and/or damage to persons or property arising from any methods, products, instructions, ideas or otherwise contained in this publication.

This publication is designed to provide accurate and authoritative information with regard to the subject matter covered herein. It is sold with the clear understanding that the Publisher is not engaged in rendering legal or any other professional services. If legal or any other expert assistance is required, the services of a competent person should be sought. FROM A DECLARATION OF PARTICIPANTS JOINTLY ADOPTED BY A COMMITTEE OF THE AMERICAN BAR ASSOCIATION AND A COMMITTEE OF PUBLISHERS.

LIBRARY OF CONGRESS CATALOGING-IN-PUBLICATION DATA
Available upon request.
ISBN: 978-1-60692-728-1

Published by Nova Science Publishers, Inc. ✛ New York

CONTENTS

Preface		vii
Chapter 1	Guideline for Isolation Precautions: Preventing Transmission of Infectious Agents in Healthcare Settings 2007 *Jane D. Siegel, Emily Rhinehart, Marguerite Jackson, Linda Chiarello*	1
Chapter 2	Health-Care-Associated Infections in Hospitals: Leadership Needed from HHS to Prioritize Prevention Practices and Improve Data on these Infections *United States Government Accountability Office*	233
Chapter 3	Health-Care-Associated Infections in Hospitals: An Overview of State Reporting Programs and Individual Hospital Initiatives to Reduce Certain Infections *United States Government Accountability Office*	291
Chapter 4	Health-Care-Associated Infections in Hospitals: Number Associated with Medical Devices Unknown, but Experts Report Provider Practices as a Significant Factor *United States Government Accountability Office*	341
Index		355

PREFACE

Hospital-acquired infections (HAIs), also known as health-care–associated infections, encompass almost all clinically evident infections that do not originate from a patient's original admitting diagnosis. Within hours after admission, a patient's flora begins to acquire characteristics of the surrounding bacterial pool. Most infections that become clinically evident after 48 hours of hospitalization are considered hospital-acquired. Infections that occur after the patient's discharge from the hospital can be considered to have a nosocomial origin if the organisms were acquired during the hospital stay. This new book presents a set of chapters detailing the depth of the problems as well as suggesting remedies.

In: Hospital-Acquired Infections
Editor: Julia B. Wilcox, pp. 1-235

ISBN: 978-1-60692-728-1
© 2009 Nova Science Publishers, Inc.

Chapter 1

GUIDELINE FOR ISOLATION PRECAUTIONS: PREVENTING TRANSMISSION OF INFECTIOUS AGENTS IN HEALTHCARE SETTINGS 2007[*]

Jane D. Siegel, Emily Rhinehart, Marguerite Jackson, Linda Chiarello

The Healthcare Infection Control Practices Advisory Committee

EXECUTIVE SUMMARY

The *Guideline for Isolation Precautions: Preventing Transmission of Infectious Agents in Healthcare Settings 2007* updates and expands the *1996 Guideline for Isolation Precautions in Hospitals*. The following developments led to revision of the 1996 guideline:

1. The transition of healthcare delivery from primarily acute care hospitals to other healthcare settings (e.g., home care, ambulatory care, free-standing specialty care sites, long-term care) created a need for recommendations that can be applied in all healthcare settings using common principles of

---

[*] The authors and HICPAC gratefully acknowledge Dr. Larry Strausbaugh for his many contributions and valued guidance in the preparation of this guideline. *Suggested citation: Siegel JD, Rhinehart E, Jackson M, Chiarello L, and the Healthcare Infection Control Practices Advisory Committee, 2007 Guideline for Isolation Precautions: Preventing Transmission of Ifnectious Agents in Healthcare Settings, June 2007* http://www.cdc.gov/ncidod/ dhqp/pdf/isolation2007.pdf

infection control practice, yet can be modified to reflect setting-specific needs. Accordingly, the revised guideline addresses the spectrum of healthcare delivery settings. Furthermore, the term "nosocomial infections" is replaced by "healthcare- associated infections" (HAIs) to reflect the changing patterns in healthcare delivery and difficulty in determining the geographic site of exposure to an infectious agent and/or acquisition of infection.

2. The emergence of new pathogens (e.g., SARS-CoV associated with the severe acute respiratory syndrome [SARS], Avian influenza in humans), renewed concern for evolving known pathogens (e.g., *C. difficile,* noroviruses, community- associated MRSA [CA-MRSA]), development of new therapies (e.g., gene therapy), and increasing concern for the threat of bioweapons attacks, established a need to address a broader scope of issues than in previous isolation guidelines.

3. The successful experience with Standard Precautions, first recommended in the 1996 guideline, has led to a reaffirmation of this approach as the foundation for preventing transmission of infectious agents in all healthcare settings. New additions to the recommendations for Standard Precautions are Respiratory Hygiene/Cough Etiquette and safe injection practices, including the use of a mask when performing certain high-risk, prolonged procedures involving spinal canal punctures (e.g., myelography, epidural anesthesia). The need for a recommendation for Respiratory Hygiene/Cough Etiquette grew out of observations during the SARS outbreaks where failure to implement simple source control measures with patients, visitors, and healthcare personnel with respiratory symptoms may have contributed to SARS coronavirus (SARS-CoV) transmission. The recommended practices have a strong evidence base. The continued occurrence of outbreaks of hepatitis B and hepatitis C viruses in ambulatory settings indicated a need to re-iterate safe injection practice recommendations as part of Standard Precautions. The addition of a mask for certain spinal injections grew from recent evidence of an associated risk for developing meningitis caused by respiratory flora.

4. The accumulated evidence that environmental controls decrease the risk of life- threatening fungal infections in the most severely immunocompromised patients (allogeneic hematopoietic stem-cell transplant patients) led to the update on the components of the Protective Environment (PE).

5. Evidence that organizational characteristics (e.g., nurse staffing levels and composition, establishment of a safety culture) influence healthcare personnel adherence to recommended infection control practices, and

therefore are important factors in preventing transmission of infectious agents, led to a new emphasis and recommendations for administrative involvement in the development and support of infection control programs.

6   Continued increase in the incidence of HAIs caused by multidrug-resistant organisms (MDROs) in all healthcare settings and the expanded body of knowledge concerning prevention of transmission of MDROs created a need for more specific recommendations for surveillance and control of these pathogens that would be practical and effective in various types of healthcare settings.

This document is intended for use by infection control staff, healthcare epidemiologists, healthcare administrators, nurses, other healthcare providers, and persons responsible for developing, implementing, and evaluating infection control programs for healthcare settings across the continuum of care. The reader is referred to other guidelines and websites for more detailed information and for recommendations concerning specialized infection control problems.

Parts I - III: Review of the Scientific Data Regarding Transmission of Infectious Agents in Healthcare Settings Part I reviews the relevant scientific literature that supports the recommended prevention and control practices. As with the 1996 guideline, the modes and factors that influence transmission risks are described in detail. New to the section on transmission are discussions of bioaerosols and of how droplet and airborne transmission may contribute to infection transmission. This became a concern during the SARS outbreaks of 2003, when transmission associated with aerosol-generating procedures was observed. Also new is a definition of "epidemiologically important organisms" that was developed to assist in the identification of clusters of infections that require investigation (i.e. multidrug-resistant organisms, *C. difficile)*. Several other pathogens that hold special infection control interest (i.e., norovirus, SARS, Category A bioterrorist agents, prions, monkeypox, and the hemorrhagic fever viruses) also are discussed to present new information and infection control lessons learned from experience with these agents. This section of the guideline also presents information on infection risks associated with specific healthcare settings and patient populations.

Part II updates information on the basic principles of hand hygiene, barrier precautions, safe work practices and isolation practices that were included in previous guidelines. However, new to this guideline, is important information on healthcare system components that influence transmission risks, including those under the influence of healthcare administrators. An important administrative priority that is described is the need for appropriate infection control staffing to meet the ever-expanding role of infection control professionals in the modern, complex healthcare system. Evidence presented also demonstrates another administrative concern, the importance of nurse staffing levels, including numbers of appropriately trained nurses in ICUs for preventing HAIs. The role of the clinical microbiology laboratory in supporting infection control is described to emphasize the need for this service in healthcare facilites. Other factors that influence transmission risks are discussed i.e., healthcare worker adherence to recommended infection control practices, organizational safety culture or climate, education and training

Discussed for the first time in an isolation guideline is surveillance of healthcare-associated infections. The information presented will be useful to new infection control professionals as well as persons involved in designing or responding to state programs for public reporting of HAI rates.

Part III describes each of the categories of precautions developed by the Healthcare Infection Control Practices Advisory Committee (HICPAC) and the Centers for Disease Control and Prevention (CDC) and provides guidance for their application in various healthcare settings. The categories of Transmission-Based Precautions are unchanged from those in the 1996 guideline: Contact, Droplet, and Airborne. One important change is the recommendation to don the indicated personal protective equipment (gowns, gloves, mask) *upon entry into the patient's room* for patients who are on Contact and/or Droplet Precautions since the nature of the interaction with the patient cannot be predicted with certainty and contaminated environmental surfaces are important sources for transmission of pathogens.

In addition, the Protective Environment (PE) for allogeneic hematopoietic stem cell transplant patients, described in previous guidelines, has been updated.

Tables, Appendices, and other Information

There are several tables that summarize important information: 1) a summary of the evolution of this document; 2) guidance on using empiric isolation precautions according to a clinical syndrome; 3) a summary of infection control recommendations for category A agents of bioterrorism; 4) components of Standard Precautions and recommendations for their application; 5) components of the Protective Environment; and 6) a glossary of definitions used in this guideline. New in this guideline is a figure that shows a recommended sequence for donning and removing personal protective equipment used for isolation precautions to optimize safety and prevent self-contamination during removal.

Appendix A: Type and Duration of Precautions Recommended for Selected Infections and Conditions

Appendix A consists of an updated alphabetical list of most infectious agents and clinical conditions for which isolation precautions are recommended. A preamble to the Appendix provides a rationale for recommending the use of one or more Transmission-Based Precautions, in addition to Standard Precautions, based on a review of the literature and evidence demonstrating a real or potential risk for person-to-person transmission in healthcare settings.The type and duration of recommended precautions are presented with additional comments concerning the use of adjunctive measures or other relevant considerations to prevent transmission of the specific agent. Relevant citations are included.

Pre- Publication of the Guideline on Preventing Transmission of MDROs

New to this guideline is a comprehensive review and detailed recommendations for prevention of transmission of MDROs. This portion of the guideline was published electronically in October 2006 and updated in November, 2006 (Siegel JD, Rhinehart E, Jackson M, Chiarello L and HICPAC. Management of Multidrug-Resistant Organisms in Healthcare Settings 2006 www.cdc.gov/ncidod/dhqp/pdf/ar/mdroGuideline2006.pdf), and is considered a part of the Guideline for Isolation Precautions. This section provides a detailed review of the complex topic of MDRO control in healthcare settings and is intended to provide a context for evaluation of MDRO at individual healthcare settings. A rationale and institutional requirements for developing an effective MDRO control program are summarized. Although the focus of this guideline is on measures to prevent *transmission* of MDROs in healthcare settings, information concerning the judicious use of antimicrobial agents is presented since such practices are intricately related to the size of the reservoir of MDROs which in turn influences transmission (e.g. colonization pressure). There are two tables that summarize recommended prevention and control practices using the following seven categories of interventions to control MDROs: administrative measures, education of healthcare personnel, judicious antimicrobial use, surveillance, infection control precautions, environmental measures, and decolonization. Recommendations for each category apply to and are adapted for the various healthcare settings. With the increasing incidence and prevalence of MDROs, all healthcare facilities must prioritize effective control of MDRO transmission.

Facilities should identify prevalent MDROs at the facility, implement control measures, assess the effectiveness of control programs, and demonstrate decreasing MDRO rates. A set of intensified MDRO prevention interventions is presented to be added 1) if the incidence of transmission of a target MDRO is NOT decreasing despite implementation of basic MDRO infection control measures, and 2) when the *first* case(s) of an epidemiologically important MDRO is identified within a healthcare facility.

Summary

This updated guideline responds to changes in healthcare delivery and addresses new concerns about transmission of infectious agents to patients and healthcare workers in the United States and infection control. The primary objective of the guideline is to improve the safety of the nation's healthcare delivery system by reducing the rates of HAIs.

Abbreviations Used in the Guideline

AIIR	Airborne infection isolation room
CDC	Centers for Disease Control and Prevention
CF	Cystic fibrosis
CJD	Creutzfeld-Jakob Disease
CLSI	Clinical Laboratory Standards Institute
ESBL	Extended spectrum beta-lactamases
FDA	Food and Drug Administration
HAI	Healthcare-associated infections
HBV	Hepatitis B virus
HCV	Hepatitis C virus
HEPA	High efficiency particulate air [filtration]
HICPAC	Healthcare Infection Control Practices Advisory Committee
HIV	Human immunodeficiency virus
HCW	Healthcare worker
HSCT	Hematopoetic stem-cell transplant
ICU	Intensive care unit
LTCF	Long-term care facility
MDRO	M ultidrug-resistant organism
M DR-GNB	M ultidrug-resistant gram-negative bacilli

MRSA	Meth ici ll in-resistant *Staphylococcus aureus*
NCCLS	National Committee for Clinical Laboratory Standards
NICU	Neonatal intensive care unit
NIOSH	National Institute for Occupational Safety and Health, CDC
NNIS	National Nosocomial Infection Surveillance
NSSP	Nonsuscepti ble *Streptococcus pneumoniae*
OSHA	Occupational Safety and Health Administration
PICU	Pediatric intensive care unit
PPE	Personal protective equipment
RSV	Respiratory syncytial virus
SARS	Severe acquired respiratory syndrome
vCJD	variant Creutzfeld-Jakob Disease
VRE	Vancomyci n-resistant enterococci
WHO	World Health Organization

PART I: REVIEW OF SCIENTIFIC DATA REGARDING TRANSMISSION OF INFECTIOUS AGENTS IN HEALTHCARE SETTINGS

I.A. Evolution of the 2007 Document

The *Guideline for Isolation Precautions: Preventing Transmission of Infectious Agents in Healthcare Settings 2007* builds upon a series of isolation and infection prevention documents promulgated since 1970. These previous documents are summarized and referenced in Table 1 and in Part I of the *1996 Guideline for Isolation Precautions in Hospitals*[1].

Objectives and Methods

The objectives of this guideline are to 1) provide infection control recommendations for all components of the healthcare delivery system, including hospitals, long-term care facilities, ambulatory care, home care and hospice; 2) reaffirm Standard Precautions as the foundation for preventing transmission during patient care in all healthcare settings; 3) reaffirm the importance of implementing Transmission-Based Precautions based on the clinical presentation or syndrome and likely pathogens until the infectious etiology has been determined (Table 2); and 4) provide epidemiologically sound and, whenever possible, evidence-based recommendations.

This guideline is designed for use by individuals who are charged with administering infection control programs in hospitals and other healthcare settings. The information also will be useful for other healthcare personnel, healthcare administrators, and anyone needing information about infection control measures to prevent transmission of infectious agents. Commonly used abbreviations are provided on page 11 and terms used in the guideline are defined in the Glossary (page 137).

Med-line and Pub Med were used to search for relevant studies published in English, focusing on those published since 1996. Much of the evidence cited for preventing transmission of infectious agents in healthcare settings is derived from studies that used "quasi-experimental designs", also referred to as nonrandomized, pre- post-intervention study designs[2]. Although these types of studies can provide valuable information regarding the effectiveness of various interventions, several factors decrease the certainty of attributing improved outcome to a specific intervention. These include: difficulties in controlling for important confounding variables; the use of multiple interventions during an outbreak; and results that are explained by the statistical principle of regression to the mean, (e.g., improvement over time without any intervention)[3]. Observational studies remain relevant and have been used to evaluate infection control interventions[4,5]. The quality of studies, consistency of results and correlation with results from randomized, controlled trials when available were considered during the literature review and assignment of evidence-based categories (See Part IV: Recommendations) to the recommendations in this guideline. Several authors have summarized properties to consider when evaluating studies for the purpose of determining if the results should change practice or in designing new studies[2,6,7].

Changes or Clarifications in Terminology

This guideline contains four changes in terminology from the 1996 guideline:

- The term *nosocomial infection* is retained to refer only to infections acquired in hospitals. The term *healthcare-associated infection* (HAI) is used to refer to infections associated with healthcare delivery in any setting (e.g., hospitals, long-term care facilities, ambulatory settings, home care). This term reflects the inability to determine with certainty where the pathogen is acquired since patients may be colonized with or exposed to potential pathogens outside of the healthcare setting, before receiving health care, or may develop infections caused by those pathogens when exposed to the conditions associated with delivery of healthcare.

Additionally, patients frequently move among the various settings within a healthcare system[8].
- A new addition to the practice recommendations for Standard Precautions is *Respiratory Hygiene/Cough Etiquette*. While Standard Precautions generally apply to the recommended practices of healthcare personnel during patient care, Respiratory Hygiene/Cough Etiquette applies broadly to all persons who enter a healthcare setting, including healthcare personnel, patients and visitors. These recommendations evolved from observations during the SARS epidemic that failure to implement basic source control measures with patients, visitors, and healthcare personnel with signs and symptoms of respiratory tract infection may have contributed to SARS coronavirus (SARS-CoV) transmission. This concept has been incorporated into CDC planning documents for SARS and pandemic influenza[9,10].
- The term *"Airborne Precautions"* has been supplemented with the term *"Airborne Infection Isolation Room (AIIR)"* for consistency with the *Guidelines for Environmental Infection Control in Healthcare Facilities*[11], the *Guidelines for Preventing the Transmission of Mycobacterium tuberculosis in Health-Care Settings 2005[12]* and the American Institute of Architects (AIA) guidelines for design and construction of hospitals, 2006 [13]
- A set of prevention measures termed *Protective Environment* has been added to the precautions used to prevent HAIs. These measures, which have been defined in other guidelines , consist of engineering and design interventions that decrease the risk of exposure to environmental fungi for severely immunocompromised allogeneic hematiopoietic stem cell transplant (HSCT) patients during their highest risk phase, usually the first 100 days post transplant, or longer in the presence of graft-versus-host disease[11,13-15]. Recommendations for a Protective Environment apply only to acute care hospitals that provide care to HSCT patients.

Scope

This guideline, like its predecessors, focuses primarily on interactions between patients and healthcare providers. The Guidelines for the Prevention of MDRO Infection were published separately in November 2006, and are available online at www.cdc.gov/ncidod/dhqp/index.html. Several other H ICPAC guidelines to prevent transmission of infectious agents associated with healthcare delivery are cited; e.g., *Guideline for Hand Hygiene*, *Guideline for Environmental Infection Control*, *Guideline for Prevention of Healthcare-*

Associated Pneumonia, and *Guideline for Infection Control in Healthcare Personnel* [11,14,16,17]. In combination, these provide comprehensive guidance on the primary infection control measures for ensuring a safe environment for patients and healthcare personnel.

This guideline does not discuss in detail specialized infection control issues in defined populations that are addressed elsewhere, (e.g., *Recommendations for Preventing Transmission of Infections among Chronic Hemodialysis Patients , Guidelines for Preventing the Transmission of Mycobacterium tuberculosis in Health-Care Facilities 2005, Guidelines for Infection Control in Dental Health-Care Settings and Infection Control Recommendations for Patients with Cystic Fibrosis* [12,18-20]. An exception has been made by including abbreviated guidance for a Protective Environment used for allogeneic HSCT recipients because components of the Protective Environment have been more completely defined since publication of the *Guidelines for Preventing Opportunistic Infections Among HSCT Recipients in 2000* and the *Guideline for Environmental Infection Control in Healthcare Facilities* [11,15].

I.B. Rationale for Standard and Transmission-Based Precautions in Healthcare Settings

Transmission of infectious agents within a healthcare setting requires three elements: a source (or reservoir) of infectious agents, a susceptible host with a portal of entry receptive to the agent, and a mode of transmission for the agent. This section describes the interrelationship of these elements in the epidemiology of HAIs.

I.B.1. Sources of Infectious Agents

Infectious agents transmitted during healthcare derive primarily from human sources but inanimate environmental sources also are implicated in transmission. Human reservoirs include patients [20-28], healthcare personnel [29-35,17,36-39], and household members and other visitors [40-45]. Such source individuals may have active infections, may be in the asymptomatic and/or incubation period of an infectious disease, or may be transiently or chronically colonized with pathogenic microorganisms, particularly in the respiratory and gastrointestinal tracts. The endogenous flora of patients (e.g., bacteria residing in the respiratory or gastrointestinal tract) also are the source of HAIs [46-54].

I.B.2. Susceptible Hosts

Infection is the result of a complex interrelationship between a potential host and an infectious agent. Most of the factors that influence infection and the occurrence and severity of disease are related to the host. However, characteristics of the host-agent interaction as it relates to pathogenicity, virulence and antigenicity are also important, as are the infectious dose, mechanisms of disease production and route of exposure [55]. There is a spectrum of possible outcomes following exposure to an infectious agent. Some persons exposed to pathogenic microorganisms never develop symptomatic disease while others become severely ill and even die. Some individuals are prone to becoming transiently or permanently colonized but remain asymptomatic. Still others progress from colonization to symptomatic disease either immediately following exposure, or after a period of asymptomatic colonization. The immune state at the time of exposure to an infectious agent, interaction between pathogens, and virulence factors intrinsic to the agent are important predictors of an individuals' outcome. Host factors such as extremes of age and underlying disease (e.g. diabetes[56,57]), human immunodeficiency virus/acquired immune deficiency syndrome [HIV/AIDS] [58,59], malignancy, and transplants [18, 60, 61] can increase susceptibility to infection as do a variety of medications that alter the normal flora (e.g., antimicrobial agents, gastric acid suppressants, corticosteroids, antirejection drugs, antineoplastic agents, and immunosuppressive drugs). Surgical procedures and radiation therapy impair defenses of the skin and other involved organ systems. Indwelling devices such as urinary catheters, endotracheal tubes, central venous and arterial catheters [62-64] and synthetic implants facilitate development of HAIs by allowing potential pathogens to bypass local defenses that would ordinarily impede their invasion and by providing surfaces for development of bioflms that may facilitate adherence of microorganisms and protect from antimicrobial activity [65] . Some infections associated with invasive procedures result from transmission within the healthcare facility; others arise from the patient's endogenous flora [46-50] . High-risk patient populations with noteworthy risk factors for infection are discussed further in Sections I.D, I.E., and I.F.

I.B.3. Modes of Transmission

Several classes of pathogens can cause infection, including bacteria, viruses, fungi, parasites, and prions. The modes of transmission vary by type of organism and some infectious agents may be transmitted by more than one route: some are transmitted primarily by direct or indirect contact, (e.g., *Herpes simplex* virus [HSV], respiratory syncytial virus, *Staphylococcus aureus*), others by the droplet, (e.g., influenza virus, *B. pertussis*) or airborne routes (e.g., *M.*

tuberculosis). Other infectious agents, such as bloodborne viruses (e.g., hepatitis B and C viruses [HBV, HCV] and HIV are transmitted rarely in healthcare settings, via percutaneous or mucous membrane exposure. Importantly, not all infectious agents are transmitted from person to person. These are distinguished in Appendix A. The three principal routes of transmission are summarized below.

I.B.3.A. Contact Transmission

The most common mode of transmission, contact transmission is divided into two subgroups: direct contact and indirect contact.

I.B.3.A.I. Direct Contact Transmission

Direct transmission occurs when microorganisms are transferred from one infected person to another person without a contaminated intermediate object or person. Opportunities for direct contact transmission between patients and healthcare personnel have been summarized in the Guideline for Infection Control in Healthcare Personnel, 1998 [17] and include:

- blood or other blood-containing body fluids from a patient directly enters a caregiver's body through contact with a mucous membrane 66 or breaks (i.e., cuts, abrasions) in the skin [67].
- mites from a scabies-infested patient are transferred to the skin of a caregiver while he/she is having direct ungloved contact with the patient's skin [68, 69].
- a healthcare provider develops herpetic whitlow on a finger after contact with HSV when providing oral care to a patient without using gloves or HSV is transmitted to a patient from a herpetic whitlow on an ungloved hand of a healthcare worker (HCW) [70, 71].

I.B.3.A.II. Indirect Contact Transmission

Indirect transmission involves the transfer of an infectious agent through a contaminated intermediate object or person. In the absence of a point-source outbreak, it is difficult to determine how indirect transmission occurs. However, extensive evidence cited in the Guideline for Hand Hygiene in Health-Care Settings suggests that the contaminated hands of healthcare personnel are important contributors to indirect contact transmission [16] . Examples of opportunities for indirect contact transmission include:

- Hands of healthcare personnel may transmit pathogens after touching an infected or colonized body site on one patient or a contaminated

inanimate object, if hand hygiene is not performed before touching another patient.[72, 73].
- Patient-care devices (e.g., electronic thermometers, glucose monitoring devices) may transmit pathogens if devices contaminated with blood or body fluids are shared between patients without cleaning and disinfecting between patients [74 75-77].
- Shared toys may become a vehicle for transmitting respiratory viruses (e.g., respiratory syncytial virus [24, 78, 79] or pathogenic bacteria (e.g., *Pseudomonas aeruginosa* [80]) among pediatric patients.
- Instruments that are inadequately cleaned between patients before disinfection or sterilization (e.g., endoscopes or surgical instruments) [81-85] or that have manufacturing defects that interfere with the effectiveness of reprocessing [86, 87] may transmit bacterial and viral pathogens.

Clothing, uniforms, laboratory coats, or isolation gowns used as personal protective equipment (PPE), may become contaminated with potential pathogens after care of a patient colonized or infected with an infectious agent, (e.g., MRSA [88], VRE [89], and C. *difficile* [90]. Although contaminated clothing has not been implicated directly in transmission, the potential exists for soiled garments to transfer infectious agents to successive patients.

I.B.3.B. Droplet Transmission

Droplet transmission is, technically, a form of contact transmission, and some infectious agents transmitted by the droplet route also may be transmitted by the direct and indirect contact routes. However, in contrast to contact transmission, respiratory droplets carrying infectious pathogens transmit infection when they travel directly from the respiratory tract of the infectious individual to susceptible mucosal surfaces of the recipient, generally over short distances, necessitating facial protection. Respiratory droplets are generated when an infected person coughs, sneezes, or talks [91, 92] or during procedures such as suctioning, endotracheal intubation, [93-96], cough induction by chest physiotherapy [97] and cardiopulmonary resuscitation [98, 99]. Evidence for droplet transmission comes from epidemiological studies of disease outbreaks [100-103], experimental studies [104] and from information on aerosol dynamics [91, 105]. Studies have shown that the nasal mucosa, conjunctivae and less frequently the mouth, are susceptible portals of entry for respiratory viruses [106]. The maximum distance for droplet transmission is currently unresolved, although pathogens transmitted by the droplet route have not been transmitted through the air over long distances, in contrast to the airborne pathogens discussed below. Historically, the area of defined risk has been a distance of <3 feet around the patient and is based on epidemiologic and simulated studies of selected infections [103, 104]. Using this distance for donning masks has been effective in preventing transmission of infectious agents via the droplet route. However, experimental studies with smallpox [107, 108] and investigations during the global SARS outbreaks of 2003 [101] suggest that droplets from patients with these two infections could reach persons located 6 feet or more from their source. It is likely that the distance droplets travel depends on the velocity and mechanism by which respiratory droplets are propelled from the source, the density of respiratory secretions, environmental factors such as temperature and humidity, and the ability of the pathogen to maintain infectivity over that distance [105]. Thus, a distance of <3 feet around the patient is best viewed as an *example* of what is meant by "a short distance from a patient" and should not be used as the sole *criterion* for deciding when a mask should be donned to protect from droplet exposure. Based on these considerations, it may be prudent to don a mask when within 6 to 10 feet of the patient or upon entry into the patient's room, especially when exposure to emerging or highly virulent pathogens is likely. More studies are needed to improve understanding of droplet transmission under various circumstances.

Droplet size is another variable under discussion. Droplets traditionally have been defined as being >5 μm in size. Droplet nuclei, particles arising from desiccation of suspended droplets, have been associated with airborne transmission and defined as <5 μm in size [105], a reflection of the pathogenesis of pulmonary tuberculosis which is not generalizeable to other organisms. Observations of particle dynamics have demonstrated that a range of droplet sizes, including those with diameters of 30μm or greater, can remain suspended in the air [109]. The behavior of droplets and droplet nuclei affect recommendations for preventing transmission. Whereas fine airborne particles containing pathogens that are able to remain infective may transmit infections over long distances, requiring AIIR to prevent its dissemination within a facility; organisms transmitted by the droplet route do not remain infective over long distances, and therefore do not require special air handling and ventilation. Examples of infectious agents that are transmitted via the droplet route include *Bordetella pertussis* [110], influenza virus [23], adenovirus [111], rhinovirus [104], *Mycoplasma pneumoniae* [112], SARS-associated coronavirus (SARS-CoV) [21, 96, 113], group A streptococcus [114], and *Neisseria meningitidis* [95, 103, 115]. Although respiratory syncytial virus may be transmitted by the droplet route, direct contact with infected respiratory secretions is the most important determinant of transmission and consistent adherence to

Standard plus Contact Precautions prevents transmission in healthcare settings [24, 116, 117].

Rarely, pathogens that are not transmitted routinely by the droplet route are dispersed into the air over short distances. For example, although *S. aureus* is transmitted most frequently by the contact route, viral upper respiratory tract infection has been associated with increased dispersal of *S. aureus* from the nose into the air for a distance of 4 feet under both outbreak and experimental conditions and is known as the "cloud baby" and "cloud adult" phenomenon [118-120].

I.B.3.C. Airborne Transmission

Airborne transmission occurs by dissemination of either airborne droplet nuclei or small particles in the respirable size range containing infectious agents that remain infective over time and distance (e.g., spores of *Aspergillus* spp, and *Mycobacterium tuberculosis*). Microorganisms carried in this manner may be dispersed over long distances by air currents and may be inhaled by susceptible individuals who have not had face-to-face contact with (or been in the same room with) the infectious individual [121-124]. Preventing the spread of pathogens that are transmitted by the airborne route requires the use of special air handling and ventilation systems (e.g., AIIRs) to contain and then safely remove the infectious agent [11, 12]. Infectious agents to which this applies include *Mycobacterium tuberculosis* [124-127], rubeola virus (measles) [122], and varicella-zoster virus (chickenpox) [123]. In addition, published data suggest the possibility that variola virus (smallpox) may be transmitted over long distances through the air under unusual circumstances and AIIRs are recommended for this agent as well; however, droplet and contact routes are the more frequent routes of transmission for smallpox [108, 128, 129]. In addition to AIIRs, respiratory protection with NIOSH certified N95 or higher level respirator is recommended for healthcare personnel entering the AIIR to prevent acquisition of airborne infectious agents such as *M. tuberculosis* [12].

For certain other respiratory infectious agents, such as influenza [130, 131] and rhinovirus [104], and even some gastrointestinal viruses (e.g., norovirus [132] and rotavirus [133]) there is some evidence that the pathogen may be transmitted via small-particle aerosols, under natural and experimental conditions. Such transmission has occurred over distances longer than 3 feet but within a defined airspace (e.g., patient room), suggesting that it is unlikely that these agents remain viable on air currents that travel long distances. AIIRs are not required routinely to prevent transmission of these agents. Additional issues concerning examples of small particle aerosol transmission of agents that are most frequently transmitted by the droplet route are discussed below.

I.B.3.D. Emerging Issues Concerning Airborne Transmission of Infectious Agents

I.B.3.D.I. Transmission from Patients

The emergence of SARS in 2002, the importation of monkeypox into the United States in 2003, and the emergence of avian influenza present challenges to the assignment of isolation categories because of conflicting information and uncertainty about possible routes of transmission. Although SARS-CoV is transmitted primarily by contact and/or droplet routes, airborne transmission over a limited distance (e.g. within a room), has been suggested, though not proven [134-141]. This is true of other infectious agents such as influenza virus [130] and noroviruses [132, 142, 143]. Influenza viruses are transmitted primarily by close contact with respiratory droplets [23, 102] and acquisition by healthcare personnel has been prevented by Droplet Precautions, even when positive pressure rooms were used in one center [144] However, inhalational transmission could not be excluded in an outbreak of influenza in the passengers and crew of a single aircraft [130]. Observations of a protective effect of UV lights in preventing influenza among patients with tuberculosis during the influenza pandemic of 1957-'58 have been used to suggest airborne transmission [145, 146.]

In contrast to the strict interpretation of an airborne route for transmission (i.e., long distances beyond the patient room environment), short distance transmission by small particle aerosols generated under specific circumstances (e.g., during endotracheal intubation) to persons in the immediate area near the patient has been demonstrated. Also, aerosolized particles <100 m can remain suspended in air when room air current velocities exceed the terminal settling velocities of the particles [109]. SARS-CoV transmission has been associated with endotracheal intubation, noninvasive positive pressure ventilation, and cardio-pulmonary resuscitation [93, 94, 96, 98, 141]. Although the most frequent routes of transmission of noroviruses are contact and food and waterborne routes, several reports suggest that noroviruses may be transmitted through aerosolization of infectious particles from vomitus or fecal material [142, 143, 147, 148]. It is hypothesized that the aerosolized particles are inhaled and subsequently swallowed.

Roy and Milton proposed a new classification for aerosol transmission when evaluating routes of SARS transmission: 1) *obligate*: under natural conditions, disease occurs following transmission of the agent only through inhalation of small particle aerosols (e.g., tuberculosis); 2) *preferential*: natural infection results from transmission through multiple routes, but small particle aerosols are the predominant route (e.g. measles, varicella); and 3) *opportunistic*: agents that naturally cause disease through other routes, but under special circumstances may be transmitted via fine particle aerosols [149] . This conceptual framework can explain rare occurrences of airborne transmission of agents that are transmitted most frequently by other routes (e.g., smallpox, SARS, influenza, noroviruses). Concerns about unknown or possible routes of transmission of agents associated with severe disease and no known treatment often result in more extreme prevention strategies than may be necessary; therefore, recommended precautions could change as the epidemiology of an emerging infection is defined and controversial issues are resolved.

I.B.3.D.II. Transmission from the Environment

Some airborne infectious agents are derived from the environment and do not usually involve person-toperson transmission. For example, anthrax spores present in a finely milled powdered preparation can be aerosolized from contaminated environmental surfaces and inhaled into the respiratory tract [150, 151] . Spores of environmental fungi (e.g., *Aspergillus spp.*) are ubiquitous in the environment and may cause disease in immunocompromised patients who inhale aerosolized (e.g., via construction dust) spores [152, 153] . As a rule, neither of these organisms is subsequently transmitted from infected patients. However, there is one well- documented report of person-to-person transmission of *Aspergillus* sp. in the ICU setting that was most likey due to the aerosolization of spores during wound debridement [154] . A Protective Environment refers to isolation practices designed to decrease the risk of exposure to environmental fungal agents in allogeneic HSCT patients [11, 14, 15, 155-158].

Environmental sources of respiratory pathogens (eg. Legionella) transmitted to humans through a common aerosol source is distinct from direct patient-topatient transmission.

I.B.3.E. Other Sources of Infection

Transmission of infection from sources other than infectious individuals include those associated with *common environmental sources or vehicles* (e.g. contaminated food, water, or medications (e.g. intravenous fluids). Although *Aspergillus* spp. have been recovered from hospital water systems [159] , the role of water as a reservoir for i m mu nosu ppressed patients remains uncertain. *Vectorborne transmission* of infectious agents from mosquitoes, flies, rats, and other vermin also can occur in healthcare settings. Prevention of vector borne transmission is not addressed in this document.

I.C. Infectious Agents of Special Infection Control Interest for Healthcare Settings

Several infectious agents with important infection control implications that either were not discussed extensively in previous isolation guidelines or have emerged recently are discussed below. These are epidemiologically important organisms (e.g., *C. difficile*), agents of bioterrorism, prions, SARS-CoV, monkeypox, noroviruses, and the hemorrhagic fever viruses. Experience with these agents has broadened the understanding of modes of transmission and effective preventive measures. These agents are included for purposes of information and, for some (i.e., SARS-CoV, monkeypox), because of the lessons that have been learned about preparedness planning and responding effectively to new infectious agents.

I.C.1. Epidemiologically Important Organisms

Any infectious agents transmitted in healthcare settings may, under defined conditions, become targeted for control because it is or has become epidemiologically important. *C. difficile* is specifically discussed below because of wide recognition of its current importance in U.S. healthcare facilities. In determining what constitutes an "epidemiologically important organism", the following characteristics apply:

- A propensity for transmission within healthcare facilities based on published reports and the occurrence of temporal or geographic clusters of > 2 patients, (e.g., *C.difficile*, norovirus, respiratory syncytial virus (RSV), influenza, rotavirus, *Enterobacter* spp; *Serratia* spp., group A streptococcus). A single case of healthcare-associated invasive disease caused by certain pathogens (e.g., group A streptococcus post-operatively [160], in burn units [161], or in a LTCF [162]; *Legionella* sp. [14, 163], *Aspergillus* sp. [164]) is generally considered a trigger for investigation and enhanced control measures because of the risk of additional cases and severity of illness associated with these infections. Antimicrobial resistance
- Resistance to first-line therapies (e.g., MRSA, VISA, VRSA, VRE, ESBL-producing organisms).
- Common and uncommon microorganisms with unusual patterns of resistance within a facility (e.g., the first isolate of *Burkholderia cepacia* complex or *Ralstonia* spp. in non-CF patients or a quinolone-resistant strain of *Pseudomonas aeruginosa* in a facility).

- Difficult to treat because of innate or acquired resistance to multiple classes of antimicrobial agents (e.g., *Stenotrophomonas maltophilia, Acinetobacter spp.*).
- Association with serious clinical disease, increased morbidity and mortality (e.g., MRSA and MSSA, group A streptococcus)
- A newly discovered or reemerging pathogen

I.C.1 .A. C.Difficile

C. difficile is a spore-forming gram positive anaerobic bacillus that was first isolated from stools of neonates in 1935 [165] and identified as the most commonly identified causative agent of antibiotic-associated diarrhea and pseudomembranous colitis in 1977 [166] . This pathogen is a major cause of healthcare-associated diarrhea and has been responsible for many large outbreaks in healthcare settings that were extremely difficult to control. Important factors that contribute to healthcare-associated outbreaks include environmental contamination, persistence of spores for prolonged periods of time, resistance of spores to routinely used disinfectants and antiseptics, hand carriage by healthcare personnel to other patients, and exposure of patients to frequent courses of antimicrobial agents [167] . Antimicrobials most frequently associated with increased risk of *C. difficile* include third generation cephalosporins, clindamycin, vancomycin, and fluoroquinolones.

Since 2001, outbreaks and sporadic cases of *C. difficile* with increased morbidity and mortality have been observed in several U.S. states, Canada, England and the Netherlands [168-172] . The same strain of *C. difficile* has been implicated in these outbreaks [173] . This strain, toxinotype III, North American PFGE type 1, and PCR-ribotype 027 (NAP1/027). has been found to hyperproduce toxin A (16 fold increase) and toxin B (23 fold increase) compared with isolates from 12 different pulsed-field gel electrophoresisPFGE types. A recent survey of U.S. infectious disease physicians found that 40% perceived recent increases in the incidence and severity of *C. difficile* disease[174]. Standardization of testing methodology and surveillance definitions is needed for accurate comparisons of trends in rates among hospitals [175] . It is hypothesized that the incidence of disease and apparent heightened transmissibility of this new strain may be due, at least in part, to the greater production of toxins A and B, increasing the severity of diarrhea and resulting in more environmental contamination. Considering the greater morbidity, mortality, length of stay, and costs associated with *C. difficile* disease in both acute care and long term care facilities, control of this pathogen is now even more important than previously. Prevention of transmission focuses on syndromic application of Contact Precautions for patients with diarrhea, accurate identification of patients, environmental measures (e.g., rigorous cleaning of patient rooms) and consistent hand hygiene. Use of soap and water, rather than alcohol based handrubs, for mechanical removal of spores from hands, and a bleach-containing disinfectant (5000 ppm) for environmental disinfection, may be valuable when there is transmission in a healthcare facility. See Appendix A for specific recommendations.

I.C.1. B. Multidrug-Resistant Organisms (MDROs)

In general, MDROs are defined as microorganisms – predominantly bacteria – that are resistant to one or more classes of antimicrobial agents[176]. Although the names of certain MDROs suggest resistance to only one agent (e.g., methicillin-resistant *Staphylococcus aureus* [MRSA], vancomycin resistant enterococcus [VRE]), these pathogens are usually resistant to all but a few commercially available antimicrobial agents. This latter feature defines MDROs that are considered to be epidemiologically important and deserve special attention in healthcare facilities[177]. Other MDROs of current concern include mu ltid rug-resistant *Streptococcus pneumoniae* (MDRSP) which is resistant to penicillin and other broad-spectrum agents such as macrolides and fluroqui nolones, multidrug-resistant gram-negative bacilli (MDR- GNB), especially those producing extended spectrum beta-lactamases (ESBLs); and strains of *S. aureus* that are intermediate or resistant to vancomycin (i.e., VISA and VRSA)[178-197, 198].

MDROs are transmitted by the same routes as antimicrobial susceptible infectious agents. Patient-to-patient transmission in healthcare settings, usually via hands of HCWs, has been a major factor accounting for the increase in MDRO incidence and prevalence, especially for MRSA and VRE in acute care facilities[199-201] . Preventing the emergence and transmission of these pathogens requires a comprehensive approach that includes administrative involvement and measures (e.g., nurse staffing, communication systems, performance improvement processes to ensure adherence to recommended infection control measures), education and training of medical and other healthcare personnel, judicious antibiotic use, comprehensive surveillance for targeted MDROs, application of infection control precautions during patient care, environmental measures (e.g., cleaning and disinfection of the patient care environment and equipment, dedicated single-patient-use of non-critical equipment), and decolonization therapy when appropriate.

The prevention and control of MDROs is a national priority - one that requires that all healthcare facilities and agencies assume responsibility and participate in community-wide control programs [176, 177]. A detailed discussion of this topic and recommendations for prevention was published in 2006 may be found at http://www.cdc.gov/ncidod/dhqp/pdf/ar/mdro Guideline2006.pdf

I.C.2. Agents of Bioterrorism

CDC has designated the agents that cause anthrax, smallpox, plague, tularemia, viral hemorrhagic fevers, and botulism as Category A (high priority) because these agents can be easily disseminated environmentally and/or transmitted from person to person; can cause high mortality and have the potential for major public health impact; might cause public panic and social disruption; and require special action for public health preparedness[202]. General information relevant to infection control in healthcare settings for Category A agents of bioterrorism is summarized in Table 3. Consult www.bt.cdc.gov for additional, updated Category A agent information as well as information concerning Category B and C agents of bioterrorism and updates. Category B and C agents are important but are not as readily disseminated and cause less morbidity and mortality than Category A agents.

Healthcare facilities confront a different set of issues when dealing with a suspected bioterrorism event as compared with other communicable diseases. An understanding of the epidemiology, modes of transmission, and clinical course of each disease, as well as carefully drafted plans that provide an approach and relevant websites and other resources for disease-specific guidance to healthcare, administrative, and support personnel, are essential for responding to and managing a bioterrorism event. Infection control issues to be addressed include: 1) identifying persons who may be exposed or infected; 2) preventing transmission among patients, healthcare personnel, and visitors; 3) providing treatment, chemoprophylaxis or vaccine to potentially large numbers of people; 4) protecting the environment including the logistical aspects of securing sufficient numbers of AIIRs or designating areas for patient cohorts when there are an insufficient number of AIIRs available;5) providing adequate quantities of appropriate personal protective equipment; and 6) identifying appropriate staff to care for potentially infectious patients (e.g., vaccinated healthcare personnel for care of patients with smallpox). The response is likely to differ for exposures resulting from an intentional release compared with naturally occurring disease because of the large number persons that can be exposed at the same time and possible differences in pathogenicity.

A variety of sources offer guidance for the management of persons exposed to the most likely agents of bioterrorism. Federal agency websites (e.g., http://www.usamriid.army.mil/publicationspage. html , www.bt.cdc.gov) and state and county health department web sites should be consulted for the most up-to-date information. Sources of information on specific agents include: anthrax [203]; smallpox [204-206]; plague [207, 208]; botulinum toxin [209]; tularemia [210]; and hemorrhagic fever viruses: [211, 212].

I.C.2.A. Pre-Event Administration of Smallpox (Vaccinia) Vaccine to Healthcare Personnel

Vaccination of personnel in preparation for a possible smallpox exposure has important infection control implications [213-215] . These include the need for meticulous screening for vaccine contraindications in persons who are at increased risk for adverse vaccinia events; containment and monitoring of the vaccination site to prevent transmission in the healthcare setting and at home; and the management of patients with vaccinia-related adverse events [216, 217] . The pre-event U.S. smallpox vaccination program of 2003 is an example of the effectiveness of carefully developed recommendations for both screening potential vaccinees for contraindications and vaccination site care and monitoring. Approximately 760,000 individuals were vaccinated in the Department of Defense and 40,000 in the civilian or public health populations from December 2002 to February 2005, including approximately 70,000 who worked in healthcare settings. There were no cases of eczema vaccinatum, progressive vaccinia, fetal vaccinia, or contact transfer of vaccinia in healthcare settings or in military workplaces [218, 219] . Outside the healthcare setting, there were 53 cases of contact transfer from military vaccinees to close personal contacts (e.g., bed partners or contacts during participation in sports such as wrestling [220]) . All contact transfers were from individuals who were not following recommendations to cover their vaccination sites. Vaccinia virus was confirmed by culture or PCR in 30 cases, and two of the confirmed cases resulted from tertiary transfer. All recipients, including one breast-fed infant, recovered without complication. Subsequent studies using viral culture and PCR techniques have confirmed the effectiveness of semipermeable dressings to contain vaccinia [221-224] . This experience emphasizes the importance of ensuring that newly vaccinated healthcare personnel adhere to recommended vaccination-site care, especially if they are to care for high-risk patients. Recommendations for pre-event smallpox vaccination of healthcare personnel and vaccinia-related infection control recommendations are published in the MMWR [216, 225] with updates posted on the CDC bioterrorism web site [205].

I.C.3. Prions

Creutzfeldt-Jakob disease (CJD) is a rapidly progressive, degenerative, neurologic disorder of humans with an incidence in the United States of approximately 1 person/million population/year [226, 227] (http://www.cdc.gov/ncidod/dvrd/cjd/). CJD is believed to be caused by a transmissible proteinaceous infectious agent termed a prion. Infectious prions are isoforms of a host-encoded glycoprotein known as the prion protein. The incubation period (i.e., time between exposure and and onset of symptoms) varies from two years to many decades. However, death typically occurs within 1 year of the onset of symptoms. Approximately 85% of CJD cases occur sporadically with no known environmental source of infection and 10% are familial. Iatrogenic transmission has occurred with most resulting from treatment with human cadaveric pituitary-derived growth hormone or gonadotropin [228, 229], from implantation of contaminated human dura mater grafts [230] or from corneal transplants [231]) . Transmission has been linked to the use of contaminated neurosurgical instruments or stereotactic electroencephalogram electrodes [232, 233 , 234 , 235.]

Prion diseases in animals include scrapie in sheep and goats, bovine spongiform encephalopathy (BSE, or "mad cow disease") in cattle, and chronic wasting disease in deer and elk [236] . BSE, first recognized in the United Kingdom (UK) in 1986, was associated with a major epidemic among cattle that had consumed contaminated meat and bone meal.

The possible transmission of BSE to humans causing variant CJD (vCJD) was first described in 1996 and subsequently found to be associated with consumption of BSE-contaminated cattle products primarily in the United Kingdom. There is strong epidemiologic and laboratory evidence for a causal association between the causative agent of BSE and vCJD [237] . Although most cases of vCJD have been reported from the UK, a few cases also have been reported from Europe, Japan, Canada, and the United States. Most vCJD cases worldwide lived in or visited the UK during the years of a large outbreak of BSE (1980-96) and may have consumed contaminated cattle products during that time (http://www.cdc.gov/ncidod/dvrd/bse/index.htm). Although there has been no indigenously acquired vCJD in the United States, the sporadic occurrence of BSE in cattle in North America has heightened awareness of the possibility that such infections could occur and have led to increased surveillance activities. Updated information may be found on the following website: http://www.cdc.gov/ncidod/ dvrd/vcjd/index.htm. The public health impact of prion diseases has been reviewed [238].

vCJD in humans has different clinical and pathologic characteristics from sporadic or classic CJD [239] , including the following: 1) younger median age at death: 28 (range 16-48) vs. 68 years; 2) longer duration of illness: median 14 months vs. 4-6 months; 3) increased frequency of sensory symptoms and early psychiatric symptoms with delayed onset of frank neurologic signs; and 4) detection of prions in tonsillar and other lymphoid tissues from vCJD patients but not from sporadic CJD patients [240]. Similar to sporadic CJD, there have been no reported cases of direct human-to-human transmission of vCJD by casual or environmental contact, droplet, or airborne routes. Ongoing blood safety surveillance in the U.S. has not detected sporadic CJD transmission through blood transfusion [241-243]. However, bloodborne transmission of vCJD is believed to have occurred in two UK patients [244, 245]. The following FDA websites provide information on steps that are being taken in the US to protect the blood supply from CJD and vCJD: http://www.fda.gov/cber/gdlns/cjdvcjd.htm; http://www.fda.gov/cber/gdlns/cjdvcjdq&a.htm.

Standard Precautions are used when caring for patients with suspected or confirmed CJD or vCJD. However, special precautions are recommended for tissue handling in the histology laboratory and for conducting an autopsy, embalming, and for contact with a body that has undergone autopsy [246]. Recommendations for reprocessing surgical instruments to prevent transmission of CJD in healthcare settings have been published by the World Health Organization (WHO) and are currently under review at CDC.

Questions concerning notification of patients potentially exposed to CJD or vCJD through contaminated instruments and blood products from patients with CJD or vCJD or at risk of having vCJD may arise. The risk of transmission associated with such exposures is believed to be extremely low but may vary based on the specific circumstance. Therefore consultation on appropriate options is advised. The United Kingdom has developed several documents that clinicians and patients in the US may find useful (http://www.hpa.org.uk/infections/topics az/cjd/ information documents. htm).

I.C.4. Severe Acute Respiratory Syndrome (SARS)

SARS is a newly discovered respiratory disease that emerged in China late in 2002 and spread to several countries [135, 140]; Mainland China, Hong Kong, Hanoi, Singapore, and Toronto were affected significantly. SARS is caused by SARS CoV, a previously unrecognized member of the coronavirus family [247, 248]. The incubation period from exposure to the onset of symptoms is 2 to 7 days but can be as long as 10 days and uncommonly even longer [249]. The illness is initially difficult to distinguish from other common respiratory infections. Signs and symptoms usually include fever >38.0°C and chills and rigors, sometimes accompanied by headache, myalgia, and mild to severe respiratory symptoms. Radiographic finding of atypical pneumonia is an important clinical indicator of possible SARS. Compared with adults, children have been affected less frequently, have milder disease, and are less likely to transmit SARS-CoV [135, 249-251]. The overall case fatality rate is approximately 6.0%; underlying disease and advanced age increase the risk of mortality (www.who.int/csr/sarsarchive/2003 05 07a/en/).

Outbreaks in healthcare settings, with transmission to large numbers of healthcare personnel and patients have been a striking feature of SARS; undiagnosed, infectious patients and visitors were important initiators of these outbreaks [21, 252-254]. The relative contribution of potential modes of transmission is not precisely known. There is ample evidence for droplet and contact transmission [96, 101, 113]; however, opportunistic airborne transmission cannot be excluded [101, 135-139, 149, 255]. For example, exposure to aerosol-generating procedures (e.g., endotracheal intubation, suctioning) was associated with transmission of infection to large numbers of healthcare personnel outside of the United States [93, 94, 96, 98, 253]. Therefore, aerosolization of small infectious particles generated during these and other similar procedures could be a risk factor for transmission to others within a multi-bed room or shared airspace. A review of the infection control literature generated from the SARS outbreaks of 2003 concluded that the greatest risk of transmission is to those who have close contact, are not properly trained in use of protective infection control procedures, do not consistently use PPE; and that N95 or higher respirators may offer additional protection to those exposed to aerosol-generating procedures and high risk activities [256, 257]. Organizational and individual factors that affected adherence to infection control practices for SARS also were identified [257].

Control of SARS requires a coordinated, dynamic response by multiple disciplines in a healthcare setting [9]. Early detection of cases is accomplished by screening persons with symptoms of a respiratory infection for history of travel to areas experiencing community transmission or contact with SARS patients, followed by implementation of Respiratory Hygiene/Cough Etiquette (i.e., placing a mask over the patient's nose and mouth) and physical separation from other patients in common waiting areas. The precise combination of precautions to protect healthcare personnel has not been determined. At the time of this publication, CDC recommends Standard Precautions, with emphasis on the use of hand hygiene, Contact Precautions with emphasis on environmental cleaning due to the detection of SARS CoV RNA by PCR on surfaces in rooms occupied by SARS patients [138, 254, 258], Airborne Precautions, including use of fit-tested NIOSH-approved N95 or higher level respirators, and eye protection [259]. In Hong Kong, the use of Droplet and Contact Precautions, which included use of a mask but not a respirator, was effective in protecting healthcare personnel [113]. However, in Toronto, consistent use of an N95 respirator was slightly more protective than a mask [93]. It is noteworthy that there was no transmission of SARS-CoV to public hospital workers in Vietnam despite inconsistent use of infection control measures, including use of PPE, which suggests other factors (e.g., severity of disease, frequency of high risk procedures or events, environmental features) may influence opportunities for transmission [260].

SARS-CoV also has been transmitted in the laboratory setting through breaches in recommended laboratory practices. Research laboratories where SARS-CoV was under investigation were the source of most cases reported after the first series of outbreaks in the winter and spring of 2003 [261, 262]. Studies of the SARS outbreaks of 2003 and transmissions that occurred in the laboratory re-affirm the effectiveness of recommended infection control precautions and highlight the importance of consistent adherence to these measures.

Lessons from the SARS outbreaks are useful for planning to respond to future public health crises, such as pandemic influenza and bioterrorism events. Surveillance for cases among patients and healthcare personnel, ensuring availability of adequate supplies and staffing, and limiting access to healthcare facilities were important factors in the response to SARS that have been summarized [9]. Guidance for infection control precautions in various settings is available at www.cdc.gov/ncidod/sars.

I.C.5. Monkeypox

Monkeypox is a rare viral disease found mostly in the rain forest countries of Central and West Africa. The disease is caused by an orthopoxvirus that is similar in appearance to smallpox but causes a milder disease. The only recognized outbreak of human monkeypox in the United States was detected in June 2003 after several people became ill following contact with sick pet prairie dogs. Infection in the prairie dogs was subsequently traced to their contact with a shipment of animals from Africa, including giant Gambian rats [263]. This outbreak demonstrates the importance of recognition and prompt reporting of unusual disease presentations by clinicians to enable prompt identification of the etiology; and the potential of epizootic diseases to spread from animal reservoirs to humans through personal and occupational exposure [264].

Limited data on transmission of monkeypox are available. Transmission from infected animals and humans is believed to occur primarily through direct contact with lesions and respiratory secretions; airborne transmission from animals to humans is unlikely but cannot be excluded, and may have occurred in veterinary practices (e.g., during administration of nebulized medications to ill prairie dogs [265]). Among humans, four instances of monkeypox transmission within hospitals have been reported in Africa among children, usually related to sharing the same ward or bed [266, 267]. Additional recent literature documents transmission of Congo Basin monkeypox in a hospital compound for an extended number of generations [268].

There has been no evidence of airborne or any other person-to-person transmission of monkeypox in the United States, and no new cases of monkeypox have been identified since the outbreak in June 2003 [269]. The outbreak strain is a clade of monkeypox distinct from the Congo Basin clade and may have different epidemiologic properties (including human-to-human transmission potential) from monkeypox strains of the Congo Basin [270]; this awaits further study. Smallpox vaccine is 85% protective against Congo Basin monkeypox [271]. Since there is an associated case fatality rate of <10%, administration of smallpox vaccine within 4 days to individuals who have had direct exposure to patients or animals with monkeypox is a reasonable consideration [272]. For the most current information on monkeypox, see www.cdc.gov/ncidod/monkeypox/clinicians.htm.

I.C.6. Noroviruses

Noroviruses, formerly referred to as Norwalk-like viruses, are members of the *Caliciviridae* family. These agents are transmitted via contaminated food or water and from person-to-person, causing explosive outbreaks of gastrointestinal disease [273]. Environmental contamination also has been documented as a contributing factor in ongoing transmission during outbreaks [274, 275]. Although noroviruses cannot be propagated in cell culture, DNA detection by molecular diagnostic techniques has facilitated a greater appreciation of their role in outbreaks of gastrointestinal disease [276]. Reported outbreaks in hospitals [132, 142, 277], nursing homes [275, 278-283], cruise ships [284, 285] hotels [143, 147], schools [148], and large crowded shelters established for hurricane evacuees [286], demonstrate their highly contagious nature, the disruptive impact they have in healthcare facilities and the community, and the difficulty of controlling outbreaks in settings where people share common facilites and space. Of note, there is nearly a 5 fold increase in the risk to patients in outbreaks where a patient is the index case compared with exposure of patients during outbreaks where a staff member is the index case [287].

The average incubation period for gastroenteritis caused by noroviruses is 12-48 hours and the clinical course lasts 12-60 hours [273]. Illness is characterized by acute onset of nausea, vomiting, abdominal cramps, and/or diarrhea. The disease is largely self-limited; rarely, death caused by severe dehydration can occur, particularly among the elderly with debilitating health conditions.

The epidemiology of norovirus outbreaks shows that even though primary cases may result from exposure to a fecally-contaminated food or water, secondary and tertiary cases often result from person-to-person transmission that is facilitated by contamination of fomites [273, 288] and dissemination of infectious particles, especially during the process of vomiting [132, 142, 143, 147, 148, 273, 279, 280] . Widespread, persistent and inapparent contamination of the environment and fomites can make outbreaks extremely difficult to control [147, 275, 284] .These clinical observations and the detection of norovirus DNA on horizontal surfaces 5 feet above the level that might be touched normally suggest that, under certain circumstances, aerosolized particles may travel distances beyond 3 feet [147] . It is hypothesized that infectious particles may be aerosolized from vomitus, inhaled, and swallowed. In addition, individuals who are responsible for cleaning the environment may be at increased risk of infection. Development of disease and transmission may be facilitated by the low infectious dose (i.e., <100 viral particles) [289] and the resistance of these viruses to the usual cleaning and disinfection agents (i.e., may survive < 10 ppm chlorine) [290-292] . An alternate phenolic agent that was shown to be effective against feline calicivirus was used for environmental cleaning in one outbreak [275, 293] . There are insufficient data to determine the efficacy of alcohol-based hand rubs against noroviruses when the hands are not visibly soiled [294] . Absence of disease in certain individuals during an outbreak may be explained by protection from infection conferred by the B histo-blood group antigen [295] . Consultation on outbreaks of gastroenteritis is available through CDC's Division of Viral and Rickettsial Diseases [296].

I.C.7. Hemorrhagic Fever Viruses (HFV)

The hemorrhagic fever viruses are a mixed group of viruses that cause serious disease with high fever, skin rash, bleeding diathesis, and in some cases, high mortality; the disease caused is referred to as viral hemorrhagic fever (VHF). Among the more commonly known HFVs are Ebola and Marburg viruses (Filoviridae), Lassa virus (Arenaviridae), Crimean-Congo hemorrhagic fever and Rift Valley Fever virus (Bunyaviridae), and Dengue and Yellow fever viruses (Flaviviridae) [212, 297] . These viruses are transmitted to humans via contact with infected animals or via arthropod vectors. While none of these viruses is endemic in the United States, outbreaks in affected countries provide potential opportunities for importation by infected humans and animals. Furthermore, there are concerns that some of these agents could be used as bioweapons [212] . Person-to-person transmission is documented for Ebola, Marburg, Lassa and Crimean-Congo hemorrhagic fever viruses. In resource-limited healthcare settings, transmission of these agents to healthcare personnel, patients and visitors has been described and in some outbreaks has accounted for a large proportion of cases [298-300]. Transmissions within households also have occurred among individuals who had direct contact with ill persons or their body fluids, but not to those who did not have such contact [301].

Evidence concerning the transmission of HFVs has been summarized [212, 302]. Person-to-person transmission is associated primarily with direct blood and body fluid contact. Percutaneous exposure to contaminated blood carries a particularly high risk for transmission and increased mortality [303, 304]. The finding of large numbers of Ebola viral particles in the skin and the lumina of sweat glands has raised concern that transmission could occur from direct contact with intact skin though epidemiologic evidence to support this is lacking [305]. Postmortem handling of infected bodies is an important risk for transmission [301, 306, 307]. In rare situations, cases in which the mode of transmission was unexplained among individuals with no known direct contact, have led to speculation that airborne transmission could have occurred [298]. However, airborne transmission of naturally occurring HFVs in humans has not been seen. In one study of airplane passengers exposed to an in-flight index case of Lassa fever, there was no transmission to any passengers [308].

In the laboratory setting, animals have been infected experimentally with Marburg or Ebola viruses via direct inoculation of the nose, mouth and/or conjunctiva [309, 310] and by using mechanically generated virus-containing aerosols [311, 312]. Transmission of Ebola virus among laboratory primates in an animal facility has been described [313]. Secondarily infected animals were in individual cages and separated by approximately 3 meters. Although the possibility of airborne transmission was suggested, the authors were not able to exclude droplet or indirect contact transmission in this incidental observation.

Guidance on infection control precautions for HVFs that are transmitted personto-person have been published by CDC [1, 211] and by the Johns Hopkins Center for Civilian Biodefense Strategies [212]. The most recent recommendations at the time of publication of this document were posted on the CDC website on 5/19/05 [314]. Inconsistencies among the various recommendations have raised questions about the appropriate precautions to use in U.S. hospitals. In less developed countries, outbreaks of HFVs have been controlled with basic hygiene, barrier precautions, safe injection practices, and safe burial practices [299, 306]. The preponderance of evidence on HFV transmission indicates that Standard, Contact and Droplet Precautions with eye protection are effective in protecting healthcare personnel and visitors who may attend an infected patient. Single gloves are adequate for routine patient care; double-gloving is advised during invasive procedures (e.g., surgery) that pose an increased risk for blood exposure. Routine eye protection (i.e. goggles or face shield) is particularly important. Fluid-resistant gowns should be worn for all patient contact. Airborne Precautions are not required for routine patient care; however, use of AIIRs is prudent when procedures that could generate infectious aerosols are performed (e.g., endotracheal intubation, bronchoscopy, suctioning, autopsy procedures involving oscillating saws). N95 or higher level respirators may provide added protection for individuals in a room during aerosol-generating procedures (Table 3, Appendix A). When a patient with a syndrome consistent with hemorrhagic fever also has a history of travel to an endemic area, precautions are initiated upon presentation and then modified as more information is obtained (Table 2). Patients with hemorrhagic fever syndrome in the setting of a suspected bioweapon attack should be managed using Airborne Precautions, including AIIRs, since the epidemiology of a potentially weaponized hemorrhagic fever virus is unpredictable.

I.D. Transmission Risks Associated with Specific Types of Healthcare Settings

Numerous factors influence differences in transmission risks among the various healthcare settings. These include the population characteristics (e.g., increased susceptibility to infections, type and prevalence of indwelling devices), intensity of care, exposure to environmental sources, length of stay, and frequency of interaction between patients/residents with each other and with HCWs. These factors, as well as organizational priorities, goals, and resources, influence how different healthcare settings adapt transmission prevention guidelines to meet their specific needs [315, 316]. Infection control management decisions are informed by data regarding institutional experience/epidemiology, trends in community and institutional HAIs, local, regional, and national epidemiology, and emerging infectious disease threats.

I.D.1. Hospitals

Infection transmission risks are present in all hospital settings. However, certain hospital settings and patient populations have unique conditions that predispose patients to infection and merit special mention. These are often sentinel sites for the emergence of new transmission risks that may be unique to that setting or present opportunities for transmission to other settings in the hospital.

I.D.1.A. Intensive Care Units

Intensive care units (ICUs) serve patients who are immunocompromised by disease state and/or by treatment modalities, as well as patients with major trauma, respiratory failure and other life-threatening conditions (e.g., myocardial infarction, congestive heart failure, overdoses, strokes, gastrointestinal bleeding, renal failure, hepatic failure, multi-organ system failure, and the extremes of age). Although ICUs account for a relatively small proportion of hospitalized patients, infections acquired in these units accounted for >20% of all HAIs [317] . In the National Nosocomial Infection Surveillance (NNIS) system, 26.6% of HAIs were reported from ICU and high risk nursery (NICU) patients in 2002 (NNIS, unpublished data). This patient population has increased susceptibility to colonization and infection, especially with MDROs and *Candida* sp. [318, 319] , because of underlying diseases and conditions, the invasive medical devices and technology used in their care (e.g. central venous catheters and other intravascular devices, mechanical ventilators, extracorporeal membrane oxygenation (ECMO), hemodialysis/-filtration, pacemakers, implantable left ventricular assist devices), the frequency of contact with healthcare personnel, prolonged length of stay, and prolonged exposure to antimicrobial agents [320-331] . Furthermore, adverse patient outcomes in this setting are more severe and are associated with a higher mortality [332] . Outbreaks associated with a variety of bacterial, fungal and viral pathogens due to common- source and person-to-person transmissions are frequent in adult and pediatric ICUs [31, 333-336, 337, 338].

I.D.1.B. Burn Units

Burn wounds can provide optimal conditions for colonization, infection, and transmission of pathogens; infection acquired by burn patients is a frequent cause of morbidity and mortality [320, 339, 340] . In patients with a burn injury involving >30% of the total body surface area (TBSA), the risk of invasive burn wound infection is particularly high [341, 342] . Infections that occur in patients with burn injury involving <30% TBSA are usually associated with the use of invasive devices. Meth ici ll in-susceptible *Staphylococcus aureus*, M RSA, enterococci, including VRE, gram-negative bacteria, and candida are prevalent pathogens in burn infections [53, 340, 343-350] and outbreaks of these organisms have been reported [351-354] . Shifts over time in the predominance of pathogens causing infections among burn patients often lead to changes in burn care practices [343, 355-358] . Burn wound infections caused by *Aspergillus* sp. or other environmental molds may result from exposure to supplies contaminated during construction [359] or to dust generated during construction or other environmental disruption [360].

Hydrotherapy equipment is an important environmental reservoir of gram-negative organisms. Its use for burn care is discouraged based on demonstrated associations between use of contaminated hydrotherapy equipment and infections. Burn wound infections and colonization, as well as bloodstream infections, caused by multidrug-resistant *P. aeruginosa* [361], *A. baumannii* [362], and MRSA [352] have been associated with hydrotherapy; excision of burn wounds in operating rooms is preferred.

Advances in burn care, specifically early excision and grafting of the burn wound, use of topical antimicrobial agents, and institution of early enteral feeding, have led to decreased infectious complications. Other advances have included prophylactic antimicrobial usage, selective digestive decontamination (SDD), and use of antimicrobial-coated catheters (ACC), but few epidemiologic studies and no efficacy studies have been performed to show the relative benefit of these measures.[357]

There is no consensus on the most effective infection control practices to prevent transmission of infections to and from patients with serious burns (e.g., single- bed rooms [358], laminar flow [363] and high efficiency particulate air filtration [HEPA] [360] or maintaining burn patients in a separate unit without exposure to patients or equipment from other units [364]). There also is controversy regarding the need for and type of barrier precautions for routine care of burn patients. One retrospective study demonstrated efficacy and cost effectiveness of a simplified barrier isolation protocol for wound colonization, emphasizing handwashing and use of gloves, caps, masks and plastic impermeable aprons (rather than isolation gowns) for direct patient contact [365]. However, there have been no studies that define the most effective combination of infection control precautions for use in burn settings. Prospective studies in this area are needed.

I.D.1.C. Pediatrics

Studies of the epidemiology of HAIs in children have identified unique infection control issues in this population [63, 64, 366-370]. Pediatric intensive care unit (PICU) patients and the lowest birthweight babies in the high- risk nursery (HRN) monitored in the NNIS system have had high rates of central venous catheter-associated bloodstream infections [64, 320, 369-372]. Additionally, there is a high prevalence of community-acquired infections among hospitalized infants and young children who have not yet become immune either by vaccination or by natural infection. The result is more patients and their sibling visitors with transmissible infections present in pediatric healthcare settings, especially during seasonal epidemics (e.g., pertussis [36, 40, 41], respiratory viral infections including those caused by RSV [24], influenza viruses [373], parainfluenza virus [374], human metapneumovirus [375], and adenoviruses [376]; rubeola [measles] [34], varicella [chickenpox] [377], and rotavirus [38, 378]).

Close physical contact between healthcare personnel and infants and young children (eg. cuddling, feeding, playing, changing soiled diapers, and cleaning copious uncontrolled respiratory secretions) provides abundant opportunities for transmission of infectious material. Practices and behaviors such as congregation of children in play areas where toys and bodily secretions are easily shared and family members rooming-in with pediatric patients can further increase the risk of transmission. Pathogenic bacteria have been recovered from toys used by hospitalized patients [379]; contaminated bath toys were implicated in an outbreak of multidrug-resistant *P. aeruginosa* on a pediatric oncology unit [80]. In addition, several patient factors increase the likelihood that infection will result from exposure to pathogens in healthcare settings (e.g., immaturity of the neonatal immune system, lack of previous natural infection and resulting immunity, prevalence of patients with congenital or acquired immune deficiencies, congenital anatomic anomalies, and use of life-saving invasive devices in neontal and pediatric intensive care units) [63] . There are theoretical concerns that infection risk will increase in association with innovative practices used in the NICU for the purpose of improving developmental outcomes, Such factors include co-bedding [380] and kangaroo care [381] that may increase opportunity for skin-to-skin exposure of multiple gestation infants to each other and to their mothers, respectively; although infection risk smay actually be reduced among infants receiving kangaroo care [382] . Children who attend child care centers [383, 384] and pediatric rehabilitation units [385] may increase the overall burden of antimicrobial resistance (eg. by contributing to the reservoir of community-associated MRSA [CA-MRSA]) [386-391]. Patients in chronic care facilities may have increased rates of colonization with resistant GNBs and may be sources of introduction of resistant organisms to acute care settings [50].

I.D.2. Non-Acute Healthcare Settings

Healthcare is provided in various settings outside of hospitals including facilities, such as long-term care facilities (LTCF) (e.g. nursing homes), homes for the developmentally disabled, settings where behavioral health services are provided, rehabilitation centers and hospices[392] .

In addition, healthcare may be provided in nonhealthcare settings such as workplaces with occupational health clinics, adult day care centers, assisted living facilities, homeless shelters, jails and prisons, school clinics and infirmaries. Each of these settings has unique circumstances and population risks to consider when designing and implementing an infection control program. Several of the most common settings and their particular challenges are discussed below. While this Guideline does not address each setting, the principles and strategies provided may be adapted and applied as appropriate.

I.D.2.A. Long-Term Care

The designation LTCF applies to a diverse group of residential settings, ranging from institutions for the developmentally disabled to nursing homes for the elderly and pediatric chronic-care facilities [393-395]. Nursing homes for the elderly predominate numerically and frequently represent longterm care as a group of facilities. Approximately 1.8 million Americans reside in the nation's 16,500 nursing homes [396]. Estimates of HAI rates of 1.8 to 13.5 per 1000 resident-care days have been reported with a range of 3 to 7 per 1000 resident-care days in the more rigorous studies [397-401]. The infrastructure described in the Department of Veterans Affairs nursing home care units is a promising example for the development of a nationwide HAI surveillance system for LTCFs [402].

LCTFs are different from other healthcare settings in that elderly patients at increased risk for infection are brought together in one setting and remain in the facility for extended periods of time; for most residents, it is their home. An atmosphere of community is fostered and residents share common eating and living areas, and participate in various facility-sponsored activities [403, 404]. Since able residents interact freely with each other, controlling transmission of infection in this setting is challenging [405]. Residents who are colonized or infected with certain microorganisms are, in some cases, restricted to their room. However, because of the psychosocial risks associated with such restriction, it has been recommended that psychosocial needs be balanced with infection control needs in the LTCF setting [406-409]. Documented LTCF outbreaks have been caused by various viruses (e.g., influenza virus [35, 410-412], rhinovirus [413], adenovirus (conjunctivitis) [414], norovirus [278, 279 275, 281]) and bacteria, including group A streptococcus [162], *B. pertussis* [415], non-susceptible *S. pneumoniae* [197, 198], other MDROs, and *Clostridium difficile* [416]) These pathogens can lead to substantial morbidity and mortality, and increased medical costs; prompt detection and implementation of effective control measures are required.

Risk factors for infection are prevalent among LTCF residents [395, 417, 418]. Age- related declines in immunity may affect responses to immunizations for influenza and other infectious agents, and increase susceptibility to tuberculosis. Immobility, incontinence, dysphagia, underlying chronic diseases, poor functional status, and age-related skin changes increase susceptibility to urinary, respiratory and cutaneous and soft tissue infections, while malnutrition can impair wound healing [419-423]. Medications (e.g., drugs that affect level of consciousness, immune function, gastric acid secretions, and normal flora, including antimicrobial therapy) and invasive devices (e.g., urinary catheters and feeding tubes) heighten susceptibility to infection and colonization in LTCF residents [424-426]. Finally, limited functional status and total dependence on healthcare personnel for activities of daily living have been identified as independent risk factors for infection [401, 417, 427] and for colonization with MRSA [428, 429] and ESBL-producing *K. pneumoniae* [430]. Several position papers and review articles have been published that provide guidance on various aspects of infection control and antimicrobial resistance in LTCFs [406-408, 431-436]. The Centers for Medicare and Medicaid Services (CMS) have established regulations for the prevention of infection in LTCFs [437].

Because residents of LTCFs are hospitalized frequently, they can transfer pathogens between LTCFs and healthcare facilities in which they receive care [8, 438-441]. This is also true for pediatric long-term care populations. Pediatric chronic care facilities have been associated with importing extended-spectrum cephalosporin-resistant, gram-negative bacilli into one PICU [50]. Children from pediatric rehabilitation units may contribute to the reservoir of community-associated MRSA [385, 389-391].

I.D.2.B. Ambulatory Care

In the past decade, healthcare delivery in the United States has shifted from the acute, inpatient hospital to a variety of ambulatory and community-based settings, including the home. Ambulatory care is provided in hospital-based outpatient clinics, nonhospital-based clinics and physician offices, public health clinics, free-standing dialysis centers, ambulatory surgical centers, urgent care centers, and many others. In 2000, there were 83 million visits to hospital outpatient clinics and more than 823 million visits to physician offices [442]; ambulatory care now accounts for most patient encounters with the health care system [443]. In these settings, adapting transmission prevention guidelines is challenging because patients remain in common areas for prolonged periods waiting to be seen by a healthcare provider or awaiting admission to the hospital, examination or treatment rooms are turned around quickly with limited cleaning, and infectious patients may not be recognized immediately. Furthermore, i mmunocompromised patients often receive chemotherapy in infusion rooms where they stay for extended periods of time along with other types of patients.

There are few data on the risk of HAIs in ambulatory care settings, with the exception of hemodialysis centers [18, 444, 445]. Transmission of infections in outpatient settings has been reviewed in three publications [446-448]. Goodman and Solomon summarized 53 clusters of infections associated with the outpatient setting from 1961-1990 [446]. Overall, 29 clusters were associated with common source transmission from contaminated solutions or equipment, 14 with personto-person transmission from or involving healthcare personnel and ten associated with airborne or droplet transmission among patients and healthcare workers. Transmission of bloodborne pathogens (i.e., hepatitis B and C viruses and, rarely, HIV) in outbreaks, sometimes involving hundreds of patients, continues to occur in ambulatory settings. These outbreaks often are related to common source exposures, usually a contaminated medical device, multi-dose vial, or intravenous solution [82, 449-453]. In all cases, transmission has been attributed to failure to adhere to fundamental infection control principles, including safe injection practices and aseptic technique. This subject has been reviewed and recommended infection control and safe injection practices summarized [454].

Airborne transmission of *M.tuberculosis* and measles in ambulatory settings, most frequently emergency departments, has been reported [34, 127, 446, 448, 455-457]. Measles virus was transmitted in physician offices and other outpatient settings during an era when immunization rates were low and measles outbreaks in the community were occurring regularly [34, 122, 458]. Rubella has been transmitted in the outpatient obstetric setting [33]; there are no published reports of varicella transmission in the outpatient setting. In the ophthalmology setting, adenovirus type 8 epidemic keratoconjunctivitis has been transmitted via incompletely disinfected ophthalmology equipment and/or from healthcare workers to patients, presumably by contaminated hands [17, 446, 448, 459-462].

If transmission in outpatient settings is to be prevented, screening for potentially infectious symptomatic and asymptomatic individuals, especially those who may be at risk for transmitting airborne infectious agents (e.g., *M. tuberculosis*, varicella-zoster virus, rubeola [measles]), is necessary at the start of the initial patient encounter. Upon identification of a potentially infectious patient, implementation of prevention measures, including prompt separation of potentially infectious patients and implementation of appropriate control measures (e.g., Respiratory Hygiene/Cough Etiquette and Transmission-Based Precautions) can decrease transmission risks [9, 12]. Transmission of MRSA and VRE in outpatient settings has not been reported, but the association of CAMRSA in healthcare personnel working in an outpatient HIV clinic with environmental CA-MRSA contamination in that clinic, suggests the possibility of transmission in that setting [463]. Patient-to-patient transmission of *Burkholderia species* and

Pseudomonas aeruginosa in outpatient clinics for adults and children with cystic fibrosis has been confirmed [464, 465].

I.D.2.C. Home Care

Home care in the United States is delivered by over 20,000 provider agencies that include home health agencies, hospices, durable medical equipment providers, home infusion therapy services, and personal care and support services providers. Home care is provided to patients of all ages with both acute and chronic conditions. The scope of services ranges from assistance with activities of daily living and physical and occupational therapy to the care of wounds, infusion therapy, and chronic ambulatory peritoneal dialysis (CAPD).

The incidence of infection in home care patients, other than those associated with infusion therapy is not well studied [466-471]. However, data collection and calculation of infection rates have been accomplished for central venous catheter-associated bloodstream infections in patients receiving home infusion therapy [470-474] and for the risk of blood contact through percutaneous or mucosal exposures, demonstrating that surveillance can be performed in this setting [475]. Draft definitions for home care associated infections have been developed [476].

Transmission risks during home care are presumed to be minimal. The main transmission risks to home care patients are from an infectious healthcare provider or contaminated equipment; providers also can be exposed to an infectious patient during home visits. Since home care involves patient care by a limited number of personnel in settings without multiple patients or shared equipment, the potential reservoir of pathogens is reduced. Infections of home care providers, that could pose a risk to home care patients include infections transmitted by the airborne or droplet routes (e.g., chickenpox, tuberculosis, influenza), and skin infestations (e.g., scabies [69] and lice) and infections (e.g.,impetigo) transmitted by direct or indirect contact. There are no published data on indirect transmission of MDROs from one home care patient to another, although this is theoretically possible if contaminated equipment is transported from an infected or colonized patient and used on another patient. Of note, investigation of the first case of VISA in homecare [186] and the first 2 reported cases of VRSA [178, 180, 181, 183] found no evidence of transmission of VISA or VRSA to other home care recipients. Home health care also may contribute to antimicrobial resistance; a review of outpatient vancomycin use found 39% of recipients did not receive the antibiotic according to recommended guidelines [477].

Although most home care agencies implement policies and procedures to prevent transmission of organisms, the current approach is based on the adaptation of the *1996 Guideline for Isolation Precautions in Hospitals* [1] as well as other professional guidance [478, 479]. This issue has been very challenging in the home care industry and practice has been inconsistent and frequently not evidence-based. For example, many home health agencies continue to observe "nursing bag technique," a practice that prescribes the use of barriers between the nursing bag and environmental surfaces in the home [480] . While the home environment may not always appear clean, the use of barriers between two noncritical surfaces has been questioned [481, 482] . Opportunites exist to conduct research in home care related to infection transmission risks [483].

I.D.2.D. Other Sites of Healthcare Delivery

Facilities that are not primarily healthcare settings but in which healthcare is delivered include clinics in correctional facilities and shelters. Both settings can have suboptimal features, such as crowded conditions and poor ventilation. Economically disadvantaged individuals who may have chronic illnesses and healthcare problems related to alcoholism, injection drug use, poor nutrition, and/or inadequate shelter often receive their primary healthcare at sites such as these [484] . Infectious diseases of special concern for transmission include tuberculosis, scabies, respiratory infections (e.g., *N. meningitides, S. pneumoniae*), sexually transmitted and bloodborne diseases (e.g.,HIV, HBV, HCV, syphilis, gonorrhea), hepatitis A virus (HAV), diarrheal agents such as norovirus, and foodborne diseases [286, 485-488] . A high index of suspicion for tuberculosis and CA-MRSA in these populations is needed as outbreaks in these settings or among the populations they serve have been reported [489-497].

Patient encounters in these types of facilities provide an opportunity to deliver recommended immunizations and screen for *M. tuberculosis* infection in addition to diagnosing and treating acute illnesses [498] . Recommended infection control measures in these non-traditional areas designated for healthcare delivery are the same as for other ambulatory care settings. Therefore, these settings must be equipped to observe Standard Precautions and, when indicated, Transmission-Based Precautions.

I.E. Transmission Risks Associated with Special Patient Populations

As new treatments emerge for complex diseases, unique infection control challenges associated with special patient populations need to be addressed.

I.E.1. Immunocompromised Patients

Patients who have congenital primary immune deficiencies or acquired disease (eg. treatment-induced immune deficiencies) are at increased risk for numerous types of infections while receiving healthcare and may be located throughout the healthcare facility. The specific defects of the immune system determine the types of infections that are most likely to be acquired (e.g., viral infections are associated with T-cell defects and fungal and bacterial infections occur in patients who are neutropenic). As a general group, immunocompromised patients can be cared for in the same environment as other patients; however, it is always advisable to minimize exposure to other patients with transmissible infections such as influenza and other respiratory viruses [499, 500]. The use of more intense chemotherapy regimens for treatment of childhood leukemia may be associated with prolonged periods of neutropenia and suppression of other components of the immune system, extending the period of infection risk and raising the concern that additional precautions may be indicated for select groups [501, 502] . With the application of newer and more intense immunosuppressive therapies for a variety of medical conditions (e.g., rheumatologic disease [503, 504] , inflammatory bowel disease [505]) , immunosuppressed patients are likely to be more widely distributed throughout a healthcare facility rather than localized to single patient units (e.g. hematology-oncology). Guidelines for preventing infections in certain groups of immunocompromised patients have been published [15, 506, 507].

Published data provide evidence to support placing allogeneic HSCT patients in a Protective Environment [15, 157, 158] . Also, three guidelines have been developed that address the special requirements of these immunocompromised patients, including use of antimicrobial prophylaxis and engineering controls to create a Protective Environment for the prevention of infections caused by *Aspergillus* spp. and other environmental fungi [11, 14, 15]. As more intense chemotherapy regimens associated with prolonged periods of neutropenia or graft-versus-host disease are implemented, the period of risk and duration of environmental protection may need to be prolonged beyond the traditional 100 days [508].

I.E.2. Cystic Fibrosis Patients

Patients with cystic fibrosis (CF) require special consideration when developing infection control guidelines. Compared to other patients, CF patients require additional protection to prevent transmission from contaminated respiratory therapy equipment [509-513]. Infectious agents such as *Burkholderia cepacia* complex and *P. aeruginosa* [464, 465, 514, 515] have unique clinical and prognostic significance.

In CF patients, *B. cepacia* infection has been associated with increased morbidity and mortality [516-518], while delayed acquisition of chronic *P. aeruginosa* infection may be associated with an improved long-term clinical outcome [519, 520]. Person-to-person transmission of *B. cepacia* complex has been demonstrated among children [517] and adults [521] with CF in healthcare settings [464, 522], during various social contacts [523], most notably attendance at camps for patients with CF [524], and among siblings with CF [525]. Successful infection control measures used to prevent transmission of respiratory secretions include segregation of CF patients from each other in ambulatory and hospital settings (including use of private rooms with separate showers), environmental decontamination of surfaces and equipment contaminated with respiratory secretions, elimination of group chest physiotherapy sessions, and disbanding of CF camps [97, 526]. The Cystic Fibrosis Foundation published a consensus document with evidence-based recommendations for infection control practices for CF patients [20].

I.F. New Therapies Associated with Potentially Transmissible Infectious Agents

I.F.1. Gene Therapy
Gene therapy has has been attempted using a number of different viral vectors, including nonreplicating retroviruses, adenoviruses, adenoassociated viruses, and replication-competent strains of poxvi ruses. Unexpected adverse events have restricted the prevalence of gene therapy protocols.

The infectious hazards of gene therapy are theoretical at this time, but require meticulous surveillance due to the possible occurrence of in vivo recombination and the subsequent emergence of a transmissible genetically altered pathogen. Greatest concern attends the use of replication-competent viruses, especially vaccinia. As of the time of publication, no reports have described transmission of a vector virus from a gene therapy recipient to another individual, but surveillance is ongoing. Recommendations for monitoring infection control issues throughout the course of gene therapy trials have been published [527-529].

I.F.2. Infections Transmitted through Blood, Organs and Other Tissues
The potential hazard of transmitting infectious pathogens through biologic products is a small but ever present risk, despite donor screening. Reported infections transmitted by transfusion or transplantation include West Nile Virus infection [530] cytomegalovirus infection [531], Creutzfeldt-Jacob disease [230], hepatitis C [532], infections with *Clostridium* spp. [533] and group A streptococcus

[534], malaria [535], babesiosis [536], Chagas disease [537], lymphocytic choriomeningitis [538], and rabies [539, 540]. Therefore, it is important to consider receipt of biologic products when evaluating patients for potential sources of infection.

I.F.3. Xenotransplantation

The transplantation of nonhuman cells, tissues, and organs into humans potentially exposes patients to zoonotic pathogens. Transmission of known zoonotic infections (e.g., trichinosis from porcine tissue), constitutes one concern, but also of concern is the possibility that transplantation of nonhuman cells, tissues, or organs may transmit previously unknown zoonotic infections (xenozoonoses) to immunosuppressed human recipients. Potential infections that might accompany transplantation of porcine organs have been described [541] . Guidelines from the U.S. Public Health Service address many infectious diseases and infection control issues that surround the developing field of xenotransplantation [542]); work in this area is ongoing.

PART II: FUNDAMENTAL ELEMENTS NEEDED TO PREVENT TRANSMISSION OF INFECTIOUS AGENTS IN HEALTHCARE SETTINGS

II.A. Healthcare System Components that Influence the Effectiveness of Precautions to Prevent Transmission

II.A.1. Administrative Measures

Healthcare organizations can demonstrate a commitment to preventing transmission of infectious agents by incorporating infection control into the objectives of the organization's patient and occupational safety programs [543-547]. An infrastructure to guide, support, and monitor adherence to Standard and Transmission-Based Precautions [434, 548, 549] will facilitate fulfillment of the organization's mission and achievement of the Joint Commission on Accreditation of Healthcare Organization's patient safety goal to decrease HAIs [550] . Policies and procedures that explain how Standard and Transmission-Based Precautions are applied, including systems used to identify and communicate information about patients with potentially transmissible infectious agents, are essential to ensure the success of these measures and may vary according to the characteristics of the organization.

A key administrative measure is provision of fiscal and human resources for maintaining infection control and occupational health programs that are responsive to emerging needs. Specific components include bedside nurse [551] and infection prevention and control professional (ICP) staffing levels [552], inclusion of ICPs in facility construction and design decisions [11], clinical microbiology laboratory support [553, 554], adequate supplies and equipment including facility ventilation systems [11], adherence monitoring [555], assessment and correction of system failures that contribute to transmission [556, 557], and provision of feedback to healthcare personnel and senior administrators [434, 548, 549, 558] . The positive influence of institutional leadership has been demonstrated repeatedly in studies of HCW adherence to recommended hand hygiene practices [176, 177, 434, 548, 549, 559-564] . Healthcare administrator involvement in infection control processes can improve administrators' awareness of the rationale and resource requirements for following recommended infection control practices.

Several administrative factors may affect the transmission of infectious agents in healthcare settings: institutional culture, individual worker behavior, and the work environment. Each of these areas is suitable for performance improvement monitoring and incorporation into the organization's patient safety goals [543, 544, 546, 565].

II.A.1.A. Scope of Work and Staffing Needs for Infection Control Professionals

The effectiveness of infection surveillance and control programs in preventing nosocomial infections in United States hospitals was assessed by the CDC through the Study on the Efficacy of Nosocomial Infection Control (SENIC Project) conducted 1970-76 [566] . In a representative sample of US general hospitals, those with a trained infection control physician or microbiologist involved in an infection control program, and at least one infection control nurse per 250 beds, were associated with a 32% lower rate of four infections studied (CVC-associated bloodstream infections, ventilator-associated pneumon ias, catheter-related urinary tract infections, and surgical site infections).

Since that landmark study was published, responsibilities of ICPs have expanded commensurate with the growing complexity of the healthcare system, the patient populations served, and the increasing numbers of medical procedures and devices used in all types of healthcare settings. The scope of work of ICPs was first assessed in 1982 [567-569] by the Certification Board of Infection Control (CBIC), and has been re-assessed every five years since that time [558, 570-572] .

The findings of these task analyses have been used to develop and update the Infection Control Certification Examination, offered for the first time in 1983. With each survey, it is apparent that the role of the ICP is growing in complexity and scope, beyond traditional infection control activities in acute care hospitals. Activities currently assigned to ICPs in response to emerging challenges include: 1) surveillance and infection prevention at facilities other than acute care hospitals e.g., ambulatory clinics, day surgery centers, long term care facilities, rehabilitation centers, home care; 2) oversight of employee health services related to infection prevention, e.g. assessment of risk and administration of recommended treatment following exposure to infectious agents, tuberculosis screening, influenza vaccination, respiratory protection fit testing, and administration of other vaccines as indicated, such as smallpox vaccine in 2003; 3) preparedness planning for annual influenza outbreaks, pandemic influenza, SARS, bioweapons attacks; 4) adherence monitoring for selected infection control practices; 5) oversight of risk assessment and implementation of prevention measures associated with construction and renovation; 6) prevention of transmission of MDROs; 7) evaluation of new medical products that could be associated with increased infection risk. e.g.,intravenous infusion materials; 9) communication with the public, facility staff, and state and local health departments concerning infection control-related issues; and 10) participation in local and multi-center research projects [434, 549, 552, 558, 573, 574].

None of the CBIC job analyses addressed specific staffing requirements for the identified tasks, although the surveys did include information about hours worked; the 2001 survey included the number of ICPs assigned to the responding facilities [558] . There is agreement in the literature that 1 ICP per 250 acute care beds is no longer adequate to meet current infection control needs; a Delphi project that assessed staffing needs of infection control programs in the 21st century concluded that a ratio of 0.8 to 1.0 ICP per 100 occupied acute care beds is an appropriate level of staffingg [552] . A survey of participants in the National Nosocomial Infections Surveillance (NNIS) system found the average daily census per ICP was 115 [316] . Results of other studies have been similar: 3 per 500 beds for large acute care hospitals, 1 per 150-250 beds in long term care facilities, and 1.56 per 250 in small rural hospitals [573, 575]. The foregoing demonstrates that infection control staffing can no longer be based on patient census alone, but rather must be determined by the scope of the program, characteristics of the patient population, complexity of the healthcare system, tools available to assist personnel to perform essential tasks (e.g., electronic tracking and laboratory support for surveillance), and unique or urgent needs of the institution and community [552]. Furthermore, appropriate training is required to optimize the quality of work performed [558, 572, 576].

II.A.1.A.I. Infection Control Nurse Liaison

Designating a bedside nurse on a patient care unit as an infection control liaison or "link nurse" is reported to be an effective adjunct to enhance infection control at the unit level [577-582]. Such individuals receive training in basic infection control and have frequent communication with the ICPs, but maintain their primary role as bedside caregiver on their units. The infection control nurse liaison increases the awareness of infection control at the unit level. He or she is especially effective in implementation of new policies or control interventions because of the rapport with individuals on the unit, an understanding of unit-specific challenges, and ability to promote strategies that are most likely to be successful in that unit. This position is an adjunct to, not a replacement for, fully trained ICPs. Furthermore, the infection control liaison nurses should not be counted when considering ICP staffing.

II.A.1.B. Bedside Nurse Staffing

There is increasing evidence that the level of bedside nurse-staffing influences the quality of patient care [583, 584]. If there are adequate nursing staff, it is more likely that infection control practices, including hand hygiene and Standard and Transmission-Based Precautions, will be given appropriate attention and applied correctly and consistently [552]. A national multicenter study reported strong and consistent inverse relationships between nurse staffing and five adverse outcomes in medical patients, two of which were HAIs: urinary tract infections and pneumonia [583]. The association of nursing staff shortages with increased rates of HAIs has been demonstrated in several outbreaks in hospitals and long term care settings, and with increased transmission of hepatitis C virus in dialysis units [22, 418, 551, 585-597]. In most cases, when staffing improved as part of a comprehensive control intervention, the outbreak ended or the HAI rate declined. In two studies [590, 596], the composition of the nursing staff ("pool" or "float" vs. regular staff nurses) influenced the rate of primary bloodstream infections, with an increased infection rate occurring when the proportion of regular nurses decreased and pool nurses increased.

II.A.1.C. Clinical Microbiology Laboratory Support

The critical role of the clinical microbiology laboratory in infection control and healthcare epidemiology is described well [553, 554, 598-600] and is supported by the Infectious Disease Society of America policy statement on consolidation of clinical microbiology laboratories published in 2001 [553]. The clinical microbiology laboratory contributes to preventing transmission of infectious diseases in healthcare settings by promptly detecting and reporting epidemiologically important organisms, identifying emerging patterns of antimicrobial resistance, and assisting in assessment of the effectiveness of recommended precautions to limit transmission during outbreaks [598] . Outbreaks of infections may be recognized first by laboratorians [162]. Healthcare organizations need to ensure the availability of the recommended scope and quality of laboratory services, a sufficient number of appropriately trained laboratory staff members, and systems to promptly communicate epidemiologically important results to those who will take action (e.g., providers of clinical care, infection control staff, healthcare epidemiologists, and infectious disease consultants) [601] . As concerns about emerging pathogens and bioterrorism grow, the role of the clinical microbiology laboratory takes on even greater importance. For healthcare organizations that outsource microbiology laboratory services (e.g., ambulatory care, home care, LTCFs, smaller acute care hospitals), it is important to specify by contract the types of services (e.g., periodic institution-specific aggregate susceptibility reports) required to support infection control.

Several key functions of the clinical microbiology laboratory are relevant to this guideline:

- Antimicrobial susceptibility by testing and interpretation in accordance with current guidelines developed by the National Committee for Clinical Laboratory Standards (NCCLS), known as the Clinical and Laboratory Standards Institute (CLSI) since 2005 [602] , for the detection of emerging resistance patterns [603, 604] , and for the preparation, analysis, and distribution of periodic cumulative antimicrobial susceptibility summary reports [605-607] . While not required, clinical laboratories ideally should have access to rapid genotypic identification of bacteria and their antibiotic resistance genes [608].
- Performance of surveillance cultures when appropriate (including retention of isolates for analysis) to assess patterns of infection transmission and effectiveness of infection control interventions at the facility or organization. Microbiologists assist in decisions concerning the indications for initiating and discontinuing active surveillance programs and optimize the use of laboratory resources.
- Molecular typing, on-site or outsourced, in order to investigate and control healthcare-associated outbreaks [609].

- Application of rapid diagnostic tests to support clinical decisions involving patient treatment, room selection, and implementation of control measures including barrier precautions and use of vaccine or chemoprophylaxis agents (e.g., influenza [610-612], B. pertussis [613], RSV [614, 615], and enteroviruses [616]). The microbiologist provides guidance to limit rapid testing to clinical situations in which rapid results influence patient management decisions, as well as providing oversight of point-of-care testing performed by non-laboratory healthcare workers [617].
- Detection and rapid reporting of epidemiologically important organisms, including those that are reportable to public health agencies.
- Implementation of a quality control program that ensures testing services are appropriate for the population served, and stringently evaluated for sensitivity, specificity, applicability, and feasibility.
- Participation in a multidisciplinary team to develop and maintain an effective institutional program for the judicious use of antimicrobial agents [618, 619].

II.A.2. Institutional Safety Culture and Organizational Characteristics

Safety culture (or safety climate) refers to a work environment where a shared commitment to safety on the part of management and the workforce is understood and followed [557, 620, 621]. The authors of the Institute of Medicine Report, To Err is Human [543], acknowledge that causes of medical error are multifaceted but emphasize repeatedly the pivotal role of system failures and the benefits of a safety culture. A safety culture is created through 1) the actions management takes to improve patient and worker safety; 2) worker participation in safety planning; 3) the availability of appropriate protective equipment; 4) influence of group norms regarding acceptable safety practices; and 5) the organization's socialization process for new personnel. Safety and patient outcomes can be enhanced by improving or creating organizational characteristics within patient care units as demonstrated by studies of surgical ICUs [622, 623]. Each of these factors has a direct bearing on adherence to transmission prevention recommendations [257]. Measurement of an institutional culture of safety is useful for designing improvements in healthcare [624, 625]. Several hospital-based studies have linked measures of safety culture with both employee adherence to safe practices and reduced exposures to blood and body fluids [626-632]. One study of hand hygiene practices concluded that improved adherence requires integration of infection control into the organization's safety culture [561]. Several hospitals that are part of the Veterans Administration Healthcare System have taken specific steps toward improving the safety culture, including error reporting mechanisms, performing root cause analysis on problems identified, providing safety incentives, and employee education. [633-635].

II.A.3. Adherence of Healthcare Personnel to Recommended Guidelines

Adherence to recommended infection control practices decreases transmission of infectious agents in healthcare settings [116, 562, 636-640]. However, several observational studies have shown limited adherence to recommended practices by healthcare personnel [559, 640-657]. Observed adherence to universal precautions ranged from 43% to 89% [641, 642, 649, 651, 652]. However, the degree of adherence depended frequently on the practice that was assessed and, for glove use, the circumstance in which they were used. Appropriate glove use has ranged from a low of 15% [645] to a high of 82% [650]. However, 92% and 98% adherence with glove use have been reported during arterial blood gas collection and resuscitation, respectively, procedures where there may be considerable blood contact [643, 656]. Differences in observed adherence have been reported among occupational groups in the same healthcare facility [641] and between experienced and nonexperienced professionals [645]. In surveys of healthcare personnel, self-reported adherence was generally higher than that reported in observational studies. Furthermore, where an observational component was included with a self-reported survey, self-perceived adherence was often greater than observed adherence [657]. Among nurses and physicians, increasing years of experience is a negative predictor of adherence [645, 651]. Education to improve adherence is the primary intervention that has been studied. While positive changes in knowledge and attitude have been demonstrated, [640, 658], there often has been limited or no accompanying change in behavior [642, 644]. Self-reported adherence is higher in groups that have received an educational intervention [630, 659]. Educational interventions that incorporated videotaping and performance feedback were successful in improving adherence during the period of study; the long-term effect of these interventions is not known [654].The use of videotape also served to identify system problems (e.g., communication and access to personal protective equipment) that otherwise may not have been recognized.

Use of engineering controls and facility design concepts for improving adherence is gaining interest. While introduction of automated sinks had a negative impact on consistent adherence to hand washing [660], use of electronic monitoring and voice prompts to remind healthcare workers to perform hand hygiene, and improving accessibility to hand hygiene products, increased adherence and contributed to a decrease in HAIs in one study [661]. More information is needed regarding how technology might improve adherence.

Improving adherence to infection control practices requires a multifaceted approach that incorporates continuous assessment of both the individual and the work environment [559, 561]. Using several behavioral theories, Kretzer and Larson concluded that a single intervention (e.g., a handwashing campaign or putting up new posters about transmission precautions) would likely be ineffective in improving healthcare personnel adherence [662]. Improvement requires that the organizational leadership make prevention an institutional priority and integrate infection control practices into the organization's safety culture [561]. A recent review of the literature concluded that variations in organizational factors (e.g., safety climate, policies and procedures, education and training) and individual factors (e.g., knowledge, perceptions of risk, past experience) were determinants of adherence to infection control guidelines for protection against SARS and other respiratory pathogens [257].

II.B. Surveillance for Healthcare-Associated Infections (HAIs)

Surveillance is an essential tool for case-finding of single patients or clusters of patients who are infected or colonized with epidemiologically important organisms (e.g., susceptible bacteria such as *S. aureus, S. pyogenes* [Group A streptococcus] or Enterobacter-Klebsiella spp; MRSA, VRE, and other MDROs; *C. difficile*; RSV; influenza virus) for which transmission-based precautions may be required. Surveillance is defined as the ongoing, systematic collection, analysis, interpretation, and dissemination of data regarding a health-related event for use in public health action to reduce morbidity and mortality and to improve health [663]. The work of Ignaz Semmelweis that described the role of person-to-person transmission in puerperal sepsis is the earliest example of the use of surveillance data to reduce transmission of infectious agents [664]. Surveillance of both process measures and the infection rates to which they are linked are important for evaluating the effectiveness of infection prevention efforts and identifying indications for change [555, 665-668].

The Study on the Efficacy of Nosocomial Infection Control (SENIC) found that different combinations of infection control practices resulted in reduced rates of nosocomial surgical site infections, pneumonia, urinary tract infections, and bacteremia in acute care hospitals [566]; however, surveillance was the only component essential for reducing all four types of HAIs. Although a similar study has not been conducted in other healthcare settings, a role for surveillance and the need for novel strategies have been described in LTCFs [398, 434, 669, 670] and in home care [470-473] . The essential elements of a surveillance system are: 1) standardized definitions; 2) identification of patient populations at risk for infection; 3) statistical analysis (e.g. risk-adjustment, calculation of rates using appropriate denominators, trend analysis using methods such as statistical process control charts); and 4) feedback of results to the primary caregivers [671-676] . Data gathered through surveillance of high-risk populations, device use, procedures, and/or facility locations (e.g., ICUs) are useful for detecting transmission trends [671-673] . Identification of clusters of infections should be followed by a systematic epidemiologic investigation to determine commonalities in persons, places, and time; and guide implementation of interventions and evaluation of the effectiveness of those interventions.

Targeted surveillance based on the highest risk areas or patients has been preferred over facility-wide surveillance for the most effective use of resources [673, 676]. However, surveillance for certain epidemiologically important organisms may need to be facility-wide. Surveillance methods will continue to evolve as healthcare delivery systems change [392, 677] and user-friendly electronic tools become more widely available for electronic tracking and trend analysis [674, 678, 679] . Individuals with experience in healthcare epidemiology and infection control should be involved in selecting software packages for data aggregation and analysis to assure that the need for efficient and accurate HAI surveillance will be met. Effective surveillance is increasingly important as legislation requiring public reporting of HAI rates is passed and states work to develop effective systems to support such legislation [680].

II.C. Education of HCWs, Patients, and Families

Education and training of healthcare personnel are a prerequisite for ensuring that policies and procedures for Standard and Transmission-Based Precautions are understood and practiced. Understanding the scientific rationale for the precautions will allow HCWs to apply procedures correctly, as well as safely modify precautions based on changing requirements, resources, or healthcare settings [14, 655, 681-688]. In one study, the likelihood of HCWs developing SARS was strongly associated with less than 2 hours of infection control training and lack of understanding of infection control procedures [689]. Education about the important role of vaccines (e.g., influenza, measles, varicella, pertussis, pneumococcal) in protecting healthcare personnel, their patients, and family members can help improve vaccination rates [690-693].

Education on the principles and practices for preventing transmission of infectious agents should begin during training in the health professions and be provided to anyone who has an opportunity for contact with patients or medical equipment (e.g., nursing and medical staff; therapists and technicians, including respiratory, physical, occupational, radiology, and cardiology personnel; phlebotomists; housekeeping and maintenance staff; and students). In healthcare facilities, education and training on Standard and Transmission-Based Precautions are typically provided at the time of orientation and should be repeated as necessary to maintain competency; updated education and training are necessary when policies and procedures are revised or when there is a special circumstance, such as an outbreak that requires modification of current practice or adoption of new recommendations. Education and training materials and methods appropriate to the HCW's level of responsibility, individual learning habits, and language needs, can improve the learning experience [658, 694-702].

Education programs for healthcare personnel have been associated with sustained improvement in adherence to best practices and a related decrease in device-associated HAIs in teaching and non-teaching settings [639, 703] and in medical and surgical ICUs {Coopersmith, 2002 #2149; Babcock, 2004 #2126; Berenholtz, 2004 #2289; www.ihi.org/IHI/Programs/Campaign, #2563}. Several studies have shown that, in addition to targeted education to improve specific practices, periodic assessment and feedback of the HCWs knowledge,and adherence to recommended practices are necessary to achieve the desired changes and to identify continuing education needs [562, 704-708] . Effectiveness of this approach for isolation practices has been demonstrated for control of RSV [116, 684].

Patients, family members, and visitors can be partners in preventing transmission of infections in healthcare settings [9, 42, 709-711] . Information about Standard Precautions, especially hand hygiene, Respiratory Hygiene/Cough Etiquette, vaccination (especially against influenza) and other routine infection prevention strategies may be incorporated into patient information materials that are provided upon admission to the healthcare facility. Additional information about Transmission-Based Precautions is best provided at the time they are initiated. Fact sheets, pamphlets, and other printed material may include information on the rationale for the additional precautions, risks to household members, room assignment for Transmission-Based Precautions purposes, explanation about the use of personal protective equipment by HCWs, and directions for use of such equipment by family members and visitors. Such information may be particularly helpful in the home environment where household members often have primary responsibility for adherence to recommended infection control practices. Healthcare personnel must be available and prepared to explain this material and answer questions as needed.

II.D. Hand Hygiene

Hand hygiene has been cited frequently as the single most important practice to reduce the transmission of infectious agents in healthcare settings [559, 712, 713] and is an essential element of Standard Precautions. The term "hand hygiene" includes both handwashing with either plain or antiseptic-containing soap and water, and use of alcohol-based products (gels, rinses, foams) that do not require the use of water. In the absence of visible soiling of hands, approved alcohol-based products for hand disinfection are preferred over antimicrobial or plain soap and water because of their superior microbiocidal activity, reduced drying of the skin, and convenience [559]. Improved hand hygiene practices have been associated with a sustained decrease in the incidence of MRSA and VRE infections primarily in the ICU [561, 562, 714-717] . The scientific rationale, indications, methods, and products for hand hygiene are summarized in other publications [559, 717].

The effectiveness of hand hygiene can be reduced by the type and length of fingernails [559, 718, 719] . Individuals wearing artifical nails have been shown to harbor more pathogenic organisms, especially gram negative bacilli and yeasts, on the nails and in the subungual area than those with native nails [720, 721] . In 2002, CDC/HICPAC recommended (Category IA) that artificial fingernails and extenders not be worn by healthcare personnel who have contact with high-risk patients (e.g., those in ICUs, ORs) due to the association with outbreaks of gram- negative bacillus and candidal infections as confirmed by molecular typing of isolates [30, 31, 559, 722-725] .The need to restrict the wearing of artificial fingernails by all healthcare personnel who provide direct patient care or by healthcare personnel who have contact with other high risk groups (e.g., oncology, cystic fibrosis patients), has not been studied, but has been recommended by some experts [20] . At this time such decisions are at the discretion of an individual facility's infection control program. There is less evidence that jewelry affects the quality of hand hygiene. Although hand contamination with potential pathogens is increased with ring-wearing [559, 726] , no studies have related this practice to HCW-to-patient transmission of pathogens.

II.E. Personal Protective Equipment (PPE) for Healthcare Personnel

PPE refers to a variety of barriers and respirators used alone or in combination to protect mucous membranes, airways, skin, and clothing from contact with infectious agents. The selection of PPE is based on the nature of the patient interaction and/or the likely mode(s) of transmission. Guidance on the use of PPE is discussed in Part III. A suggested procedure for donning and removing PPE that will prevent skin or clothing contamination is presented in the Figure. Designated containers for used disposable or reusable PPE should be placed in a location that is convenient to the site of removal to facilitate disposal and containment of contaminated materials. Hand hygiene is always the final step after removing and disposing of PPE. The following sections highlight the primary uses and methods for selecting this equipment.

II.E.1. Gloves

Gloves are used to prevent contamination of healthcare personnel hands when 1) anticipating direct contact with blood or body fluids, mucous membranes, nonintact skin and other potentially infectious material; 2) having direct contact with patients who are colonized or infected with pathogens transmitted by the contact route e.g., VRE, MRSA, RSV [559, 727, 728]; or 3) handling or touching visibly or potentially contaminated patient care equipment and environmental surfaces [72, 73, 559]. Gloves can protect both patients and healthcare personnel from exposure to infectious material that may be carried on hands [73]. The extent to which gloves will protect healthcare personnel from transmission of bloodborne pathogens (e.g., HIV, HBV, HCV) following a needlestick or other pucture that penetrates the glove barrier has not been determined. Although gloves may reduce the volume of blood on the external surface of a sharp by 4686% [729], the residual blood in the lumen of a hollowbore needle would not be affected; therefore, the effect on transmission risk is unknown.

Gloves manufactured for healthcare purposes are subject to FDA evaluation and clearance [730]. Nonsterile disposable medical gloves made of a variety of materials (e.g., latex, vinyl, nitrile) are available for routine patient care [731]. The selection of glove type for non-surgical use is based on a number of factors, including the task that is to be performed, anticipated contact with chemicals and chemotherapeutic agents, latex sensitivity, sizing, and facility policies for creating a latex-free environment [17, 732-734]. For contact with blood and body fluids during non-surgical patient care, a single pair of gloves generally provides adequate barrier protection [734]. However, there is considerable variability among gloves; both the quality of the manufacturing process and type of material influence their barrier effectiveness [735]. While there is little difference in the barrier properties of unused intact gloves [736], studies have shown repeatedly that vinyl gloves have higher failure rates than latex or nitrile gloves when tested under simulated and actual clinical conditions [731, 735-738]. For this reason either latex or nitrile gloves are preferable for clinical procedures that require manual dexterity and/or will involve more than brief patient contact. It may be necessary to stock gloves in several sizes. Heavier, reusable utility gloves are indicated for non-patient care activities, such as handling or cleaning contaminated equipment or surfaces [11, 14, 739].

During patient care, transmission of infectious organisms can be reduced by adhering to the principles of working from "clean" to "dirty", and confining or limiting contamination to surfaces that are directly needed for patient care. It may be necessary to change gloves during the care of a single patient to prevent cross-contamination of body sites [559, 740]. It also may be necessary to change gloves if the patient interaction also involves touching portable computer keyboards or other mobile equipment that is transported from room to room. Discarding gloves between patients is necessary to prevent transmission of infectious material. Gloves must not be washed for subsequent reuse because microorganisms cannot be removed reliably from glove surfaces and continued glove integrity cannot be ensured. Furthermore, glove reuse has been associated with transmission of MRSA and gram-negative bacilli [741-743].

When gloves are worn in combination with other PPE, they are put on last. Gloves that fit snugly around the wrist are preferred for use with an isolation gown because they will cover the gown cuff and provide a more reliable continuous barrier for the arms, wrists, and hands. Gloves that are removed properly will prevent hand contamination (Figure). Hand hygiene following glove removal further ensures that the hands will not carry potentially infectious material that might have penetrated through unrecognized tears or that could contaminate the hands during glove removal [559, 728, 741].

II.E.2. Isolation Gowns

Isolation gowns are used as specified by Standard and Transmission-Based Precautions, to protect the HCW's arms and exposed body areas and prevent contamination of clothing with blood, body fluids, and other potentially infectious material [24, 88, 262, 744-746]. The need for and type of isolation gown selected is based on the nature of the patient interaction, including the anticipated degree of contact with infectious material and potential for blood and body fluid penetration of the barrier. The wearing of isolation gowns and other protective apparel is mandated by the OSHA Bloodborne Pathogens Standard [739]. Clinical and laboratory coats or jackets worn over personal clothing for comfort and/or purposes of identity are not considered PPE.

When applying Standard Precautions, an isolation gown is worn only if contact with blood or body fluid is anticipated. However, when Contact Precautions are used (i.e., to prevent transmission of an infectious agent that is not interrupted by Standard Precautions alone and that is associated with environmental contamination), donning of both gown and gloves upon room entry is indicated to address unintentional contact with contaminated environmental surfaces [54, 72, 73, 88]. The routine donning of isolation gowns upon entry into an intensive care unit or other high-risk area does not prevent or influence potential colonization or infection of patients in those areas [365, 747-750].

Isolation gowns are always worn in combination with gloves, and with other PPE when indicated. Gowns are usually the first piece of PPE to be donned. Full coverage of the arms and body front, from neck to the mid-thigh or below will ensure that clothing and exposed upper body areas are protected. Several gown sizes should be available in a healthcare facility to ensure appropriate coverage for staff members. Isolation gowns should be removed before leaving the patient care area to prevent possible contamination of the environment outside the patient's room. Isolation gowns should be removed in a manner that prevents contamination of clothing or skin (Figure). The outer, "contaminated", side of the gown is turned inward and rolled into a bundle, and then discarded into a designated container for waste or linen to contain contamination.

II.E.3. Face Protection: Masks, Goggles, Face Shields

II.E.3.A. *Masks*

Masks are used for three primary purposes in healthcare settings: 1) placed on healthcare personnel to protect them from contact with infectious material from patients e.g., respiratory secretions and sprays of blood or body fluids, consistent with Standard Precautions and Droplet Precautions; 2) placed on healthcare personnel when engaged in procedures requiring sterile technique to protect patients from exposure to infectious agents carried in a healthcare worker's mouth or nose, and 3) placed on coughing patients to limit potential dissemination of infectious respiratory secretions from the patient to others (i.e., Respiratory Hygiene/Cough Etiquette). Masks may be used in combination with goggles to protect the mouth, nose and eyes, or a face shield may be used instead of a mask and goggles, to provide more complete protection for the face, as discussed below. *Masks should not be confused with particulate respirators that are used to prevent inhalation of small particles that may contain infectious agents transmitted via the airborne route as described below.*

The mucous membranes of the mouth, nose, and eyes are susceptible portals of entry for infectious agents, as can be other skin surfaces if skin integrity is compromised (e.g., by acne, dermatitis) [66, 751-754]. Therefore, use of PPE to protect these body sites is an important component of Standard Precautions. The protective effect of masks for exposed healthcare personnel has been demonstrated [93, 113, 755, 756]. Procedures that generate splashes or sprays of blood, body fluids, secretions, or excretions (e.g., endotracheal suctioning, bronchoscopy, invasive vascular procedures) require either a face shield (disposable or reusable) or mask and goggles [93-95, 96, 113, 115, 262, 739, 757]. The wearing of masks, eye protection, and face shields in specified circumstances when blood or body fluid exposures are likely to occur is mandated by the OSHA Bloodborne Pathogens Standard [739]. Appropriate PPE should be selected based on the anticipated level of exposure.

Two mask types are available for use in healthcare settings: surgical masks that are cleared by the FDA and required to have fluid-resistant properties, and procedure or isolation masks [758] #2688. No studies have been published that compare mask types to determine whether one mask type provides better protection than another. Since procedure/isolation masks are not regulated by the FDA, there may be more variability in quality and performance than with surgical masks. Masks come in various shapes (e.g., molded and non-molded), sizes, filtration efficiency, and method of attachment (e.g., ties, elastic, ear loops). Healthcare facilities may find that different types of masks are needed to meet individual healthcare personnel needs.

II.E.3.B. Goggles, Face Shields

Guidance on eye protection for infection control has been published [759]. The eye protection chosen for specific work situations (e.g., goggles or face shield) depends upon the circumstances of exposure, other PPE used, and personal vision needs. Personal eyeglasses and contact lenses are NOT considered adequate eye protection (www.cdc.gov/niosh/topics/eye/eye-infectious.html). NIOSH states that, eye protection must be comfortable, allow for sufficient peripheral vision, and must be adjustable to ensure a secure fit. It may be necessary to provide several different types, styles, and sizes of protective equipment. Indirectly-vented goggles with a manufacturer's anti-fog coating may provide the most reliable practical eye protection from splashes, sprays, and respiratory droplets from multiple angles. Newer styles of goggles may provide better indirect airflow properties to reduce fogging, as well as better peripheral vision and more size options for fitting goggles to different workers. Many styles of goggles fit adequately over prescription glasses with minimal gaps. While effective as eye protection, goggles do not provide splash or spray protection to other parts of the face.

The role of goggles, in addition to a mask, in preventing exposure to infectious agents transmitted via respiratory droplets has been studied only for RSV. Reports published in the mid-1980s demonstrated that eye protection reduced occupational transmission of RSV [760, 761]. Whether this was due to preventing hand-eye contact or respiratory droplet-eye contact has not been determined. However, subsequent studies demonstrated that RSV transmission is effectively prevented by adherence to Standard plus Contact Precautions and that for this virus routine use of goggles is not necessary [24, 116, 117, 684, 762]. It is important to remind healthcare personnel that even if Droplet Precautions are not recommended for a specific respiratory tract pathogen, protection for the eyes, nose and mouth by using a mask and goggles, or face shield alone, is necessary when it is likely that there will be a splash or spray of any respiratory secretions or other body fluids as defined in Standard Precautions

Disposable or non-disposable face shields may be used as an alternative to goggles [759]. As compared with goggles, a face shield can provide protection to other facial areas in addition to the eyes. Face shields extending from chin to crown provide better face and eye protection from splashes and sprays; face shields that wrap around the sides may reduce splashes around the edge of the shield.

Removal of a face shield, goggles and mask can be performed safely after gloves have been removed, and hand hygiene performed. The ties, ear pieces and/or headband used to secure the equipment to the head are considered "clean" and therefore safe to touch with bare hands. The front of a mask, goggles and face shield are considered contaminated (Figure).

II.E.4. Respiratory Protection

The subject of respiratory protection as it applies to preventing transmission of airborne infectious agents, including the need for and frequency of fit-testing is under scientific review and was the subject of a CDC workshop in 2004 [763]. Respiratory protection currently requires the use of a respirator with N95 or higher filtration to prevent inhalation of infectious particles. Information about respirators and respiratory protection programs is summarized in the *Guideline for Preventing Transmission of Mycobacterium tuberculosis in Health-care Settings, 2005* (CDC.MMWR 2005; 54: RR-1 7 [12]).

Respiratory protection is broadly regulated by OSHA under the general industry standard for respiratory protection (29CFR1910.134)[764] which requires that U.S. employers in all employment settings implement a program to protect employees from inhalation of toxic materials. OSHA program components include medical clearance to wear a respirator; provision and use of appropriate respirators, including fit-tested NIOSH-certified N95 and higher particulate filtering respirators; education on respirator use and periodic re-evaluation of the respiratory protection program. When selecting particulate respirators, models with inherently good fit characteristics (i.e., those expected to provide protection factors of 10 or more to 95% of wearers) are preferred and could theoretically relieve the need for fit testing [765, 766] . Issues pertaining to respiratory protection remain the subject of ongoing debate. Information on various types of respirators may be found at www.cdc.gov/niosh/npptl/respirators/respsars.html and in published studies [765, 767, 768]. A user-seal check (formerly called a "fit check") should be performed by the wearer of a respirator each time a respirator is donned to minimize air leakage around the facepiece [769] . The optimal frequency of fit-testng has not been determined; re-testing may be indicated if there is a change in facial features of the wearer, onset of a medical condition that would affect respiratory function in the wearer, or a change in the model or size of the initially assigned respirator [12].

Respiratory protection was first recommended for protection of preventing U.S. healthcare personnel from exposure to *M. tuberculosis* in 1989. That recommendation has been maintained in two successive revisions of the Guidelines for Prevention of Transmission of Tuberculosis in Hospitals and other Healthcare Settings [12, 126] . The incremental benefit from respirator use, in addition to administrative and engineering controls (i.e., AIIRs, early recognition of patients likely to have tuberculosis and prompt placement in an AIIR, and maintenance of a patient with suspected tuberculosis in an AIIR until no longer infectious), for preventing transmission of airborne infectious agents (e.g., *M. tuberculosis)* is undetermined. Although some studies have demonstrated effective prevention of *M. tuberculosis* transmission in hospitals where surgical masks, instead of respirators, were used in conjunction with other administrative and engineering controls [637, 770, 771] , CDC currently recommends N95 or higher level respirators for personnel exposed to patients with suspected or confirmed tuberculosis. Currently this is also true for other diseases that could be transmitted through the airborne route, including SARS [262] and smallpox [108, 129, 772] , until inhalational transmission is better defined or healthcare-specific protective equipment more suitable for for preventing infection are developed. Respirators are also currently recommended to be worn during the performance of aerosol-generating procedures (e.g., intubation, bronchoscopy, suctioning) on patients with SARS Co-V infection, avian influenza and pandemic influenza (See Appendix A).

Although Airborne Precautions are recommended for preventing airborne transmission of measles and varicella-zoster viruses, there are no data upon which to base a recommendation for respiratory protection to protect susceptible personnel against these two infections; transmission of varicella-zoster virus has been prevented among pediatric patients using negative pressure isolation alone [773]. Whether respiratory protection (i.e., wearing a particulate respirator) would enhance protection from these viruses has not been studied. Since the majority of healthcare personnel have natural or acquired immunity to these viruses, only immune personnel generally care for patients with these infections [774-777]. Although there is no evidence to suggest that masks are not adequate to protect healthcare personnel in these settings, for purposes of consistency and simplicity, or because of difficulties in ascertaining immunity, some facilities may require the use of respirators for entry into all AIIRs, regardless of the specific infectious agent.

Procedures for safe removal of respirators are provided (Figure). In some healthcare settings, particulate respirators used to provide care for patients with *M. tuberculosis* are reused by the same HCW. This is an acceptable practice providing the respirator is not damaged or soiled, the fit is not compromised by change in shape, and the respirator has not been contaminated with blood or body fluids. There are no data on which to base a recommendation for the length of time a respirator may be reused.

II.F. Safe Work Practices to Prevent HCW Exposure to Bloodborne Pathogens

II.F.1. Prevention of Needlesticks and Other Sharps-Related Injuries

Injuries due to needles and other sharps have been associated with transmission of HBV, HCV and HIV to healthcare personnel [778, 779]. The prevention of sharps injuries has always been an essential element of Universal and now Standard Precautions [1, 780]. These include measures to handle needles and other sharp devices in a manner that will prevent injury to the user and to others who may encounter the device during or after a procedure. These measures apply to routine patient care and do not address the prevention of sharps injuries and other blood exposures during surgical and other invasive procedures that are addressed elsewhere [781-785].

Since 1991, when OSHA first issued its Bloodborne Pathogens Standard to protect healthcare personnel from blood exposure, the focus of regulatory and legislative activity has been on implementing a hierarchy of control measures. This has included focusing attention on removing sharps hazards through the development and use of engineering controls. The federal Needlestick Safety and Prevention Act signed into law in November, 2000 authorized OSHA's revision of its Bloodborne Pathogens Standard to more explicitly require the use of safety-engineered sharp devices [786] . CDC has provided guidance on sharps injury prevention [787, 788], including for the design, implementation and evaluation of a comprehensive sharps injury prevention program .[789]

II.F.2. Prevention of Mucous Membrane Contact

Exposure of mucous membranes of the eyes, nose and mouth to blood and body fluids has been associated with the transmission of bloodborne viruses and other infectious agents to healthcare personnel [66, 752, 754, 779]. The prevention of mucous membrane exposures has always been an element of Universal and now Standard Precautions for routine patient care [1, 753] and is subject to OSHA bloodborne pathogen regulations. Safe work practices, in addition to wearing PPE, are used to protect mucous membranes and non-intact skin from contact with potentially infectious material. These include keeping gloved and ungloved hands that are contaminated from touching the mouth, nose, eyes, or face; and positioning patients to direct sprays and splatter away from the face of the caregiver. Careful placement of PPE before patient contact will help avoid the need to make PPE adjustments and possible face or mucous membrane contamination during use.

In areas where the need for resuscitation is unpredictable, mouthpieces, pocket resuscitation masks with one-way valves, and other ventilation devices provide an alternative to mouth-to-mouth resuscitation, preventing exposure of the caregiver's nose and mouth to oral and respiratory fluids during the procedure.

II.F.2.A. Precautions During Aerosol-Generating Procedures

The performance of procedures that can generate small particle aerosols (aerosol-generating procedures), such as bronchoscopy, endotracheal intubation, and open suctioning of the respiratory tract, have been associated with transmission of infectious agents to healthcare personnel, including *M. tuberculosis* [790], SARSCoV [93, 94, 98] and *N. meningitides*[95]. Protection of the eyes, nose and mouth, in addition to gown and gloves, is recommended during performance of these procedures in accordance with Standard Precautions. Use of a particulate respirator is recommended during aerosol-generating procedures when the aerosol is likely to contain *M. tuberculosis*, SARS-CoV, or avian or pandemic influenza viruses.

II.G. Patient Placement

II.G.1. Hospitals and Long-Term Care Settings

Options for patient placement include single patient rooms, two patient rooms, and multi-bed wards. Of these, single patient rooms are prefered when there is a concern about transmission of an infectious agent. Although some studies have failed to demonstrate the efficacy of single patient rooms to prevent HAIs [791], other published studies, including one commissioned by the American Institute of Architects and the Facility Guidelines Institute, have documented a beneficial relationship between private rooms and reduction in infectious and noninfectious adverse patient outcomes [792, 793]. The AIA notes that private rooms are the trend in hospital planning and design. However, most hospitals and long-term care facilities have multi-bed rooms and must consider many competing priorities when determining the appropriate room placement for patients (e.g., reason for admission; patient characteristics, such as age, gender, mental status; staffing needs; family requests; psychosocial factors; reimbursement concerns). In the absence of obvious infectious diseases that require specified airborne infection isolation rooms (e.g., tuberculosis, SARS, chickenpox), the risk of transmission of infectious agents is not always considered when making placement decisions. When there are only a limited number of single-patient rooms, it is prudent to prioritize them for those patients who have conditions that facilitate transmission of infectious material to other patients (e.g., draining wounds, stool incontinence, uncontained secretions) and for those who are at increased risk of acquisition and adverse outcomes resulting from HAI (e.g., immunosuppression, open wounds, indwelling catheters, anticipated prolonged length of stay, total dependence on HCWs for activities of daily living)[15, 24, 43, 430, 794, 795].

Single-patient rooms are always indicated for patients placed on Airborne Precautions and in a Protective Environment and are preferred for patients who require Contact or Droplet Precautions [23, 24, 410, 435, 796, 797]. During a suspected or proven outbreak caused by a pathogen whose reservoir is the gastrointestinal tract, use of single patient rooms with private bathrooms limits opportunities for transmission, especially when the colonized or infected patient has poor personal hygiene habits, fecal incontinence, or cannot be expected to assist in maintaining procedures that prevent transmission of microorganisms (e.g., infants, children, and patients with altered mental status or developmental delay). In the absence of continued transmission, it is not necessary to provide a private bathroom for patients colonized or infected with enteric pathogens as long as personal hygiene practices and Standard Precautions, especially hand hygiene and appropriate environmental cleaning, are maintained. Assignment of a dedicated commode to a patient,and cleaning and disinfecting fixtures and equipment that may have fecal contamination (e.g., bathrooms, commodes [798], scales used for weighing diapers) and the adjacent surfaces with appropriate agents may be especially important when a single-patient room can not be used since environmental contamination with intestinal tract pathogens is likely from both continent and incontinent patients [54, 799]. Results of several studies to determine the benefit of a single-patient room to prevent transmission of *Clostridium difficile* are inconclusive [167, 800-802]. Some studies have shown that being in the same room with a colonized or infected patient is not necessarily a risk factor for transmission [791, 803-805]. However, for children, the risk of healthcare-associated diarrhea is increased with the increased number of patients per room [806]. Thus, patient factors are important determinants of infection transmission risks, and the need for a single-patient room and/or private bathroom for any patient is best determined on a case-by-case basis.

Cohorting is the practice of grouping together patients who are colonized or infected with the same organism to confine their care to one area and prevent contact with other patients. Cohorts are created based on clinical diagnosis, microbiologic confirmation when available, epidemiology, and mode of transmission of the infectious agent. It is generally preferred not to place severely immunosuppressed patients in rooms with other patients. Cohorting has been used extensively for managing outbreaks of MDROs including MRSA [22, 807], VRE [638, 808, 809], MDR-ESBLs [810]; *Pseudomonas aeruginosa* [29]; methicillin-susceptible *Staphylococcus aureus* [811]; RSV [812, 813]; adenovirus keratoconjunctivitis [814]; rotavirus [815]; and SARS [816]. Modeling studies provide additional support for cohorting patients to control outbreaks Talon [817-819]. However, cohorting often is implemented only after routine infection control measures have failed to control an outbreak.

Assigning or cohorting healthcare personnel to care only for patients infected or colonized with a single target pathogen limits further transmission of the target pathogen to uninfected patients [740, 819] but is difficult to achieve in the face of current staffing shortages in hospitals [583] and residential healthcare sites [820-822]. However, when continued transmission is occurring after implementing routine infection control measures and creating patient cohorts, cohorting of healthcare personnel may be beneficial.

During the seasons when RSV, human metapneumovirus [823], parainfluenza, influenza, other respiratory viruses [824], and rotavirus are circulating in the community, cohorting based on the presenting clinical syndrome is often a priority in facilities that care for infants and young children [825]. For example, during the respiratory virus season, infants may be cohorted based soley on the clinical diagnosis of bronchiolitis due to the logistical difficulties and costs associated with requiring microbiologic confirmation prior to room placement, and the predominance of RSV during most of the season. However, when available, single patient rooms are always preferred since a common clinical presentation (e.g., bronchiolitis), can be caused by more than one infectious agent [823, 824, 826]. Furthermore, the inability of infants and children to contain body fluids, and the close physical contact that occurs during their care, increases infection transmission risks for patients and personnel in this setting [24, 795].

II.G.2. Ambulatory Settings

Patients actively infected with or incubating transmissible infectious diseases are seen frequently in ambulatory settings (e.g., outpatient clinics, physicians' offices, emergency departments) and potentially expose healthcare personnel and other patients, family members and visitors [21, 34, 127, 135, 142, 827]. In response to the global outbreak of SARS in 2003 and in preparation for pandemic influenza, healthcare providers working in outpatient settings are urged to implement source containment measures (e.g., asking couging patients to wear a surgical mask or cover their coughs with tissues) to prevent transmission of respiratory infections, beginning at the point of initial patient encounter [9, 262, 828] as described below in section III.A.1 .a. Signs can be posted at the entrance to facilities or at the reception or registration desk requesting that the patient or individuals accompanying the patient promptly inform the receptionist if there are symptoms of a respiratory infection (e.g., cough, flu-like illness, increased production of respiratory secretions). The presence of diarrhea, skin rash, or known or suspected exposure to a transmissible disease (e.g., measles, pertussis, chickenpox, tuberculosis) also could be added. Placement of potentially infectious patients without delay in an examination room limits the number of exposed individuals, e.g., in the common waiting area.

In waiting areas, maintaining a distance between symptomatic and non-symptomatic patients (e.g., >3 feet), in addition to source control measures, may limit exposures. However, infections transmitted via the airborne route (e.g., *M tuberculosis*, measles, chickenpox) require additional precautions [12, 125, 829]. Patients suspected of having such an infection can wear a surgical mask for source containment, if tolerated, and should be placed in an examination room, preferably an AIIR, as soon as possible. If this is not possible, having the patient wear a mask and segregate him/herself from other patients in the waiting area will reduce opportunities to expose others. Since the person(s) accompanying the patient also may be infectious, application of the same infection control precautions may need to be extended to these persons if they are symptomatic [21, 252, 830] . For example, family members accompanying children admitted with suspected *M. tuberculosis* have been found to have unsuspected pulmonary tuberculosis with cavitary lesions, even when asymptomatic [42, 831].

Patients with underlying conditions that increase their susceptibility to infection (e.g., those who are immunocompromised [43, 44] or have cystic fibrosis [20]) require special efforts to protect them from exposures to infected patients in common waiting areas. By informing the receptionist of their infection risk upon arrival, appropriate steps may be taken to further protect them from infection. In some cystic fibrosis clinics, in order to avoid exposure to other patients who could be colonized with *B. cepacia*, patients have been given beepers upon registration so that they may leave the area and receive notification to return when an examination room becomes available [832].

II.G.3. Home Care

In home care, the patient placement concerns focus on protecting others in the home from exposure to an infectious household member. For individuals who are especially vulnerable to adverse outcomes associated with certain infections, it may be beneficial to either remove them from the home or segregate them within the home. Persons who are not part of the household may need to be prohibited from visiting during the period of infectivity. For example, if a patient with pulmonary tuberculosis is contagious and being cared for at home, very young children (<4 years of age) [833] and immunocompromised persons who have not yet been infected should be removed or excluded from the household. During the SARS outbreak of 2003, segregation of infected persons during the communicable phase of the illness was beneficial in preventing household transmission [249, 834].

II.H. Transport of Patients

Several principles are used to guide transport of patients requiring Transmission-Based Precautions. In the inpatient and residential settings these include 1) limiting transport of such patients to essential purposes, such as diagnostic and therapeutic procedures that cannot be performed in the patient's room; 2) when transport is necessary, using appropriate barriers on the patient (e.g., mask, gown, wrapping in sheets or use of impervious dressings to cover the affected area(s) when infectious skin lesions or drainage are present, consistent with the route and risk of transmission; 3) notifying healthcare personnel in the receiving area of the impending arrival of the patient and of the precautions necessary to prevent transmission; and 4) for patients being transported outside the facility, informing the receiving facility and the medi-van or emergency vehicle personnel in advance about the type of Transmission-Based Precautions being used. For tuberculosis, additional precautions may be needed in a small shared air space such as in an ambulance [12].

II.I. Environmental Measures

Cleaning and disinfecting non-critical surfaces in patient-care areas are part of Standard Precautions. In general, these procedures do not need to be changed for patients on Transmission-Based Precautions. The cleaning and disinfection of all patient-care areas is important for frequently touched surfaces, especially those closest to the patient, that are most likely to be contaminated (e.g., bedrails, bedside tables, commodes, doorknobs, sinks, surfaces and equipment in close proximity to the patient) [11, 72, 73, 835] . The frequency or intensity of cleaning may need to change based on the patient's level of hygiene and the degree of environmental contamination and for certain for infectious agents whose reservoir is the intestinal tract [54]. This may be especially true in LTCFs and pediatric facilities where patients with stool and urine incontinence are encountered more frequently. Also, increased frequency of cleaning may be needed in a Protective Environment to minimize dust accumulation [11]. Special recommendations for cleaning and disinfecting environmental surfaces in dialysis centers have been published [18] . In all healthcare settings, administrative, staffing and scheduling activities should prioritize the proper cleaning and disinfection of surfaces that could be implicated in transmission. During a suspected or proven outbreak where an environmental reservoir is suspected, routine cleaning procedures should be reviewed, and the need for additional trained cleaning staff should be assessed. Adherence should be monitored and reinforced to promote consistent and correct cleaning is performed.

EPA-registered disinfectants or detergents/disinfectants that best meet the overall needs of the healthcare facility for routine cleaning and disinfection should be selected [11, 836] . In general, use of the existing facility detergent/disinfectant according to the manufacturer's recommendations for amount, dilution, and contact time is sufficient to remove pathogens from surfaces of rooms where colonized or infected individuals were housed. This includes those pathogens that are resistant to multiple classes of antimicrobial agents (e.g., *C. difficile*, VRE, MRSA, MDR-GNB [11, 24, 88, 435, 746, 796, 837]). Most often, environmental reservoirs of pathogens during outbreaks are related to a failure to follow recommended procedures for cleaning and disinfection rather than the specific cleaning and disinfectant agents used [838-841].

Certain pathogens (e.g., rotavirus, noroviruses, *C. difficile*) may be resistant to some routinely used hospital disinfectants [275, 292, 842-847] .The role of specific disinfectants in limiting transmission of rotavirus has been demonstrated experimentally [842]. Also, since *C. difficile* may display increased levels of spore production when exposed to non-chlorine-based cleaning agents, and the spores are more resistant than vegetative cells to commonly used surface disinfectants, some investigators have recommended the use of a 1:10 dilution of 5.25% sodium hypochlorite (household bleach) and water for routine environmental disinfection of rooms of patients with *C. difficile* when there is continued transmission [844, 848]. In one study, the use of a hypochlorite solution was associated with a decrease in rates of C. difficile infections [847]. The need to change disinfectants based on the presence of these organisms can be determined in consultation with the infection control committee [11, 847, 848]. Detailed recommendations for disinfection and sterilization of surfaces and medical equipment that have been in contact with prion-containing tissue or high risk body fluids, and for cleaning of blood and body substance spills, are available in the Guidelines for Environmental Infection Control in Health-Care Facilities [11] and in the Guideline for Disinfection and Sterilization [848].

II.J. Patient Care Equipment and Instruments/Devices

Medical equipment and instruments/devices must be cleaned and maintained according to the manufacturers' instructions to prevent patient-to-patient transmission of infectious agents [86, 87, 325, 849]. Cleaning to remove organic material must always precede high level disinfection and sterilization of critical and semi-critical instruments and devices because residual proteinacous material reduces the effectiveness of the disinfection and sterilization processes [836, 848]. Noncritical equipment, such as commodes, intravenous pumps, and ventilators, must be thoroughly cleaned and disinfected before use on another patient. All such equipment and devices should be handled in a manner that will prevent HCW and environmental contact with potentially infectious material. It is important to include computers and personal digital assistants (PDAs) used in patient care in policies for cleaning and disinfection of non-critical items. The literature on contamination of computers with pathogens has been summarized [850] and two reports have linked computer contamination to colonization and infections in patients [851, 852]. Although keyboard covers and washable keyboards that can be easily disinfected are in use, the infection control benefit of those items and optimal management have not been determined.

In all healthcare settings, providing patients who are on Transmission-Based Precautions with dedicated noncritical medical equipment (e.g., stethoscope, blood pressure cuff, electronic thermometer) has been beneficial for preventing transmission [74, 89, 740, 853, 854]. When this is not possible, disinfection after use is recommended. Consult other guidelines for detailed guidance in developing specific protocols for cleaning and reprocessing medical equipment and patient care items in both routine and special circumstances [11, 14, 18, 20, 740, 836, 848].

In home care, it is preferable to remove visible blood or body fluids from durable medical equipment before it leaves the home. Equipment can be cleaned on-site using a detergent/disinfectant and, when possible, should be placed in a single plastic bag for transport to the reprocessing location [20, 739].

II.K. Textiles and Laundry

Soiled textiles, including bedding, towels, and patient or resident clothing may be contaminated with pathogenic microorganisms. However, the risk of disease transmission is negligible if they are handled, transported, and laundered in a safe manner [11, 855, 856]. Key principles for handling soiled laundry are 1) not shaking the items or handling them in any way that may aerosolize infectious agents; 2) avoiding contact of one's body and personal clothing with the soiled items being handled; and 3) containing soiled items in a laundry bag or designated bin. When laundry chutes are used, they must be maintained to minimize dispersion of aerosols from contaminated items [11]. The methods for handling, transporting, and laundering soiled textiles are determined by organizational policy and any applicable regulations [739]; guidance is provided in the Guidelines for Environmental Infection Control [11]. Rather than rigid rules and regulations, hygienic and common sense storage and processing of clean textiles is recommended [11, 857]. When laundering occurs outside of a healthcare facility, the clean items must be packaged or completely covered and placed in an enclosed space during transport to prevent contamination with outside air or construction dust that could contain infectious fungal spores that are a risk for immunocompromised patients [11].

Institutions are required to launder garments used as personal protective equipment and uniforms visibly soiled with blood or infective material [739]. There are few data to determine the safety of home laundering of HCW uniforms, but no increase in infection rates was observed in the one published study [858] and no pathogens were recovered from home- or hospital-laundered scrubs in another study [859]. In the home, textiles and laundry from patients with potentially transmissible infectious pathogens do not require special handling or separate laundering, and may be washed with warm water and detergent [11, 858, 859].

II.L. Solid Waste

The management of solid waste emanating from the healthcare environment is subject to federal and state regulations for medical and non-medical waste [860, 861] . No additional precautions are needed for non-medical solid waste that is being removed from rooms of patients on Transmission-Based Precautions. Solid waste may be contained in a single bag (as compared to using two bags) of sufficient strength. [862].

II.M. Dishware and Eating Utensils

The combination of hot water and detergents used in dishwashers is sufficient to decontaminate dishware and eating utensils. Therefore, no special precautions are needed for dishware (e.g., dishes, glasses, cups) or eating utensils; reusable dishware and utensils may be used for patients requiring Transmission-Based Precautions. In the home and other communal settings, eating utensils and drinking vessels that are being used should not be shared, consistent with principles of good personal hygiene and for the purpose of preventing transmission of respiratory viruses, *Herpes simplex* virus, and infectious agents that infect the gastrointestinal tract and are transmitted by the fecal/oral route (e.g., hepatitis A virus, noroviruses). If adequate resources for cleaning utensils and dishes are not available, disposable products may be used.

II.N. Adjunctive Measures

Important adjunctive measures that are not considered primary components of programs to prevent transmission of infectious agents, but improve the effectiveness of such programs, include 1) antimicrobial management programs; 2) postexposure chemoprophylaxis with antiviral or antibacterial agents; 3) vaccines used both for pre and postexposure prevention; and 4) screening and restricting visitors with signs of transmissible infections. Detailed discussion of judicious use of antimicrobial agents is beyond the scope of this document; however the topic is addressed in the MDRO section (Management of Multidrug-Resistant Organisms in Healthcare Settings 2006. www.cdc.gov/ncidod/dhqp/pdf/ar/mdroGuideline2006.pdf).

II.N.1. Chemoprophylaxis

Antimicrobial agents and topical antiseptics may be used to prevent infection and potential outbreaks of selected agents. Infections for which postexposure chemoprophylaxis is recommended under defined conditions include *B. pertussis* [17, 863], *N. meningitidis* [864], *B. anthracis* after environmental exposure to aeosolizable material [865], influenza virus [611], HIV [866], and group A streptococcus [160]. Orally administered antimicrobials may also be used under defined circumstances for MRSA decolonization of patients or healthcare personnel [867].

Another form of chemoprophylaxis is the use of topical antiseptic agents. For example, triple dye is used routinely on the umbilical cords of term newborns to reduce the risk of colonization, skin infections, and omphalitis caused by *S. aureus*, including MRSA, and group A streptococcus [868, 869]. Extension of the use of triple dye to low birth weight infants in the NICU was one component of a program that controlled one longstanding MRSA outbreak [22]. Topical antiseptics are also used for decolonization of healthcare personnel or selected patients colonized with MRSA, using mupirocin as discussed in the MDRO guideline [870 867, 871-873].

II.N.2. Immunoprophylaxis

Certain immunizations recommended for susceptible healthcare personnel have decreased the risk of infection and the potential for transmission in healthcare facilities [17, 874]. The OSHA mandate that requires employers to offer hepatitis B vaccination to HCWs played a substantial role in the sharp decline in incidence of occupational HBV infection [778, 875]. The use of varicella vaccine in healthcare personnel has decreased the need to place susceptible HCWs on administrative leave following exposure to patients with varicella [775]. Also, reports of healthcare-associated transmission of rubella in obstetrical clinics [33, 876] and measles in acute care settings [34] demonstrate the importance of immunization of susceptible healthcare personnel against childhood diseases. Many states have requirements for HCW vaccination for measles and rubella in the absence of evidence of immunity. Annual influenza vaccine campaigns targeted to patients and healthcare personnel in LTCFs and acute-care settings have been instrumental in preventing or limiting institutional outbreaks and increasing attention is being directed toward improving influenza vaccination rates in healthcare personnel [35, 611, 690, 877, 878, 879].

Transmission of *B. pertussis* in healthcare facilities has been associated with large and costly outbreaks that include both healthcare personnel and patients [17, 36, 41, 100, 683, 827, 880, 881]. HCWs who have close contact with infants with pertussis are at particularly high risk because of waning immunity and, until 2005, the absence of a vaccine that could be used in adults. However, two acellular pertussis vaccines were licensed in the United States in 2005, one for use in individuals aged 11-18 and one for use in ages 10-64 years [882]. Provisional ACIP recommendations at the time of publication of this document include adolescents and adults, especially those with contact with infants < 12 months of age and healthcare personnel with direct patient contact [883-884].

Immunization of children and adults will help prevent the introduction of vaccine- preventable diseases into healthcare settings. The recommended immunization schedule for children is published annually in the January issues of the *Morbidity Mortality Weekly Report* with interim updates as needed [885, 886]. An adult immunization schedule also is available for healthy adults and those with special immunization needs due to high risk medical conditions [887].

Some vaccines are also used for postexposure prophylaxis of susceptible individuals, including varicella [888], influenza [611], hepatitis B [778], and smallpox [225] vaccines [17, 874]. In the future, administration of a newly developed *S. aureus* conjugate vaccine (still under investigation) to selected patients may provide a novel method of preventing healthcare-associated *S. aureus*, including MRSA, infections in high-risk groups (e.g., hemodialysis patients and candidates for selected surgical procedures) [889, 890].

Immune globulin preparations also are used for postexposure prophylaxis of certain infectious agents under specified circumstances (e.g., varicella-zoster virus [VZIG], hepatitis B virus [HBIG], rabies [RIG], measles and hepatitis A virus [IG] [17, 833, 874]). The RSV monoclonal antibody preparation, Palivizumab, may have contributed to controlling a nosocomial outbreak of RSV in one NICU, but there is insufficient evidence to support a routine recommendation for its use in this setting [891].

II.N. 3. Management of Visitors

II.N.3.A. Visitors as Sources of Infection

Visitors have been identified as the source of several types of HAIs (e.g., pertussis [40, 41], *M. tuberculosis* [42, 892], influenza, and other respiratory viruses [24, 43, 44, 373] and SARS [21, 252-254]). However, effective methods for visitor screening in healthcare settings have not been studied. Visitor screening is especially important during community outbreaks of infectious diseases and for high risk patient units. Sibling visits are often encouraged in birthing centers, post partum rooms and in pediatric inpatient units, ICUs, and in residential settings for children; in hospital settings, a child visitor should visit only his or her own sibling. Screening of visiting siblings and other children before they are allowed into clinical areas is necessary to prevent the introduction of childhood illnesses and common respiratory infections.

Screening may be passive through the use of signs to alert family members and visitors with signs and symptoms of communicable diseases not to enter clinical areas. More active screening may include the completion of a screening tool or questionnaire which elicits information related to recent exposures or current symptoms. That information is reviewed by the facility staff and the visitor is either permitted to visit or is excluded [833].

Family and household members visiting pediatric patients with pertussis and tuberculosis may need to be screened for a history of exposure as well as signs and symptoms of current infection. Potentially infectious visitors are excluded until they receive appropriate medical screening, diagnosis, or treatment. If exclusion is not considered to be in the best interest of the patient or family (i.e., primary family members of critically or terminally ill patients), then the symptomatic visitor must wear a mask while in the healthcare facility and remain in the patient's room, avoiding exposure to others, especially in public waiting areas and the cafeteria.

Visitor screening is used consistently on HSCT units [15, 43]. However, considering the experience during the 2003 SARS outbreaks and the potential for pandemic influenza, developing effective visitor screening systems will be beneficial [9]. Education concerning Respiratory Hygiene/Cough Etiquette is a useful adjunct to visitor screening.

II.N.3.B. Use of Barrier Precautions by Visitors

The use of gowns, gloves, or masks by visitors in healthcare settings has not been addressed specifically in the scientific literature. Some studies included the use of gowns and gloves by visitors in the control of MDRO's, but did not perform a separate analysis to determine whether their use by visitors had a measurable impact [893-895]. Family members or visitors who are providing care or having very close patient contact (e.g., feeding, holding) may have contact with other patients and could contribute to transmission if barrier precautions are not used correctly. Specific recommendations may vary by facility or by unit and should be determined by the level of interaction.

PART III: PRECAUTIONS TO PREVENT TRANSMISSION OF INFECTIOUS AGENTS

There are two tiers of HICPAC/CDC precautions to prevent transmission of infectious agents, Standard Precautions and Transmission-Based Precautions. Standard Precautions are intended to be applied to the care of all patients in all healthcare settings, regardless of the suspected or confirmed presence of an infectious agent. *Implementation of Standard Precautions constitutes the primary strategy for the prevention of healthcare-associated transmission of infectious agents among patients and healthcare personnel.* Transmission-Based Precautions are for patients who are known or suspected to be infected or colonized with infectious agents, including certain epidemiologically important pathogens, which require additional control measures to effectively prevent transmission. Since the infecting agent often is not known at the time of admission to a healthcare facility, Transmission-Based Precautions are used empirically, according to the clinical syndrome and the likely etiologic agents at the time, and then modified when the pathogen is identified or a transmissible infectious etiology is ruled out. Examples of this syndromic approach are presented in Table 2. The HICPAC/CDC Guidelines also include recommendations for creating a Protective Environment for allogeneic HSCT patients.

The specific elements of Standard and Transmission-Based Precautions are discussed in Part II of this guideline. In Part III, the circumstances in which Standard Precautions, Transmission-Based Precautions, and a Protective Environment are applied are discussed. See Tables 4 and 5 for summaries of the key elements of these sets of precautions

III.A. Standard Precautions

Standard Precautions combine the major features of Universal Precautions (UP) [780, 896] and Body Substance Isolation (BSI) [640] and are based on the principle that all blood, body fluids, secretions, excretions except sweat, nonintact skin, and mucous membranes may contain transmissible infectious agents. Standard Precautions include a group of infection prevention practices that apply to all patients, regardless of suspected or confirmed infection status, in any setting in which healthcare is delivered (Table 4). These include: hand hygiene; use of gloves, gown, mask, eye protection, or face shield, depending on the anticipated exposure; and safe injection practices. Also, equipment or items in the patient environment likely to have been contaminated with infectious body fluids must be handled in a manner to prevent transmission of infectious agents (e.g. wear gloves for direct contact, contain heavily soiled equipment, properly clean and disinfect or sterilize reusable equipment before use on another patient).

The application of Standard Precautions during patient care is determined by the nature of the HCW-patient interaction and the extent of anticipated blood, body fluid, or pathogen exposure. For some interactions (e.g., performing venipuncture), only gloves may be needed; during other interactions (e.g., intubation), use of gloves, gown, and face shield or mask and goggles is necessary. Education and training on the principles and rationale for recommended practices are critical elements of Standard Precautions because they facilitate appropriate decision-making and promote adherence when HCWs are faced with new circumstances [655, 681-686] . An example of the importance of the use of Standard Precautions is intubation, especially under emergency circumstances when infectious agents may not be suspected, but later are identified (e.g., SARS-CoV, *N. meningitides*). The application of Standard Precautions is described below and summarized in Table 4. Guidance on donning and removing gloves, gowns and other PPE is presented in the Figure. Standard Precautions are also intended to protect patients by ensuring that healthcare personnel do not carry infectious agents to patients on their hands or via equipment used during patient care.

III.A.1. New Elements of Standard Precautions

Infection control problems that are identified in the course of outbreak investigations often indicate the need for new recommendations or reinforcement of existing infection control recommendations to protect patients. Because such recommendations are considered a standard of care and may not be included in other guidelines, they are added here to Standard Precautions. Three such areas of practice that have been added are: Respiratory Hygiene/Cough Etiquette, safe injection practices, and use of masks for insertion of catheters or injection of material into spinal or epidural spaces via lumbar puncture procedures (e.g., myelogram, spinal or epidural anesthesia). While most elements of Standard Precautions evolved from Universal Precautions that were developed for protection of healthcare personnel, these new elements of Standard Precautions focus on protection of patients.

III.A.1.A. Respiratory Hygiene/Cough Etiquette

The transmission of SARSCoV in emergency departments by patients and their family members during the widespread SARS outbreaks in 2003 highlighted the need for vigilance and prompt implementation of infection control measures at the first point of encounter within a healthcare setting (e.g., reception and triage areas in emergency departments, outpatient clinics, and physician offices) [21, 254, 897] . The strategy proposed has been termed Respiratory Hygiene/Cough Etiquette [9, 828] and is intended to be incorporated into infection control practices as a new component of Standard Precautions. The strategy is targeted at patients and accompanying family members and friends with undiagnosed transmissible respiratory infections, and applies to any person with signs of illness including cough, congestion, rhinorrhea, or increased production of respiratory secretions when entering a healthcare facility [40, 41, 43]. The term *cough etiquette* is derived from recommended source control measures for *M. tuberculosis* [12, 126].

The elements of Respiratory Hygiene/Cough Etiquette include 1) education of healthcare facility staff, patients, and visitors; 2) posted signs, in language(s) appropriate to the population served, with instructions to patients and accompanying family members or friends; 3) source control measures (e.g., covering the mouth/nose with a tissue when coughing and prompt disposal of used tissues, using surgical masks on the coughing person when tolerated and appropriate); 4) hand hygiene after contact with respiratory secretions; and 5) spatial separation, ideally >3 feet, of persons with respiratory infections in common waiting areas when possible. Covering sneezes and coughs and placing masks on coughing patients are proven means of source containment that prevent infected persons from dispersing respiratory secretions into the air [107, 145, 898, 899] . Masking may be difficult in some settings, (e.g., pediatrics, in which case, the emphasis by necessity may be on cough etiquette [900]. Physical proximity of <3 feet has been associated with an increased risk for transmission of infections via the droplet route (e.g., *N. meningitidis* [103] and group A streptococcus [114] and therefore supports the practice of distancing infected persons from others who are not infected. The effectiveness of good hygiene practices, especially hand hygiene, in preventing transmission of viruses and reducing the incidence of respiratory infections both within and outside [901-903] healthcare settings is summarized in several reviews [559, 717, 904].

These measures should be effective in decreasing the risk of transmission of pathogens contained in large respiratory droplets (e.g., influenza virus [23], adenovi rus [111], *B. pertussis* [827] and *Mycoplasma pneumoniae* [112] . Although fever will be present in many respiratory infections, patients with pertussis and mild upper respiratory tract infections are often afebrile. Therefore, the absence of fever does not always exclude a respiratory infection. Patients who have asthma, allergic rhinitis, or chronic obstructive lung disease also may be coughing and sneezing. While these patients often are not infectious, cough etiquette measures are prudent.

Healthcare personnel are advised to observe Droplet Precautions (i.e., wear a mask) and hand hygiene when examining and caring for patients with signs and symptoms of a respiratory infection. Healthcare personnel who have a respiratory infection are advised to avoid direct patient contact, especially with high risk patients. If this is not possible, then a mask should be worn while providing patient care.

III.A.1.B. Safe Injection Practices

The investigation of four large outbreaks of HBV and HCV among patients in ambulatory care facilities in the United States identified a need to define and reinforce safe injection practices [453]. The four outbreaks occurred in a private medical practice, a pain clinic, an endoscopy clinic, and a hematology/oncology clinic. The primary breaches in infection control practice that contributed to these outbreaks were 1) reinsertion of used needles into a multiple-dose vial or solution container (e.g., saline bag) and 2) use of a single needle/syringe to administer intravenous medication to multiple patients. In one of these outbreaks, preparation of medications in the same workspace where used needle/syringes were dismantled also may have been a contributing factor. These and other outbreaks of viral hepatitis could have been prevented by adherence to basic principles of aseptic technique for the preparation and administration of parenteral medications [453, 454]. These include the use of a sterile, single-use, disposable needle and syringe for each injection given and prevention of contamination of injection equipment and medication.

Whenever possible, use of single-dose vials is preferred over multiple-dose vials, especially when medications will be administered to multiple patients.

Outbreaks related to unsafe injection practices indicate that some healthcare personnel are unaware of, do not understand, or do not adhere to basic principles of infection control and aseptic technique. A survey of US healthcare workers who provide medication through injection found that 1 % to 3% reused the same needle and/or syringe on multiple patients [905] . Among the deficiencies identified in recent outbreaks were a lack of oversight of personnel and failure to follow-up on reported breaches in infection control practices in ambulatory settings. Therefore, to ensure that all healthcare workers understand and adhere to recommended practices, principles of infection control and aseptic technique need to be reinforced in training programs and incorporated into institutional polices that are monitored for adherence [454].

III.A.1.C. Infection Control Practices for Special Lumbar Puncture Procedures

In 2004, CDC investigated eight cases of post-myelography meningitis that either were reported to CDC or identified through a survey of the Emerging Infections Network of the Infectious Disease Society of America. Blood and/or cerebrospinal fluid of all eight cases yielded streptococcal species consistent with oropharyngeal flora and there were changes in the CSF indices and clinical status indicative of bacterial meningitis. Equipment and products used during these procedures (e.g., contrast media) were excluded as probable sources of contamination. Procedural details available for seven cases determined that antiseptic skin preparations and sterile gloves had been used. However, none of the clinicians wore a face mask, giving rise to the speculation that droplet transmission of oralpharyngeal flora was the most likely explanation for these infections. Bacterial meningitis following myelogram and other spinal procedures (e.g., lumbar puncture, spinal and epidural anesthesia, intrathecal chemotherapy) has been reported previously [906-915] . As a result, the question of whether face masks should be worn to prevent droplet spread of oral flora during spinal procedures (e.g., myelogram, lumbar puncture, spinal anesthesia) has been debated [916, 917] . Face masks are effective in limiting the dispersal of oropharyngeal droplets [918] and are recommended for the placement of central venous catheters [919] . In October 2005, the Healthcare Infection Control Practices Advisory Committee (HICPAC) reviewed the evidence and concluded that there is sufficient experience to warrant the additional protection of a face mask for the individual placing a catheter or injecting material into the spinal or epidural space.

III.B. Transmission-Based Precautions

There are three categories of Transmission-Based Precautions: Contact Precautions, Droplet Precautions, and Airborne Precautions. Transmission-Based Precautions are used when the route(s) of transmission is (are) not completely interrupted using Standard Precautions alone. For some diseases that have multiple routes of transmission (e.g., SARS), more than one Transmission-Based Precautions category may be used. When used either singly or in combination, they are always used in addition to Standard Precautions. See Appendix A for recommended precautions for specific infections. When Transmission-Based Precautions are indicated, efforts must be made to counteract possible adverse effects on patients (i.e., anxiety, depression and other mood disturbances [920-922], perceptions of stigma [923] , reduced contact with clinical staff [924-926] , and increases in preventable adverse events [565] in order to improve acceptance by the patients and adherence by HCWs.

III.B.1. Contact Precautions
Contact Precautions are intended to prevent transmission of infectious agents, including epidemiologically important microorganisms, which are spread by direct or indirect contact with the patient or the patient's environment as described in I.B.3.a. The specific agents and circumstance for which Contact Precautions are indicated are found in Appendix A. The application of Contact Precautions for patients infected or colonized with MDROs is described in the 2006 HICPAC/CDC MDRO guideline [927] . Contact Precautions also apply where the presence of excessive wound drainage, fecal incontinence, or other discharges from the body suggest an increased potential for extensive environmental contamination and risk of transmission. A single- patient room is preferred for patients who require Contact Precautions. When a single-patient room is not available, consultation with infection control personnel is recommended to assess the various risks associated with other patient placement options (e.g., cohorting, keeping the patient with an existing roommate). In multi-patient rooms, >3 feet spatial separation between beds is advised to reduce the opportunities for inadvertent sharing of items between the infected/colonized patient and other patients. Healthcare personnel caring for patients on Contact Precautions wear a gown and gloves for all interactions that may involve contact with the patient or potentially contaminated areas in the patient's environment. Donning PPE upon room entry and discarding before exiting the patient room is done to contain pathogens, especially those that have been implicated in transmission through environmental contamination (e.g., VRE, *C. difficile*,

noroviruses and other intestinal tract pathogens; RSV) [54, 72, 73, 78, 274, 275, 740].

III.B.2. Droplet Precautions

Droplet Precautions are intended to prevent transmission of pathogens spread through close respiratory or mucous membrane contact with respiratory secretions as described in I.B.3.b. Because these pathogens do not remain infectious over long distances in a healthcare facility, special air handling and ventilation are not required to prevent droplet transmission. Infectious agents for which Droplet Precautions are indicated are found in Appendix A and include *B. pertussis*, influenza virus, adenovirus, rhinovirus, *N. meningitides*, and group A streptococcus (for the first 24 hours of antimicrobial therapy). A single patient room is preferred for patients who require Droplet Precautions. When a single-patient room is not available, consultation with infection control personnel is recommended to assess the various risks associated with other patient placement options (e.g., cohorting, keeping the patient with an existing roommate). Spatial separation of > 3 feet and drawing the curtain between patient beds is especially important for patients in multi-bed rooms with infections transmitted by the droplet route. Healthcare personnel wear a mask (a respirator is not necessary) for close contact with infectious patient; the mask is generally donned upon room entry. Patients on Droplet Precautions who must be transported outside of the room should wear a mask if tolerated and follow Respiratory Hygiene/Cough Etiquette.

III.B.3. Airborne Precautions

Airborne Precautions prevent transmission of infectious agents that remain infectious over long distances when suspended in the air (e.g., rubeola virus [measles], varicella virus [chickenpox], *M. tuberculosis,* and possibly SARS-CoV) as described in I.B.3.c and Appendix A. The preferred placement for patients who require Airborne Precautions is in an airborne infection isolation room (AIIR). An AIIR is a single-patient room that is equipped with special air handling and ventilation capacity that meet the American Institute of Architects/Facility Guidelines Institute (AIA/FG I) standards for AII Rs (i.e., monitored negative pressure relative to the surrounding area, 12 air exchanges per hour for new construction and renovation and 6 air exchanges per hour for existing facilities, air exhausted directly to the outside or recirculated through HEPA filtration before return) [12, 13] . Some states require the availability of such rooms in hospitals, emergency departments, and nursing homes that care for patients with *M. tuberculosis*. A respiratory protection program that includes education about use of respirators, fit-testing, and user seal checks is required in any facility with

AIIRs. In settings where Airborne Precautions cannot be implemented due to limited engineering resources (e.g., physician offices), masking the patient, placing the patient in a private room (e.g., office examination room) with the door closed, and providing N95 or higher level respirators or masks if respirators are not available for healthcare personnel will reduce the likelihood of airborne transmission until the patient is either transferred to a facility with an AIIR or returned to the home environment, as deemed medically appropriate. Healthcare personnel caring for patients on Airborne Precautions wear a mask or respirator, depending on the disease-specific recommendations (Respiratory Protection II.E.4, Table 2, and Appendix A), that is donned prior to room entry. Whenever possible, non-immune HCWs should not care for patients with vaccine-preventable airborne diseases (e.g., measles, chickenpox, and smallpox).

III.C. Syndromic and Empiric Applications of Transmission-Based Precautions

Diagnosis of many infections requires laboratory confirmation. Since laboratory tests, especially those that depend on culture techniques, often require two or more days for completion, Transmission-Based Precautions must be implemented while test results are pending based on the clinical presentation and likely pathogens. Use of appropriate Transmission-Based Precautions at the time a patient develops symptoms or signs of transmissible infection, or arrives at a healthcare facility for care, reduces transmission opportunities. While it is not possible to identify prospectively all patients needing Transmission-Based Precautions, certain clinical syndromes and conditions carry a sufficiently high risk to warrant their use empirically while confirmatory tests are pending (Table 2). Infection control professionals are encouraged to modify or adapt this table according to local conditions.

III.D. Discontinuation of Transmission-Based Precautions

Transmission- Based Precautions remain in effect for limited periods of time (i.e., while the risk for transmission of the infectious agent persists or for the duration of the illness (Appendix A). For most infectious diseases, this duration reflects known patterns of persistence and shedding of infectious agents associated with the natural history of the infectious process and its treatment. For some diseases (e.g., pharyngeal or cutaneous diphtheria, RSV), Transmission-

Based Precautions remain in effect until culture or antigen-detection test results document eradication of the pathogen and, for RSV, symptomatic disease is resolved. For other diseases, (e.g., *M. tuberculosis*) state laws and regulations, and healthcare facility policies, may dictate the duration of precautions[12]). In immunocompromised patients, viral shedding can persist for prolonged periods of time (many weeks to months) and transmission to others may occur during that time; therefore, the duration of contact and/or droplet precautions may be prolonged for many weeks [500, 928-933].

The duration of Contact Precautions for patients who are colonized or infected with MDROs remains undefined. MRSA is the only MDRO for which effective decolonization regimens are available [867] . However, carriers of MRSA who have negative nasal cultures after a course of systemic or topical therapy may resume shedding MRSA in the weeks that follow therapy [934, 935]. Although early guidelines for VRE suggested discontinuation of Contact Precautions after three stool cultures obtained at weekly intervals proved negative [740] , subsequent experiences have indicated that such screening may fail to detect colonization that can persist for >1 year [27, 936-938] . Likewise, available data indicate that colonization with VRE, MRSA [939], and possibly MDR-GNB, can persist for many months, especially in the presence of severe underlying disease, invasive devices, and recurrent courses of antimicrobial agents.

It may be prudent to assume that MDRO carriers are colonized permanently and manage them accordingly. Alternatively, an interval free of hospitalizations, antimicrobial therapy, and invasive devices (e.g., 6 or 12 months) before reculturing patients to document clearance of carriage may be used. Determination of the best strategy awaits the results of additional studies. See the 2006 HICPAC/CDC MDRO guideline [927] for discussion of possible criteria to discontinue Contact Precautions for patients colonized or infected with MDROs.

III.E. Application of Transmission-Based Precautions in Ambulatory and Home Care Settings

Although Transmission-Based Precautions generally apply in all healthcare settings, exceptions exist. For example, in home care, AIIRs are not available. Furthermore, family members already exposed to diseases such as varicella and tuberculosis would not use masks or respiratory protection, but visiting HCWs would need to use such protection. Similarly, management of patients colonized or infected with MDROs may necessitate

Contact Precautions in acute care hospitals and in some LTCFs when there is continued transmission, but the risk of transmission in ambulatory care and home care, has not been defined. Consistent use of Standard Precautions may suffice in these settings, but more information is needed.

III.F. Protective Environment

A Protective Environment is designed for allogeneic HSCT patients to minimize fungal spore counts in the air and reduce the risk of invasive environmental fungal infections (see Table 5 for specifications) [11, 13-15]. The need for such controls has been demonstrated in studies of aspergillus outbreaks associated with construction [11, 14, 15, 157, 158]. As defined by the American Insitute of Architecture [13] and presented in detail in the Guideline for Environmental Infection Control 2003 [11, 861], air quality for HSCT patients is improved through a combination of environmental controls that include 1) HEPA filtration of incoming air; 2) directed room air flow; 3) positive room air pressure relative to the corridor; 4) well-sealed rooms (including sealed walls, floors, ceilings, windows, electrical outlets) to prevent flow of air from the outside; 5) ventilation to provide >12 air changes per hour; 6) strategies to minimize dust (e.g., scrubbable surfaces rather than upholstery [940] and carpet [941], and routinely cleaning crevices and sprinkler heads); and 7) prohibiting dried and fresh flowers and potted plants in the rooms of HSCT patients. The latter is based on molecular typing studies that have found indistinguishable strains of *Aspergillus terreus* in patients with hematologic malignancies and in potted plants in the vicinity of the patients [942-944]. The desired quality of air may be achieved without incurring the inconvenience or expense of laminar airflow [15, 157]. To prevent inhalation of fungal spores during periods when construction, renovation, or other dust-generating activities that may be ongoing in and around the health-care facility, it has been advised that severely immunocompromised patients wear a high-efficiency respiratory-protection device (e.g., an N95 respirator) when they leave the Protective Environment [11, 14, 945]). The use of masks or respirators by HSCT patients when they are outside of the Protective Environment for prevention of environmental fungal infections in the absence of construction has not been evaluated. A Protective Environment does not include the use of barrier precautions beyond those indicated for Standard and Transmission-Based Precautions. No published reports support the benefit of placing solid organ transplants or other immunocompromised patients in a Protective Environment.

PART IV: RECOMMENDATIONS

These recommendations are designed to prevent transmission of infectious agents among patients and healthcare personnel in all settings where healthcare is delivered. As in other CDC/HICPAC guidelines, each recommendation is categorized on the basis of existing scientific data, theoretical rationale, applicability, and when possible, economic impact. The CDC/HICPAC system for categorizing recommendations is as follows:

Category IA Strongly recommended for implementation and strongly supported by well-designed experimental, clinical, or epidemiologic studies.

Category IB Strongly recommended for implementation and supported by some experimental, clinical, or epidemiologic studies and a strong theoretical rationale.

Category IC Required for implementation, as mandated by federal and/or state regulation or standard.

Category II Suggested for implementation and supported by suggestive clinical or epidemiologic studies or a theoretical rationale.

No recommendation; unresolved issue. Practices for which insufficient evidence or no consensus regarding efficacy exists.

I. Administrative Responsibilities

Healthcare organization administrators should ensure the implementation of recommendations in this section.

I.A. Incorporate preventing transmission of infectious agents into the objectives of the organization's patient and occupational safety programs [543-546, 561, 620, 626, 946]. *Category IB/IC*

I.B. Make preventing transmission of infectious agents a priority for the healthcare organization. Provide administrative support, including fiscal and human resources for maintaining infection control programs [434, 548, 549, 559, 561, 566, 662, 552, 562-564, 946]. *Category IB/IC*

I.B.1. Assure that individuals with training in infection control are employed by or are available by contract to all healthcare facilities so that the infection control program is managed by one or more qualified individuals [552, 566 316, 575, 947 573, 576, 946]. *Category IB/IC*

I.B.1.a. Determine the specific infection control full-time equivalents (FTEs) according to the scope of the infection control program, the complexity of the healthcare facility or system, the characteristics of the patient population, the unique or urgent needs of the facility and community, and proposed staffing levels based on survey results and recommendations from professional organizations [434, 549 552, 566 316, 569, 573, 575 948 949]. *Category IB*

I.B.2. Include prevention of healthcare-associated infections (HAI) as one determinant of bedside nurse staffing levels and composition, especially in high-risk units [585-589 590 592 593 551, 594, 595 418, 596, 597 583] .*Category IB*

I.B.3. Delegate authority to infection control personnel or their designees (e.g., patient care unit charge nurses) for making infection control decisions concerning patient placement and assignment of Transmission-Based Precautions [549 434, 857, 946]. *Category IC*

I.B.4. Involve infection control personnel in decisions on facility construction and design, determination of AIIR and Protective Environment capacity needs and environmental assessments [11, 13, 950 951 12] . *Category IB/IC*

I.B.4.a. Provide ventilation systems required for a sufficient number of AIIRs (as determined by a risk assessment) and Protective Environments in healthcare facilities that provide care to patients for whom such rooms are indicated, according to published recommendations [11-13, 15] . *Category IB/IC*

I.B.5. Involve infection control personnel in the selection and post-implementation evaluation of medical equipment and supplies and changes in practice that could affect the risk of HAI [952, 953]. *Category IC*

I.B.6. Ensure availability of human and fiscal resources to provide clinical microbiology laboratory support, including a sufficient number of medical technologists trained in microbiology, appropriate to the healthcare setting, for monitoring transmission of microorganisms, planning and conducting epidemiologic investigations, and detecting emerging pathogens. Identify resources for performing surveillance cultures, rapid diagnostic testing for viral and other selected pathogens, preparation of antimicrobial susceptibility summary reports, trend analysis, and molecular typing of clustered isolates (performed either on-site or in a reference laboratory) and use these resources according to facility-specific epidemiologic needs, in consultation with clinical microbiologists [553, 609, 610, 612, 617, 954, 614, 603, 615, 616, 605, 599, 554, 598, 606, 607] . *Category IB*

I.B.7. Provide human and fiscal resources to meet occupational health needs related to infection control (e.g., healthcare personnel immunization, post-exposure evaluation and care, evaluation and management of healthcare personnel with communicable infections [739, 12, 17, 879-881, 955, 134, 690] . *Category IB/IC*

I.B.8. In all areas where healthcare is delivered, provide supplies and equipment necessary for the consistent observance of Standard Precautions, including hand hygiene products and personal protective equipment (e.g., gloves, gowns, face and eye protection) [739, 559, 946] . *Category IB/IC*

I.B.9. Develop and implement policies and procedures to ensure that reusable patient care equipment is cleaned and reprocessed appropriately before use on another patient [11, 956, 957, 958, 959, 836, 87, 11, 960, 961] . *Category IA/IC*

I.C. Develop and implement processes to ensure oversight of infection control activities appropriate to the healthcare setting and assign responsibility for oversight of infection control activities to an individual or group within the healthcare organization that is knowledgeable about infection control [434, 549, 566] . *Category II* I.D. Develop and implement systems for early detection and management (e.g., use of appropriate infection control measures, including isolation precautions, PPE) of potentially infectious persons at initial points of patient ncounter in outpatient settings (e.g., triage areas, emergency departments, outpatient clinics, physician offices) and at the time of admission to hospitals and long-term care facilities (LTCF) [9, 122, 134, 253, 827] *Category IB*

I.E. Develop and implement policies and procedures to limit patient visitation by persons with signs or symptoms of a communicable infection. Screen visitors to high-risk patient care areas (e.g., oncology units, hematopoietic stem call transplant [HSCT] units, intensive care units, other severely immunocompromised patients) for possible infection [43 24, 41, 962, 963].*Category IB*

I.F. Identify performance indicators of the effectiveness of organization-specific measures to prevent transmission of infectious agents (Standard and Transmission-Based Precautions), establish processes to monitor adherence to those performance measures and provide feedback to staff members [704, 739, 705, 708, 666, 964, 667, 668, 555] . *Category IB*

II. Education and Training

II.A. Provide job- or task-specific education and training on preventing transmission of infectious agents associated with healthcare during orientation to the healthcare facility; update information periodically during ongoing education programs. Target all healthcare personnel for education and training, including but not limited to medical, nursing, clinical technicians, laboratory staff; property service (housekeeping), laundry, maintenance and dietary workers; students, contract staff and volunteers. Document competency initially and repeatedly, as appropriate, for the specific staff positions. Develop a system to ensure that healthcare personnel employed by outside agencies meet these education and training requirements through programs offered by the agencies or by participation in the healthcare facility's program designed for full-time personnel [126, 559, 561, 562, 655, 681-684, 686, 688, 689, 702, 893, 919, 965]. *Category IB*

II.A.1. Include in education and training programs, information concerning use of vaccines as an adjunctive infection control measure 17, 611, 690, 874. *Category IB*

II.A.2. Enhance education and training by applying principles of adult learning, using reading level and language appropriate material for the target audience, and using online educational tools available to the institution [658, 694, 695, 697, 698, 700, 966]. *Category IB*

II.B. Provide instructional materials for patients and visitors on recommended hand hygiene and Respiratory Hygiene/Cough Etiquette practices and the application of Transmission-Based Precautions [9, 709, 710, 963]. *Category II*

III. Surveillance

III.A. Monitor the incidence of epidemiologically-important organisms and targeted HAIs that have substantial impact on outcome and for which effective preventive interventions are available; use information collected through surveillance of high-risk populations, procedures, devices and highly transmissible infectious agents to detect transmission of infectious agents in the healthcare facility [566, 671, 672, 675, 687, 919, 967, 968, 673, 969, 970] *Category IA*

III.B. Apply the following epidemiologic principles of infection surveillance [671, 967, 673, 969, 663, 664]. *Category IB*

- Use standardized definitions of infection
- Use laboratory-based data (when available)
- Collect epidemiologically-important variables (e.g., patient locations and/or clinical service in hospitals and other large multi-unit facilities, population-specific risk factors [e.g., low birth-weight neonates], underlying conditions that predispose to serious adverse outcomes)
- Analyze data to identify trends that may indicated increased rates of transmission
- Feedback information on trends in the incidence and prevalence of HAIs, probable risk factors, and prevention strategies and their impact to the appropriate healthcare providers, organization administrators, and as required by local and state health authorities

III.C. Develop and implement strategies to reduce risks for transmission and evaluate effectiveness [566, 673, 684, 970, 963, 971]. *Category IB*

III.D. When transmission of epidemiologically-important organisms continues despite implementation and documented adherence to infection prevention and control strategies, obtain consultation from persons knowledgeable in infection control and healthcare epidemiology to review the situation and recommend additional measures for control [566, 247, 687]. *Category IB*

III.E. Review periodically information on community or regional trends in the incidence and prevalence of epidemiologically-important organisms (e.g., influenza, RSV, pertussis, invasive group A streptococcal disease, MRSA, VRE) (including in other healthcare facilities) that may impact transmission of organisms within the facility [398, 687, 972, 973, 974]. *Category II*

IV. Standard Precautions

Assume that every person is potentially infected or colonized with an organism that could be transmitted in the healthcare setting and apply the following infection control practices during the delivery of health care.

IV.A. Hand Hygiene

IV.A.1. During the delivery of healthcare, avoid unnecessary touching of surfaces in close proximity to the patient to prevent both contamination of clean hands from environmental surfaces and transmission of pathogens from contaminated hands to surfaces [72,7,3 739, 800, 975]{CDC, 2001 #970. *Category IB/IC*

IV.A.2. When hands are visibly dirty, contaminated with proteinaceous material, or visibly soiled with blood or body fluids, wash hands with either a nonantimicrobial soap and water or an antimicrobial soap and water [559]. *Category IA*

IV.A.3. If hands are not visibly soiled, or after removing visible material withnonantimicrobial soap and water, decontaminate hands in the clinical situations described in IV.A.2.a-f. The preferred method of hand decontamination is with an alcohol-based hand rub [562, 978]. Alternatively, hands may be washed with an antimicrobial soap and water. Frequent use of alcohol-based hand rub immediately following handwashing with nonantimicrobial soap may increase the frequency of dermatitis [559]. *Category IB* Perform hand hygiene:

IV.A.3.a. Before having direct contact with patients [664, 979]. *Category IB*

IV.A.3.b. After contact with blood, body fluids or excretions, mucous membranes, nonintact skin, or wound dressings [664]. *Category IA* IV.A.3.c. After contact with a patient's intact skin (e.g., when taking a pulse or blood pressure or lifting a patient) [167, 976, 979, 980] *Category IB*

IV.A.3.d. If hands will be moving from a contaminated-body site to a clean-body site during patient care. *Category II*

IV.A.3.e. After contact with inanimate objects (including medical equipment) in the immediate vicinity of the patient [72, 73, 88, 800, 981, 982] . *Category II*

IV.A.3.f. After removing gloves [728, 741, 742] . *Category IB*

IV.A.4. Wash hands with non-antimicrobial soap and water or with antimicrobial soap and water if contact with spores (e.g., *C. difficile* or *Bacillus anthracis*) is likely to have occurred. The physical action of washing and rinsing hands under such circumstances is recommended because alcohols, chlorhexidine, iodophors, and other antiseptic agents have poor activity against spores [559, 956, 983] *Category II*

IV.A.5. Do not wear artificial fingernails or extenders if duties include direct contact with patients at high risk for infection and associated adverse outcomes (e.g., those in ICUs or operating rooms) [30, 31, 559, 722-724] . *Category IA*

IV.A.5.a. Develop an organizational policy on the wearing of non-natural nails by healthcare personnel who have direct contact with patients outside of the groups specified above [984] . *Category II*

IV.B. Personal protective equipment (PPE) (see Figure)

IV.B.1. Observe the following principles of use:

IV.B.1.a. Wear PPE, as described in IV.B.2-4, when the nature of the anticipated patient interaction indicates that contact with blood or body fluids may occur [739, 780, 896]. *Category IB/IC*

IV.B.1 .b. Prevent contamination of clothing and skin during the process of removing PPE (see Figure). *Category II*

IV.B.1 .c. Before leaving the patient's room or cubicle, remove and discard PPE [18, 739]. *Category IB/IC*

IV.B.2. Gloves

IV.B.2.a. Wear gloves when it can be reasonably anticipated that contact with blood or other potentially infectious materials, mucous membranes, nonintact skin, or potentially contaminated intact skin (e.g., of a patient incontinent of stool or urine) could occur [18, 728, 739, 741, 780, 985]. *Category IB/IC*

IV.B.2.b. Wear gloves with fit and durability appropriate to the task [559, 731, 732, 739, 986, 987] . *Category IB*

IV.B.2.b.i. Wear disposable medical examination gloves for providing direct patient care.

IV.B.2.b.ii. Wear disposable medical examination gloves or reusable utility gloves for cleaning the environment or medical equipment.

IV.B.2.c. Remove gloves after contact with a patient and/or the surrounding environment (including medical equipment) using proper technique to prevent hand contamination (see Figure). Do not wear the same pair of gloves for the care of more than one patient. Do not wash gloves for the purpose of reuse since this practice has been associated with transmission of pathogens [559, 728, 741-743, 988]. *Category IB*

IV.B.2.d. Change gloves during patient care if the hands will move from a contaminated body-site (e.g., perineal area) to a clean body-site (e.g., face). *Category II*

IV.B.3. Gowns

IV.B.3.a. Wear a gown, that is appropriate to the task, to protect skin and prevent soiling or contamination of clothing during procedures and patient-care activities when contact with blood, body fluids, secretions, or excretions is anticipated [739, 780, 896]. *Category IB/IC*

IV.B.3.a.i. Wear a gown for direct patient contact if the patient has uncontained secretions or excretions [24, 88, 89, 739, 744] *Category IB/IC*

IV.B.3.a.ii. Remove gown and perform hand hygiene before leaving the patient's environment [24, 88, 89, 739, 744] *Category IB/IC* IV.B.3.b. Do not reuse gowns, even for repeated contacts with the same patient. *Category II*

IV.B.3.c. Routine donning of gowns upon entrance into a high risk unit (e.g., ICU, NICU, HSCT unit) is not indicated [365, 747-750]. *Category IB* IVB4. Mouth, nose, eye protection

V.B.4.a. Use PPE to protect the mucous membranes of the eyes, nose and mouth during procedures and patient-care activities that are likely to generate splashes or sprays of blood, body fluids, secretions and excretions. Select masks, goggles, face shields, and combinations of each according to the need anticipated by the task performed [113, 739, 780, 896]. *Category IB/IC*

IV.B.5. During aerosol-generating procedures (e.g., bronchoscopy, suctioning of the respiratory tract [if not using in-line suction catheters], endotracheal intubation) in patients who are not suspected of being infected with an agent for which respiratory protection is otherwise recommended (e.g., *M. tuberculosis,* SARS or hemorrhagic fever viruses), wear one of the following: a face shield that fully covers the front and sides of the face, a mask with attached shield, or a mask and goggles (in addition to gloves and gown) [95, 96, 113, 126, 93, 94, 134]. *Category IB*

IV.C. Respiratory Hygiene/Cough Etiquette

IV.C.1. Educate healthcare personnel on the importance of source control measures to contain respiratory secretions to prevent droplet and fomite transmission of respiratory pathogens, especially during seasonal outbreaks of viral respiratory tract infections (e.g., influenza, RSV, adenovirus, parainfluenza virus) in communities [14, 24, 684, 10, 262]. *Category IB*

IV.C.2. Implement the following measures to contain respiratory secretions in patients and accompanying individuals who have signs and symptoms of a respiratory infection, beginning at the point of initial encounter in a healthcare setting (e.g., triage, reception and waiting areas in emergency departments, outpatient clinics and physician offices) [20, 24, 145, 902, 989]

IV.C.2.a. Post signs at entrances and in strategic places (e.g., elevators, cafeterias) within ambulatory and inpatient settings with instructions to patients and other persons with symptoms of a respiratory infection to cover their mouths/noses when coughing or sneezing, use and dispose of tissues, and perform hand hygiene after hands have been in contact with respiratory secretions. *Category II*

IV.C.2.b. Provide tissues and no-touch receptacles (e.g.,foot-pedaloperated lid or open, plastic-lined waste basket) for disposal of tissues [20]. *Category II*

IV.C.2.c. Provide resources and instructions for performing hand hygiene in or near waiting areas in ambulatory and inpatient settings; provide conveniently-located dispensers of alcohol-based hand rubs and, where sinks are available, supplies for handwashing [559, 903]. *Category IB*

IV.C.2.d. During periods of increased prevalence of respiratory infections in the community (e.g., as indicated by increased school absenteeism, increased number of patients seeking care for a respiratory infection), offer masks to coughing patients and other symptomatic persons (e.g., persons who accompany ill patients) upon entry into the facility or medical office [126, 899, 898] and encourage them to maintain special separation, ideally a distance of at least 3 feet, from others in common waiting areas [23, 103, 111, 114, 20, 134]. *Category IB*

IV.C.2.d.i. Some facilities may find it logistically easier to institute this recommendation year-round as a standard of practice. *Category II*

IV.D. Patient placement

IV.D.1. Include the potential for transmission of infectious agents in patient-placement decisions. Place patients who pose a risk for transmission to others (e.g., uncontained secretions, excretions or wound drainage; infants with suspected viral respiratory or gastrointestinal infections) in a single-patient room when available [24, 430, 435, 796, 797, 806, 990, 410, 793]. *Category IB*

IV.D.2. Determine patient placement based on the following principles:

- Route(s) of transmission of the known or suspected infectious agent
- Risk factors for transmission in the infected patient
- Risk factors for adverse outcomes resulting from an HAI in other patients in the area or room being considered for patient-placement
- Availability of single-patient rooms
- Patient options for room-sharing (e.g., cohorting patients with the same infection) *Category II*

IV.E. Patient-care equipment and instruments/devices [956]

IV.E.1. Establish policies and procedures for containing, transporting, and handling patient-care equipment and instruments/devices that may be contaminated with blood or body fluids [18, 739, 975]. *Category IB/IC*

IV.E.2. Remove organic material from critical and semi-critical instrument/devices, using recommended cleaning agents before high level disinfection and sterilization to enable effective disinfection and sterilization processes [836, 991, 992]. *Category IA*

IV.E.3. Wear PPE (e.g., gloves, gown), according to the level of anticipated contamination, when handling patient-care equipment and instruments/devices that is visibly soiled or may have been in contact with blood or body fluids [18, 739, 975]. *Category IB/IC*

IV.F. Care of the environment 11

IV.F.1. Establish policies and procedures for routine and targeted cleaning of environmental surfaces as indicated by the level of patient contact and degree of soiling [11]. *Category II*

IV.F.2. Clean and disinfect surfaces that are likely to be contaminated with pathogens, including those that are in close proximity to the patient (e.g., bed rails, over bed tables) and frequently-touched surfaces in the patient care environment (e.g., door knobs, surfaces in and surrounding toilets in patients' rooms) on a more frequent schedule compared to that for other surfaces (e.g., horizontal surfaces in waiting rooms) [11, 73, 740, 746, 993, 994, 72, 800, 835, 995]. *Category IB*

IV.F.3. Use EPA-registered disinfectants that have microbiocidal (i.e., killing) activity against the pathogens most likely to contaminate the patient-care environment. Use in accordance with manufacturer's instructions [842-844, 956, 996]. *Category IB/IC*

IV.F.3.a. Review the efficacy of in-use disinfectants when evidence of continuing transmission of an infectious agent (e.g., rotavirus, *C. difficile,* norovirus) may indicate resistance to the in-use product and change to a more effective disinfectant as indicated [275, 842, 847]. *Category II*

IV.F.4. In facilities that provide health care to pediatric patients or have waiting areas with child play toys (e.g., obstetric/gynecology offices and clinics), establish policies and procedures for cleaning and disinfecting toys at regular intervals [379, 80]. *Category IB*

- Use the following principles in developing this policy and procedures: *Category II*
- Select play toys that can be easily cleaned and disinfected
- Do not permit use of stuffed furry toys if they will be shared
- Clean and disinfect large stationary toys (e.g., climbing equipment) at least weekly and whenever visibly soiled
- If toys are likely to be mouthed, rinse with water after disinfection; alternatively wash in a dishwasher
- When a toy requires cleaning and disinfection, do so immediately or store in a designated labeled container separate from toys that are clean and ready for use

IV.F.5. Include multi-use electronic equipment in policies and procedures for preventing contamination and for cleaning and disinfection, especially those items that are used by patients, those used during delivery of patient care, and mobile devices that are moved in and out of patient rooms frequently (e.g., daily) [850, 851, 852, 997]. *Category IB*

IV.F.5.a. No recommendation for use of removable protective covers or washable keyboards. *Unresolved issue*

IV.G. Textiles and laundry

IV.G.1. Handle used textiles and fabrics with minimum agitation to avoid contamination of air, surfaces and persons [739, 998, 999]. *Category IB/IC*

IV.G.2. If laundry chutes are used, ensure that they are properly designed, maintained, and used in a manner to minimize dispersion of aerosols from contaminated laundry [11, 13, 1000, 1001]. *Category IB/IC* IV.H. Safe injection practices The following recommendations apply to the use of needles, cannulas that replace needles, and, where applicable intravenous delivery systems [454]

IV.H.1. Use aseptic technique to avoid contamination of sterile injection equipment [1002, 1003]. *Category IA*

IV.H.2. Do not administer medications from a syringe to multiple patients, even if the needle or cannula on the syringe is changed. Needles, cannulae and syringes are sterile, single-use items; they should not be reused for another patient nor to access a medication or solution that might be used for a subsequent patient [453, 919, 1004, 1005] *Category IA*

IV.H.3. Use fluid infusion and administration sets (i.e., intravenous bags, tubing and connectors) for one patient only and dispose appropriately after use. Consider a syringe or needle/cannula contaminated once it has been used to enter or connect to a patient's intravenous infusion bag or administration set [453]. *Category IB*

IV.H.4. Use single-dose vials for parenteral medications whenever possible [453]. *Category IA*

IV.H.5. Do not administer medications from single-dose vials or ampules to multiple patients or combine leftover contents for later use [369, 453, 1005]. *Category IA*

IV.H.6. If multidose vials must be used, both the needle or cannula and syringe used to access the multidose vial must be sterile [453, 1002] *Category IA*

IV.H.7. Do not keep multidose vials in the immediate patient treatment area and store in accordance with the manufacturer's recommendations; discard if sterility is compromised or questionable [453, 1003]. *Category IA*

IV.H.8. Do not use bags or bottles of intravenous solution as a common source of supply for multiple patients [453, 1006]. *Category IB*

IV.I. Infection control practices for special lumbar puncture procedures Wear a surgical mask when placing a catheter or injecting material into the spinal canal or subdural space (i.e., during myelograms, lumbar puncture and spinal or epidural anesthesia [906, 907-909, 910, 911, 912-914, 918, 1007]. *Category IB*

IV.J. Worker safety Adhere to federal and state requirements for protection of healthcare personnel from exposure to bloodborne pathogens [739]. *Category IC*

V. Transmission-Based Precautions

V.A. General principles
V.A.1. In addition to Standard Precautions, use Transmission-Based Precautions for patients with documented or suspected infection or colonization with highly transmissible or epidemiologically-important pathogens for which additional precautions are needed to prevent transmission (see Appendix A) [24, 93, 126, 141, 306, 806, 1008]. *Category IA*

V.A.2. Extend duration of Transmission-Based Precautions, (e.g., Droplet, Contact) for immunosuppressed patients with viral infections due to prolonged shedding of viral agents that may be transmitted to others [928, 931-933, 1009-1011]. *Category IA*

V.B. Contact Precautions

V.B.1. Use Contact Precautions as recommended in Appendix A for patients with known or suspected infections or evidence of syndromes that represent an increased risk for contact transmission. For specific recommendations for use of Contact Precautions for colonization or infection with MDROs, go to the MDRO guideline: www.cdc.gov/ncidod/dhqp/pdf/ar/mdroGuideline2006.pdf [870].

V.B.2. Patient placement

V.B.2.a. In *acute care hospitals*, place patients who require Contact Precautions in a single-patient room when available [24, 687, 793, 796, 797, 806, 837, 893, 1012, 1013] *Category IB*

When single-patient rooms are in short supply, apply the following principles for making decisions on patient placement:

- Prioritize patients with conditions that may facilitate transmission (e.g., uncontained drainage, stool incontinence) for single-patient room placement. *Category II*
- Place together in the same room (cohort) patients who are infected or colonized with the same pathogen and are suitable roommates [29, 638, 808, 811-813, 815, 818, 819] *Category IB*
- If it becomes necessary to place a patient who requires Contact Precautions in a room with a patient who is not infected or colonized with the same infectious agent:

  o Avoid placing patients on Contact Precautions in the same room with patients who have conditions that may increase the risk of adverse outcome from infection or that may facilitate transmission (e.g., those who are immunocompromised, have open wounds, or have anticipated prolonged lengths of stay). *Category II*

  o Ensure that patients are physically separated (i.e., >3 feet apart) from each other. Draw the privacy curtain between beds to minimize opportunities for direct contact.) *Category II*

  o Change protective attire and perform hand hygiene between contact with patients in the same room, regardless of whether one or both patients are on Contact Precautions [728, 741, 742, 988, 1014, 1015]. *Category IB*

V.B.2.b. In *long-term care and other residential settings*, make decisions regarding patient placement on a case-by-case basis, balancing infection risks to other patients in the room, the presence of risk factors that increase the likelihood of transmission, and the potential adverse psychological impact on the infected or colonized patient [920, 921]. *Category II*

V.B.2.c. In *ambulatory settings*, place patients who require Contact Precautions in an examination room or cubicle as soon as possible [20]. *Category II*

V.B.3. Use of personal protective equipment

V.B.3.a. Gloves

Wear gloves whenever touching the patient's intact skin [24, 89, 134, 559, 746, 837] or surfaces and articles in close proximity to the patient (e.g., medical equipment, bed rails) [72, 73, 88, 837]. Don gloves upon entry into the room or cubicle. *Category IB*

V.B.3.b. Gowns

V.B.3.b.i. Wear a gown whenever anticipating that clothing will have direct contact with the patient or potentially contaminated environmental surfaces or equipment in close proximity to the patient. Don gown upon entry into the room or cubicle. Remove gown and observe hand hygiene before leaving the patient-care environment [24, 88, 134, 745, 837]. *Category IB*

V.B.3.b.ii. After gown removal, ensure that clothing and skin do not contact potentially contaminated environmental surfaces that could result in possible transfer of microorganism to other patients or environmental surfaces [72, 73]. *Category II*

V.B.4. Patient transport

V.B.4.a. In *acute care hospitals and long-term care and other residential settings*, limit transport and movement of patients outside of the room to medically-necessary purposes. *Category II*

V.B.4.b. When transport or movement in any healthcare setting is necessary, ensure that infected or colonized areas of the patient's body are contained and covered. *Category II*

V.B.4.c. Remove and dispose of contaminated PPE and perform hand hygiene prior to transporting patients on Contact Precautions. *Category II*

V.B.4.d. Don clean PPE to handle the patient at the transport destination. *Category II*

V.B.5.Patient-care equipment and instruments/devices

V. B .5.a. Handle patient-care equipment and instruments/devices according to Standard Precautions [739, 836]. *Category IB/IC*

V.B.5.b. In *acute care hospitals and long-term care and other residential settings*, use disposable noncritical patient-care equipment (e.g., blood pressure cuffs) or implement patient-dedicated use of such equipment. If common use of equipment for multiple patients is unavoidable, clean and disinfect such equipment before use on another patient [24, 88, 796, 836, 837, 1016]. *Category IB*

V.B.5.c. In *home care settings*

V.B.5.c.i. Limit the amount of non-disposable patient-care equipment brought into the home of patients on Contact Precautions. Whenever possible, leave patient-care equipment in the home until discharge from home care services. *Category II*

V. B .5.c. ii. If noncritical patient-care equipment (e.g., stethoscope) cannot remain in the home, clean and disinfect items before taking them from the home using a low- to intermediate-level disinfectant. Alternatively, place contaminated reusable items in a plastic bag for transport and subsequent cleaning and disinfection. *Category II*

V.B.5.d. In *ambulatory settings*, place contaminated reusable noncritical patient-care equipment in a plastic bag for transport to a soiled utility area for reprocessing. *Category II*

V.B.6. Environmental measures

Ensure that rooms of patients on Contact Precautions are prioritized for frequent cleaning and disinfection (e.g., at least daily) with a focus on frequently-touched surfaces (e.g., bed rails, overbed table, bedside commode, lavatory surfaces in patient bathrooms, doorknobs) and equipment in the immediate vicinity of the patient [11, 24, 88, 746, 837]. *Category IB*

V.B.7. Discontinue Contact Precautions after signs and symptoms of the infection have resolved or according to pathogen-specific recommendations in Appendix A. *Category IB*

V.C. Droplet Precautions

V.C.1. Use Droplet Precautions as recommended in Appendix A for patients known or suspected to be infected with pathogens transmitted by respiratory droplets (i.e., large-particle droplets >5μ in size) that are generated by a patient who is coughing, sneezing or talking [14, 23], Steinberg, 1969 #1708, [41, 95, 103, 111, 112, 755, 756, 989, 1017] *Category IB*

V.C.2. Patient placement

V.C.2.a. In acute care hospitals, place patients who require Droplet Precautions in a single-patient room when available *Category II* When single-patient rooms are in short supply, apply the following principles for making decisions on patient placement:

- Prioritize patients who have excessive cough and sputum production for single-patient room placement *Category II*
- Place together in the same room (cohort) patients who are infected the same pathogen and are suitable roommates [814, 816]. *Category IB*

- If it becomes necessary to place patients who require Droplet Precautions in a room with a patient who does not have the same infection:
- Avoid placing patients on Droplet Precautions in the same room with patients who have conditions that may increase the risk of adverse outcome from infection or that may facilitate transmission (e.g., those who are immunocompromised, have or have anticipated prolonged lengths of stay). *Category II*
- Ensure that patients are physically separated (i.e., >3 feet apart) from each other. Draw the privacy curtain between beds to minimize opportunities for close contact [103, 104, 410]. *Category IB*
- Change protective attire and perform hand hygiene between contact with patients in the same room, regardless of whether one patient or both patients are on Droplet Precautions [741-743, 988, 1014, 1015]. *Category IB*

V.C.2.b. In *long-term care and other residential settings*, make decisions regarding patient placement on a case-by-case basis after considering infection risks to other patients in the room and available alternatives [410]. *Category II*

V.C.2.c. In *ambulatory settings*, place patients who require Droplet Precautions in an examination room or cubicle as soon as possible. Instruct patients to follow recommendations for Respiratory Hygiene/Cough Etiquette [447, 448, 9, 828]. *Category II*

V.C.3. Use of personal protective equipment

V.C.3.a. Don a mask upon entry into the patient room or cubicle [14, 23, 41, 103, 111, 113, 115, 827]. *Category IB*

V.C.3.b. No recommendation for routinely wearing eye protection (e.g., goggle or face shield), in addition to a mask, for close contact with patients who require Droplet Precautions. *Unresolved issue*

V.C.3.c. For patients with suspected or proven SARS, avian influenza or pandemic influenza, refer to the following websites for the most current recommendations (www.cdc.gov/ncidod/sars/;www.cdc.gov/flu/avian/ ;www.pandemic xflu.gov/) [134, 1018, 1019]

V.C.4. Patient transport

V.C.4.a. In *acute care hospitals and long-term care and other residential settings*, limit transport and movement of patients outside of the room to medically-necessary purposes. *Category II*

V.C.4.b. If transport or movement in any healthcare setting is necessary, instruct patient to wear a mask and follow Respiratory Hygiene/Cough Etiquette www.cdc.gov/flu/professionals/infectioncontrol/resphygiene.htm) . *Category IB*

V.C.4.c. No mask is required for persons transporting patients on Droplet Precautions. *Category II*

V.C.4.d. Discontinue Droplet Precautions after signs and symptoms have resolved or according to pathogen-specific recommendations in Appendix A. *Category IB*

V.D. Airborne Precautions

V.D.1. Use Airborne Precautions as recommended in Appendix A for patients known or suspected to be infected with infectious agents transmitted person-to-person by the airborne route (e.g., *M tuberculosis* [12], measles [34, 122, 1020], chickenpox [123, 773, 1021], disseminated herpes zoster [1022]. *Category IA/IC*

V.D.2. Patient placement

V.D.2.a. In *acute care hospitals and long-term care settings*, place patients who require Airborne Precautions in an AIIR that has been constructed in accordance with current guidelines [11-13]. *Category IA/IC*

V.D.2.a.i. Provide at least six (existing facility) or 12 (new construction/renovation) air changes per hour.

V.D.2.a.ii. Direct exhaust of air to the outside. If it is not possible to exhaust air from an AIIR directly to the outside, the air may be returned to the air-handling system or adjacent spaces if all air is directed through HEPA filters.

V.D.2.a.iii. Whenever an AIIR is in use for a patient on Airborne Precautions, monitor air pressure daily with visual indicators (e.g., smoke tubes, flutter strips), regardless of the presence of differential pressure sensing devices (e.g., manometers) [11, 12, 1023, 1024].

V.D.2.a.iv. Keep the AIIR door closed when not required for entry and exit.

V.D.2.b. When an AIIR is not available, transfer the patient to a facility that has an available AIIR [12]. *Category II*

V.D.2.c. In the event of an outbreak or exposure involving large numbers of patients who require Airborne Precautions:

- Consult infection control professionals before patient placement to determine the safety of alternative room that do not meet engineering requirements for an AIIR.
- Place together (cohort) patients who are presumed to have the same infection(based on clinical presentation and diagnosis when known) in areas of the facility that are away from other patients, especially patients who are at increased risk for infection (e.g., immunocompromised patients).
- Use temporary portable solutions (e.g., exhaust fan) to create a negative pressure environment in the converted area of the facility.

Guideline for Isolation Precautions

Discharge air directly to the outside, away from people and air intakes, or direct all the air through HEPA filters before it is introduced to other air spaces [12] Category II

V.D.2.d. In *ambulatory settings*:

V.D.2.d.i. Develop systems (e.g., triage, signage) to identify patients with known or suspected infections that require Airborne Precautions upon entry into ambulatory settings [9, 12, 34, 127, 134]. *Category IA*

V.D.2.d.ii. Place the patient in an AIIR as soon as possible. If an AIIR is not available, place a surgical mask on the patient and place him/her in an examination room. Once the patient leaves, the room should remain vacant for the appropriate time, generally one hour, to allow for a full exchange of air [11, 12, 122]. *Category IB/IC*

V.D.2.d.iii. Instruct patients with a known or suspected airborne infection to wear a surgical mask and observe Respiratory Hygiene/Cough Etiquette. Once in an AIIR, the mask may be removed; the mask should remain on if the patient is not in an AIIR [12, 107, 145, 899]. *Category IB/IC*

V.D.3. Personnel restrictions

Restrict susceptible healthcare personnel from entering the rooms of patients known or suspected to have measles (rubeola), varicella (chickenpox), disseminated zoster, or smallpox if other immune healthcare personnel are available [17, 775]. *Category IB*

V.D.4. Use of PPE

V.D.4.a. Wear a fit-tested NIOSH-approved N95 or higher level respirator for respiratory protection when entering the room or home of a patient when the following diseases are suspected or confirmed:

- Infectious pulmonary or laryngeal tuberculosis or when infectious tuberculosis skin lesions are present and procedures that would aerosolize viable organisms (e.g., irrigation, incision and drainage, whirlpool treatments) are performed [12, 1025, 1026]. *Category IB*
- Smallpox (vaccinated and unvaccinated). Respiratory protection is recommended for all healthcare personnel, including those with a documented "take" after smallpox vaccination due to the risk of a genetically engineered virus against which the vaccine may not provide protection, or of exposure to a very large viral load (e.g., from high-risk aerosol-generating procedures, immunocompromised patients, hemorrhagic or flat smallpox [108, 129]. *Category II*

V.D.4.b. No recommendation is made regarding the use of PPE by healthcare personnel who are presumed to be immune to measles (rubeola) or varicella-zoster based on history of disease, vaccine, or serologic testing when caring for an individual with known or suspected measles, chickenpox or disseminated zoster, due to difficulties in establishing definite immunity [1027, 1028]. *Unresolved issue*

V.D.4.c. No recommendation is made regarding the type of personal protective equipment (i.e., surgical mask or respiratory protection with a N95 or higher respirator) to be worn by susceptible healthcare personnel who must have contact with patients with known or suspected measles, chickenpox or disseminated herpes zoster. *Unresolved issue*

V.D.5. Patient transport

V.D.5.a. In *acute care hospitals and long-term care and other residential settings*, limit transport and movement of patients outside of the room to medically-necessary purposes. *Category II*

V.D.5.b. If transport or movement outside an AIIR is necessary, instruct patients to wear a surgical mask, if possible, and observe Respiratory Hygiene/Cough Etiquette [12] . *Category II*

V.D.5.c. For patients with skin lesions associated with varicella or smallpox or draining skin lesions caused by *M. tuberculosis*, cover the affected areas to prevent aerosolization or contact with the infectious agent in skin lesions [108, 1025, 1026, 1029-1031]. *Category IB*

V.D.5.d. Healthcare personnel transporting patients who are on Airborne Precautions do not need to wear a mask or respirator during transport if the patient is wearing a mask and infectious skin lesions are covered. *Category II*

V.D.6. Exposure management

Immunize or provide the appropriate immune globulin to susceptible persons as soon as possible following unprotected contact (i.e., exposed) to a patient with measles, varicella or smallpox: *Category IA*

- Administer measles vaccine to exposed susceptible persons within 72 hours after the exposure or administer immune globulin within six days of the exposure event for high-risk persons in whom vaccine is contraindicated [17, 1032-1035].
- Administer varicella vaccine to exposed susceptible persons within 120 hours after the exposure or administer varicella immune globulin (VZIG or alternative product), when available, within 96 hours for high-risk persons in whom vaccine is contraindicated (e.g., immunocompromised

patients, pregnant women, newborns whose mother's varicella onset was <5 days before or within 48 hours after delivery [888, 1035-1037]).
- Administer smallpox vaccine to exposed susceptible persons within 4 days after exposure [108, 1038-1040].

V.D.7. Discontinue Airborne Precautions according to pathogen-specific recommendations in Appendix A. *Category IB*

V.D.8. Consult CDC's "Guidelines for Preventing the Transmission of *Mycobacterium tuberculosis* in Health-Care Settings, 2005" [12] and the "Guideline for Environmental Infection Control in Health-Care Facilities" [11] for additional guidance on environment strategies for preventing transmission of tuberculosis in healthcare settings. The environmental recommendations in these guidelines may be applied to patients with other infections that require Airborne Precautions.

VI. Protective Environment (Table 4)

VI.A. Place allogeneic hematopoietic stem cell transplant (HSCT) patients in a Protective Environment as described in the "Guideline to Prevent Opportunistic Infections in HSCT Patients" [15], the "Guideline for Environmental Infection Control in Health-Care Facilities" [11], and the "Guidelines for Preventing Health-Care-Associated Pneumonia, 2003" [14] to reduce exposure to environmental fungi (e.g., *Aspergillus* sp) [157, 158] *Category IB*

VI.B. No recommendation for placing patients with other medical conditions that are associated with increased risk for environmental fungal infections (e.g., aspergillosis) in a Protective Environment [11]. *Unresolved issue*

VI.C. For patients who require a Protective Environment, implement the following (see Table 5) [11, 15]

VI.C.1. Environmental controls

VI.C.1.a. Filtered incoming air using central or point-of-use high efficiency particulate (HEPA) filters capable of removing 99.97% of particles >0.3 μm in diameter [13]. *Category IB*

VI.C.1.b. Directed room airflow with the air supply on one side of the room that moves air across the patient bed and out through an exhaust on the opposite side of the room [13] . *Category IB* VI.C.1.c. Positive air pressure in room relative to the corridor (pressure differential of >12.5 Pa [0.01-in water gauge]) [13] . *Category IB*

VI.C.1.c.i. Monitor air pressure daily with visual indicators (e.g., smoke tubes, flutter strips) [11, 1024] . *Category IA*

VI.C.1.d. Well-sealed rooms that prevent infiltration of outside air [13]. *Category IB*

VI.C.1.e. At least 12 air changes per hour [13]. *Category IB*

VI.C.2. Lower dust levels by using smooth, nonporous surfaces and finishes that can be scrubbed, rather than textured material (e.g., upholstery). Wet dust horizontal surfaces whenever dust is detected and routinely clean crevices and sprinkler heads where dust may accumulate [940, 941]. *Category II*

VI.C.3. Avoid carpeting in hallways and patient rooms in areas [941]. *Category IB*

VI.C.4. Prohibit dried and fresh flowers and potted plants [942-944]. *Category II*

VI.D. Minimize the length of time that patients who require a Protective Environment are outside their rooms for diagnostic procedures and other activities [11, 158, 945]. *Category IB*

VI.E. During periods of construction, to prevent inhalation of respirable particles that could contain infectious spores, provide respiratory protection (e.g., N95 respirator) to patients who are medically fit to tolerate a respirator when they are required to leave the Protective Environment [945, 158]. *Category II*

VI.E.1.a. No recommendation for fit-testing of patients who are using respirators. *Unresolved issue*

VI.E.1.b. No recommendation for use of particulate respirators when leaving the Protective Environment in the absence of construction. *Unresolved issue*

VI.F. Use of Standard and Transmission-Based Precautions in a Protective Environment.

VI.F.1. Use Standard Precautions as recommended for all patient interactions. *Category IA*

VI.F.2. Implement Droplet and Contact Precautions as recommended for diseases listed in Appendix A. Transmission-Based precautions for viral infections may need to be prolonged because of the patient's immunocompromised state and prolonged shedding of viruses [930, 1010, 928, 932, 1011]. *Category IB*

VI.F.3. Barrier precautions, (e.g., masks, gowns, gloves) are not required for healthcare personnel in the absence of suspected or confirmed infection in the patient or if they are not indicated according to Standard Precautions [15]. *Category II*

VI.F.4. Implement Airborne Precautions for patients who require a Protective Environment room and who also have an airborne infectious disease (e.g., pulmonary or laryngeal tuberculosis, acute varicella-zoster). *Category IA*

VI.F.4.a. Ensure that the Protective Environment is designed to maintain positive pressure [13]. *Category IB*

VI.F.4.b. Use an anteroom to further support the appropriate air-balance relative to the corridor and the Protective Environment; provide independent exhaust of contaminated air to the outside or place a HEPA filter in the exhaust duct if the return air must be recirculated [13, 1041]. *Category IB*

VI.F.4.c. If an anteroom is not available, place the patient in an AIIR and use portable, industrial-grade HEPA filters in the room to enhance filtration of spores [1042]. *Category II*

APPENDIX A

Preamble The mode(s) and risk of transmission for each specific disease agent included in Appendix A were reviewed. Principle sources consulted for the development of disease-specific recommendations for Appendix A included infectious disease manuals and textbooks [833, 1043, 1044]. The published literature was searched for evidence of person-to-person transmission in healthcare and non-healthcare settings with a focus on reported outbreaks that would assist in developing recommendations for all settings where healthcare is delivered. Criteria used to assign Transmission-Based Precautions categories follow:

- A Transmission-Based Precautions category was assigned if there was strong evidence for person-to-person transmission via droplet, contact, or airborne routes in healthcare or non-healthcare settings and/or if patient factors (e.g., diapered infants, diarrhea, draining wounds) increased the risk of transmission
- Transmission-Based Precautions category assignments reflect the predominant mode(s) of transmission
- If there was no evidence for person-to-person transmission by droplet, contact or airborne routes, Standard Precautions were assigned
- If there was a low risk for person-to-person transmission and no evidence of healthcare-associated transmission, Standard Precautions were assigned
- Standard Precautions were assigned for bloodborne pathogens (e.g., hepatitis B and C viruses, human immunodeficiency virus) as per CDC recommendations for Universal Precautions issued in 1988 [780]. Subsequent experience has confirmed the efficacy of Standard Precautions to prevent exposure to infected blood and body fluid [778, 779, 866].

APPENDIX A1
TYPE AND DURATION OF PRECAUTIONS RECOMMENDED FOR SELECTED INFECTIONS AND CONDITIONS

Infection/Condition	Precautions		Comments
	Type *	Duration †	
Abscess			
Draining, major	C	DI	No dressing or containment of drainage; until drainage stops or can be contained by dressing
Draining, minor or limited	S		Dressing covers and contains drainage
Acquired human immunodeficiency syndrome (H	S		Post-exposure chemoprophylaxis for some blood exposures [866].
Actinomycosis	S		Not transmitted from person to person
Adenovirus infection (see agent-specific guidance under gastroenteritis, conjuctivitis, pneumonia)			
Amebiasis	S		Person to person transmission is rare. Transmission in settings for the mentally challenged and in a family group has been reported [1045]. Use care when handling diapered infants and mentally challenged persons [1046].
Anthrax	S		Infected patients do not generally pose a transmission risk.
Cutaneous	S		Transmission through non-intact skin contact with draining lesions possible, therefore use Contact Precautions if large amount of uncontained drainage. Handwashing with soap and water preferable to use of waterless alcohol based antiseptics since alcohol does not have sporicidal activity [983].
Pulmonary	S		Not transmitted from person to person

Infection/Condition	Precautions		
	Type *	Duration †	Comments
nvironmental: aerosolizable spore-containing powder or other substance		DE	Until decontamination of environment complete [203]. Wear respirator (N95 mask or PAPRs), protective clothing; decontaminate persons with powder on them (http://www.cdc.gov/mmwr/preview/mmwrhtml/mm5 1 35a3.htm) Hand hygiene: Handwashing for 30-60 seconds with soap and water or 2% chlorhexidene gluconate after spore contact (alcohol handrubs inactive against spores [983]. Post-exposure prophylaxis following environmental exposure: 60 days of antimicrobials (either doxycycline, ciprofloxacin, or levofloxacin) and post-exposure vaccine under IND
Antibiotic-associated colitis (see *Clostridium*			
Arthropod-borne viral encephalitides (eastern, western, Venezuelan equine encephalomyelitis; St Louis, California encephalitis; West Nile Virus) and viral fevers (dengue, yellow fever, Colorado tick fever)	S		Not transmitted from person to person except rarely by transfusion, and for West Nile virus by organ transplant, breastmilk or transplacentally [530, 1047]. Install screens in windows and doors in endemic areas Use DEET-containing mosquito repellants and clothing to cover extremities
Ascariasis	S		Not transmitted from person to person
Aspergillosis	S		Contact Precautions and Airborne Precautions if massive soft tissue infection with copious drainage and repeated irrigations required [154].
Avian influenza (see influenza, avian below)			
Babesiosis	S		Not transmitted from person to person except rarely by
Blastomycosis, North American, cutaneous or	S		Not transmitted from person to person
Botulism	S		Not transmitted from person to person

(Continued).

Infection/Condition	Precautions		Comments
	Type *	Duration †	
Bronchiolitis (see respiratory infections in infants	C	DI	Use mask according to Standard Precautions.
Brucellosis (undulant, Malta, Mediterranean fever)	S		Not transmitted from person to person except rarely via banked spermatozoa and sexual contact [1048, 1049] . Provid antimicrobial prophylaxis following laboratory exposure [1050].
Campylobacter gastroenteritis (see gastroenteritis)			
Candidiasis, all forms including mucocutaneous	S		
Cat-scratch fever (benign inoculation lymphoreticulosis)	S		Not transmitted from person to person
Cellulitis	S		
Chancroid (soft chancre) (*H. ducreyi*)	S		Transmitted sexually from person to person
Chickenpox (see varicella)			
Chlamydia trachomatis			
Conjunctivitis	S		
Genital (lymphogranuloma venereum)	S		
Pneumonia (infants < 3 mos. of age))	S		
Chlamydia pneumoniae	S		Outbreaks in institutionalized populations reported, rarely [1051],
Cholera (see gastroenteritis)			
Closed-cavity infection			
Open drain in place; limited or minor drainage	S		Contact Precautions if there is copious uncontained drainage
No drain or closed drainage system in place	S		
Clostridium			
C. botulinum	S		Not transmitted from person to person
C. difficile (see Gastroenteritis, C. difficile)	C	DI	

Condition	Precaution	Duration	Comments
C. perfringens			
Food poisoning	S		Not transmitted from person to person
Gas gangrene	S		Transmission from person to person rare; one outbreak in a surgical setting reported [1053]. Use Contact Precautions if wound drainage is extensive.
Coccidioidomycosis (valley fever)			
Draining lesions	S		Not transmitted from person to person except under extraordinary circumstances because the infectious arthroconidial form of *Coccidioides immitis* is not produced in humans [1054].
Pneumonia	S		Not transmitted from person to person except under extraordinary circumstances, (e.g., inhalation of aerosolized tissue phase endospores during necropsy, transplantation of infected lung because the infectious arthroconidial form of *Coccidioides immitis* is not produced in humans [1054, 1055].
Colorado tick fever	S		Not transmitted from person to person
Congenital rubella	C	Until 1 yr of age	Standard Precautions if nasopharyngeal and urine cultures repeatedly neg. after 3 mos. of age
Conjunctivitis			
Acute bacterial	S		
Chlamydia	S		
Gonococcal	S		
Acute viral (acute hemorrhagic)	C	DI	Adenovirus most common; enterovirus [70, 1056], Coxsackie virus A24 [1057]) also associated with community outbreaks. Highly contagious; outbreaks in eye clinics, pediatric and neonatal settings, institutional settings reported. Eye clinics should follow Standard Precautions when handling patients with conjunctivitis. Routine use of infection control measures in the handling of instruments and equipment will prevent the occurrence of outbreaks in this and other settings. [460, 814, 1058, 1059 461, 1060].

(Continued).

Infection/Condition	Precautions		Comments
	Type *	Duration †	
Corona virus associated with SARS (SARS-CoV) (see severe acute respiratory syndrome)			
Coxsackie virus disease (see enteroviral infection)			
Creutzfeldt-Jakob disease CJD, vCJD	S		Use disposable instruments or special sterilization/disinfection for surfaces, objects contaminated with neural tissue if CJD or vCJD suspected and has not been R/O; No special burial procedures 1061
Croup (see respiratory infections in infants and			
Crimean-Congo Fever (see Viral Hemorrhagic Fever)	S		
Cryptococcosis	S		Not transmitted from person to person, except rarely via tissue and corneal transplant [1062, 1063]
Cryptosporidiosis (see gastroenteritis)			
Cysticercosis	S		Not transmitted from person to person
Cytomegalovirus infection, including in neonates and immunosuppressed patients	S		No additional precautions for pregnant HCWs
Decubitus ulcer (see Pressure ulcer)			
Dengue fever	S		Not transmitted from person to person
Diarrhea, acute-infective etiology suspected (see			
Diphtheria			
Cutaneous	C	CN	Until 2 cultures taken 24 hrs. apart negative
Pharyngeal	D	CN	Until 2 cultures taken 24 hrs. apart negative
Ebola virus (see viral hemorrhagic fevers)			
Echinococcosis (hydatidosis)	S		Not transmitted from person to person

Echovirus (see enteroviral infection)			
Encephalitis or encephalomyelitis (see specific etiologic agents)			
Endometritis (endomyometritis)	S		
Enterobiasis (pinworm disease, oxyuriasis)	S		
Enterococcus species (see multidrug-resistant organisms if epidemiologically significant or vancomycin resistant)			
Enterocolitis, *C. difficile* (see *C. difficile*, gastroenteritis)			
Enteroviral infections (i.e., Group A and B Coxsackie viruses and Echo viruses) (excludes polio virus)	S		Use Contact Precautions for diapered or incontinent children for duration of illness and to control institutional outbreaks
Epiglottitis, due to *Haemophilus influenzae* type b	D	U 24 hrs	See specific disease agents for epiglottitis due to other etiologies
Epstein-Barr virus infection, including infectious	S		
Erythema infectiosum (also see Parvovirus B19)			
Escherichia coli gastroenteritis (see gastroenteritis)			
Food poisoning			
Botulism	S		Not transmitted from person to person
C. perfringens or welchii	S		Not transmitted from person to person
Staphylococcal	S		Not transmitted from person to person
Furunculosis, staphylococcal	S		Contact if drainage not controlled. Follow institutional policies if
Infants and young children	C	DI	
Gangrene (gas gangrene)	S		Not transmitted from person to person

(Continued).

Infection/Condition	Precautions		Comments
	Type *	Duration †	
Gastroenteritis	S		Use Contact Precautions for diapered or incontinent persons for the duration of illness or to control institutional outbreaks for gastroenteritis caused by all of the agents below
Adenovirus	S		Use Contact Precautions for diapered or incontinent persons for the duration of illness or to control institutional outbreaks
Campylobacter species	S		Use Contact Precautions for diapered or incontinent persons for the duration of illness or to control institutional outbreaks
Cholera (Vibrio cholerae)	S		Use Contact Precautions for diapered or incontinent persons for the duration of illness or to control institutional outbreaks
C. difficile	C	DI	Discontinue antibiotics if appropriate. Do not share electronic thermometers [853, 854]; ensure consistent environmental cleaning and disinfection. Hypochlorite solutions may be required for cleaning if transmission continues [847]. Handwashing with soap and water preferred because of the absence of sporicidal activity of alcohol in waterless antiseptic handrubs [983].
Cryptosporidium species	S		Use Contact Precautions for diapered or incontinent persons for the duration of illness or to control institutional outbreaks
E. coli			
Enteropathogenic O157:H7 and other shiga toxin-producing Strains	S		Use Contact Precautions for diapered or incontinent persons for the duration of illness or to control institutional outbreaks
Other species	S		Use Contact Precautions for diapered or incontinent persons for the duration of illness or to control institutional outbreaks

Giardia lamblia	S		Use Contact Precautions for diapered or incontinent persons for the duration of illness or to control institutional outbreaks
Noroviruses	S		Use Contact Precautions for diapered or incontinent persons for the duration of illness or to control institutional outbreaks. Persons who clean areas heavily contaminated with feces or vomitus may benefit from wearing masks since virus can be aerosolized from these body substances [142, 147 148]; ensure consistent environmental cleaning and disinfection with focus on restrooms even when apparently unsoiled [273, 1064]) . Hypochlorite solutions may be required when there is continued transmission [290-292] . Alcohol is less active, but there is no evidence that alcohol antiseptic handrubs are not effective for hand decontamination [294]. Cohorting of affected patients to separate airspaces and toilet facilities may help interrupt transmission during outbreaks.
Rotavirus	C	DI	Ensure consistent environmental cleaning and disinfection and frequent removal of soiled diapers. Prolonged shedding may occur in both immunocompetent and immunocompromised children and the elderly [932, 933]
Salmonella species (including *S. typhi*)	S		Use Contact Precautions for diapered or incontinent persons for the duration of illness or to control institutional outbreaks
Shigella species (Bacillary dysentery)	S		Use Contact Precautions for diapered or incontinent persons for the duration of illness or to control institutional outbreaks
Vibrio parahaemolyticus	S		Use Contact Precautions for diapered or incontinent persons for the duration of illness or to control institutional outbreaks
Viral (if not covered elsewhere)	S		Use Contact Precautions for diapered or incontinent persons for the duration of illness or to control institutional outbreaks
Yersinia enterocolitica	S		Use Contact Precautions for diapered or incontinent persons for the duration of illness or to control institutional outbreaks

(Continued).

Infection/Condition	Precautions		Comments
	Type *	Duration †	
German measles (see rubella; see congenital			
Giardiasis (see gastroenteritis)			
Gonococcal ophthalmia neonatorum (gonorrheal ophthalmia, acute conjunctivitis of newborn)	S		
Gonorrhea	S		
Granuloma inguinale (Donovanosis, granuloma	S		
Guillain-Barré' syndrome	S		Not an infectious condition
Haemophilus influenzae (see disease-specific			
Hand, foot, and mouth disease (see enteroviral			
Hansen's Disease (see Leprosy)			
Hantavirus pulmonary syndrome	S		Not transmitted from person to person
Helicobacter pylori	S		
Hepatitis, viral			
Type A	S		Provide hepatitis A vaccine post-exposure as recommended 1065
Diapered or incontinent patients	C		Maintain Contact Precautions in infants and children <3 years of age for duration of hospitalization; for children 3-14 yrs. of age for 2 weeks after onset of symptoms; >14 yrs. of age for 1 week after onset of symptoms [833, 1066, 1067]
Type B-HBsAg positive; acute or chronic	S		See specific recommendations for care of patients in hemodialysis centers [778]
Type C and other unspecified non-A, non-B	S		See specific recommendations for care of patients in hemodialysis centers [778]
Type D (seen only with hepatitis B)	S		

Condition	Precaution	Duration	Comments
Type E	S		Use Contact Precautions for diapered or incontinent individuals for the duration of illness [1068]
Type G	S		
Herpangina (see enteroviral infection)			
Hookworm	S		
Herpes simplex (Herpesvirus hominis)			
Encephalitis	S		
Mucocutaneous, disseminated or primary, severe	C	Until lesions dry and crusted	
Mucocutaneous, recurrent (skin, oral, genital)	S		
Neonatal	C	Until lesions dry and crusted	Also, for asymptomatic, exposed infants delivered vaginally or by C-section and if mother has active infection and membranes have been ruptured for more than 4 to 6 hrs until infant surface cultures obtained at 24-36 hrs. of age negative after 48 hrs incubation [1069, 1070]
Herpes zoster (varicella-zoster) (shingles)			
Disseminated disease in any patient Localized disease in immunocompromised patient until disseminated infection ruled out	A,C	DI	Susceptible HCWs should not enter room if immune caregivers are available; no recommendation for type of protection of immune HCWs; no recommendation for type of protection, i.e. surgical mask or respirator; for susceptible HCWs.
Localized in patient with intact immune system with lesions that can be contained/covered	S	DI	Susceptible HCWs should not provide direct patient care when other immune caregivers are available.
Histoplasmosis	S		Not transmitted from person to person
Human immunodeficiency virus (HIV)	S		Post-exposure chemoprophylaxis for some blood exposures [866].

(Continued).

Infection/Condition	Precautions		
	Type *	Duration †	Comments
Human metapneumovirus	C	DI	HAI reported [107], but route of transmission not established [823]. Assumed to be Contact transmission as for RSV since the viruses are closely related and have similar clinical manifestations and epidemiology. Wear masks according to Standard Precautions.
Impetigo	C	U 24 hrs	
Infectious mononucleosis	S		
Influenza			
Human (seasonal influenza)	D	5 days except DI in immuno compromised persons	Single patient room when available or cohort; avoid placement with high-risk patients; mask patient when transported out of room; chemoprophylaxis/vaccine to control/prevent outbreaks [611]. Use gown and gloves according to Standard Precautions. Duration of precautions especially important in pediatric settings. Duration of viral shedding (i.e. for several weeks) has been observed; implications for transmission are unknown [930].
Avian (e.g., H5N1, H7, H9 strains))			See www.cdc.gov/flu/avian/professional/infect-control.htm for avian influenza guidance.
Pandemic influenza (also a human influenza virus)	D	5 days from onset of symptoms	See http://www.pandemicflu.gov for current pandemic influenza guidance.
Kawasaki syndrome	S		Not an infectious condition
Lassa fever (see viral hemorrhagic fevers)			
Legionnaires' disease	S		Not transmitted from person to person
Leprosy	S		

Leptospirosis	S		Not transmitted from person to person
Lice			
Head (pediculosis)	C	U 4 hrs	http://www.cdc.gov/ncidod/dpd/parasites/lice/default.htm
Body	S		Transmitted person to person through infested clothing. Wear gown and gloves when removing clothing; bag and wash clothes according to CDC guidance above
Pubic	S		Transmitted person to person through sexual contact

Infection/Condition	Precautions		
	Type *	Duration †	Comments
Listeriosis (listeria monocytogenes)	S		Person-to-person transmission rare; cross-transmission in neonatal settings reported [1072, 1073 1074, 1075]
Lyme disease	S		Not transmitted from person to person
Lymphocytic choriomeningitis	S		Not transmitted from person to person
Lymphogranuloma venereum	S		
Malaria	S		Not transmitted from person to person except through transfusion rarely and through a failure to follow Standard Precautions during patient care [1076-1079]. Install screens in windows and doors in endemic areas. Use DEET-containing mosquito repellants and clothing to cover extremities
Marburg virus disease (see viral hemorrhagic			
Measles (rubeola)	A	4 days after onset of rash; DI in immune compromised	Susceptible HCWs should not enter room if immune care providers are available; no recommendation for face protection for immune HCW; no recommendation for type of face protection for susceptible HCWs, i.e., mask or respirator [1027, 1028]. For exposed susceptibles, post-exposure vaccine within 72 hrs. or immune globulin within 6 days when available [17, 1032, 1034]. Place exposed susceptible patients on Airborne Precautions and exclude susceptible healthcare personnel from duty from day 5 after first exposure to day 21 after last exposure, regardless of post-exposure vaccine.[17]

(Continued).

Infection/Condition	Precautions		Comments
	Type *	Duration †	
Melioidosis, all forms	S		Not transmitted from person to person
Meningitis			
Aseptic (nonbacterial or viral; also see enteroviral	S		Contact for infants and young children
Bacterial, gram-negative enteric, in neonates	S		
Fungal	S		
Haemophilus influenzae, type b known or	D	U 24 hrs	
Listeria monocytogenes (See Listeriosis)	S		
Neisseria meningitidis (meningococcal) known or	D	U 24 hrs	See meningococcal disease below
Streptococcus pneumoniae	S		
M. tuberculosis	S		Concurrent, active pulmonary disease or draining cutaneous lesions may necessitate addition of Contact and/or Airborne Precautions; For children, airborne precautions until active tuberculosis ruled
Other diagnosed bacterial	S		
Meningococcal disease: sepsis, pneumonia,	D	U 24 hrs	Postexposure chemoprophylaxis for household contacts, HCWs exposed to respiratory secretions; postexposure vaccine only to control outbreaks [15, 17]
Molluscum contagiosum	S		
Monkeypox	A,C	A-Until monkeypox confirmed and smallpox excluded C-Until lesions crusted	Use See www.cdc.gov/ncidod/monkeypox for most current recommendations. Transmission in hospital settings unlikely [269]. Pre- and post-exposure smallpox vaccine recommended for exposed HCWs

Mucormycosis	S	
Multidrug-resistant organisms (MDROs), infection or colonization (e.g., MRSA, VRE, VISA/VRSA, ESBLs, resistant *S. pneumoniae*)	S/C	MDROs judged by the infection control program, based on local, state, regional, or national recommendations, to be of clinical and epidemiologic significance. Contact Precautions recommended in settings with evidence of ongoing transmission, acute care settings with increased risk for transmission or wounds that cannot be contained by dressings. See recommendations for management options in Management of Multidrug-Resistant Organisms In Healthcare Settings, 2006 [870]. Contact state health department for guidance regarding new or emerging MDRO.
Mumps (infectious parotitis)	D	U 9 days After onset of swelling; susceptible HCWs should not provide care if immune caregivers are available. Note: (Recent assessment of outbreaks in healthy 18-24 year olds has indicated that salivary viral shedding occurred early in the course of illness and that 5 days of isolation after onset of parotitis may be appropriate in community settings; however the implications for healthcare personnel and high-risk patient populations remain to be clarified.)
Mycobacteria, nontuberculosis (atypical)		
Pulmonary	S	Not transmitted person-to-person
Wound	S	
Mycoplasma pneumonia	D	DI
Necrotizing enterocolitis	S	Contact Precautions when cases clustered temporally [1080-1083]
Nocardiosis, draining lesions, or other	S	Not transmitted person-to-person
Norovirus (see gastroenteritis)		
Norwalk agent gastroenteritis (see gastroenteritis)		
Orf	S	

(Continued).

Infection/Condition	Precautions		Comments
	Type *	Duration †	
Parainfluenza virus infection, respiratory in infants and young children	C	DI	Viral shedding may be prolonged in immunosuppressed patients 1009, 1010 . Reliability of antigen testing to determine when to remove patients with prolonged hospitalizations from Contact Precautions uncertain.
Parvovirus B19 (Erythema infectiosum)	D		Maintain precautions for duration of hospitalization when chronic disease occurs in an immunocompromised patient. For patients with transient aplastic crisis or red-cell crisis, maintain precautions for 7 days. Duration of precautions for immunosuppressed patients with persistently positive PCR not defined, but transmission has occurred [929].
Pediculosis (lice)	C	U 24 hrs after treatment	
Pertussis (whooping cough)	D	U 5 days	Single patient room preferred. Cohorting an option. Post-exposure chemoprophylaxis for household contacts and HCWs with prolonged exposure to respiratory secretions[863] . Recommendations for Tdap vaccine in adults under development.
Pinworm infection (Enterobiasis)	S		
Plague (Yersinia pestis)			
Bubonic	S		
Pneumonic	D	U 48 hrs	Antimicrobial prophylaxis for exposed HCW [207].
Pneumonia			
Adenovirus	D, C	DI	Outbreaks in pediatric and institutional settings reported 376, [1084-1086] . In immunocompromised hosts, extend duration of Droplet and Contact Precautions due to prolonged shedding of virus [931]
Bacterial not listed elsewhere (including gram-	S		

Infection/Condition	Precautions		Comments
	Type *	Duration †	
B. cepacia in patients with CF, including respiratory tract colonization	C	Unknown	Avoid exposure to other persons with CF; private room preferred. Criteria for D/C precautions not established. See CF Foundation guideline [20]
B. cepacia in patients without CF (see Multidrug-resistant organisms)			
Chlamydia	S		
Fungal	S		
Haemophilus influenzae, type b			
Adults	S		
Infants and children	D	U 24 hrs	
Legionella spp.	S		
Meningococcal	D	U 24 hrs	See meningococcal disease above
Multidrug-resistant bacterial (see multidrug-			
Mycoplasma (primary atypical pneumonia)	D	DI	
Pneumococcal pneumonia	S		Use Droplet Precautions if evidence of transmission within a patient care unit or facility [196-198, 1087]
Pneumocystis jiroveci (Pneumocystis carinii)	S		Avoid placement in the same room with an immunocompromised patient.
Staphylococcus aureus	S		For MRSA, see MDROs
Streptococcus, group A			
Adults	D	U 24 hrs	See streptococcal disease (group A streptococcus) below Contact precautions if skin lesions present
Infants and young children	D	U 24 hrs	Contact Precautions if skin lesions present
Varicella-zoster (See Varicella-Zoster)			
Viral			
Adults	S		

(Continued).

Infection/Condition	Precautions		Comments
	Type *	Duration †	
Infants and young children (see respiratory infectious disease, acute, or specific viral agent)			
Poliomyelitis	C	DI	
Pressure ulcer (decubitus ulcer, pressure sore)			
Major	C	DI	If no dressing or containment of drainage; until drainage stops or can be contained by dressing
Minor or limited	S		If dressing covers and contains drainage
Prion disease (See Creutzfeld-Jacob Disease)			
Psittacosis (ornithosis) (*Chlamydia psittaci*)	S		Not transmitted from person to person
Q fever	S		
Rabies	S		Person to person transmission rare; transmission via corneal, tissue and organ transplants has been reported [539, 1088]. If patient has bitten another individual or saliva has contaminated an open wound or mucous membrane, wash exposed area thoroughly and administer postexposure prophylaxis. [1089]
Rat-bite fever (Streptobacillus moniliformis disease, Spirillum minus disease)	S		Not transmitted from person to person
Relapsing fever	S		Not transmitted from person to person
Resistant bacterial infection or colonization (see multidrug-resistant organisms)			
Respiratory infectious disease, acute (if not			
Adults	S		
Infants and young children	C	DI	Also see syndromes or conditions listed in Table 2

Infection/Condition	Precautions		Comments
	Type *	Duration †	
Respiratory syncytial virus infection, in infants, young children and immunocompromised adults	C	DI	Wear mask according to Standard Precautions [24] CB [116, 117]. In immunocompromised patients, extend the duration of Contact Precautions due to prolonged shedding [928]). Reliability of antigen testing to determine when to remove patients with prolonged hospitalizations from Contact Precautions uncertain.
Reye's syndrome	S		Not an infectious condition
Rheumatic fever	S		Not an infectious condition
Rhinovirus	D	DI	Droplet most important route of transmission [104 1090]. Outbreaks have occurred in NICUs and LTCFs [413, 1091, 1092]. Add Contact Precautions if copious moist secretions and close contact likely to occur (e.g., young infants) [111, 833]
Rickettsial fevers, tickborne (Rocky Mountain spotted fever, tickborne typhus fever)	S		Not transmitted from person to person except through transfusion, rarely
Rickettsialpox (vesicular rickettsiosis)	S		Not transmitted from person to person
Ringworm (dermatophytosis, dermatomycosis, tinea)	S		Rarely, outbreaks have occurred in healthcare settings, (e.g., NICU [1093], rehabilitation hospital [1094] . Use Contact Precautions for outbreak.
Ritter's disease (staphylococcal scalded skin syndrome)	C	DI	See staphylococcal disease, scalded skin syndrome below
Rocky Mountain spotted fever	S		Not transmitted from person to person except through transfusion, rarely
Roseola infantum (exanthem subitum; caused by	S		
Rotavirus infection (see gastroenteritis)			

(Continued).

Infection/Condition	Precautions		Comments
	Type *	Duration †	
Rubella (German measles) (also see congenital rubella)	D	U 7 days after onset of rash	Susceptible HCWs should not enter room if immune caregivers are available. No recommendation for wearing face protection (e.g., a surgical mask) if immune. Pregnant women who are not immune should not care for these patients [17, 33]. Administer vaccine within three days of exposure to non-pregnant susceptible individuals. Place exposed susceptible patients on Droplet Precautions; exclude susceptible healthcare personnel from duty from day 5 after first exposure to day 21 after last exposure, regardless of post-exposure vaccine.
Rubeola (see measles)			
Salmonellosis (see gastroenteritis)			
Scabies	C	U 24	
Scalded skin syndrome, staphylococcal	C	DI	See staphylococcal disease, scalded skin syndrome below.
Schistosomiasis (bilharziasis)	S		
Severe acute respiratory syndrome (SARS)	A, D,C	DI plus 10 days after resolution of fever, provided respiratory symptoms are absent or	Airborne Precautions preferred; D if AIIR unavailable. N95 or higher respiratory protection; surgical mask if N95 unavailable; eye protection (goggles, face shield); aerosol-generating procedures and "supershedders" highest risk for transmission via small droplet nuclei and large droplets [93, 94, 96].Vigilant environmental disinfection (see www.cdc.gov/ncidod/sars)
Shigellosis (see gastroenteritis)			
Smallpox (variola; see vaccinia for management of vaccinated persons)	A,C	DI	Until all scabs have crusted and separated (3-4 weeks). Non-vaccinated HCWs should not provide care when immune HCWs are available; N95 or higher respiratory protection for susceptible and

Infection/Condition	Precautions		Comments
	Type *	Duration †	
Sporotrichosis	S		successfully vaccinated individuals; postexposure vaccine within 4 days of exposure protective [108, 129, 1038-1040.]
Spirillum minor disease (rat-bite fever)	S		Not transmitted from person to person
Staphylococcal disease (*S aureus*)			
Skin, wound, or burn			
Major	C	DI	No dressing or dressing does not contain drainage adequately
Minor or limited	S		Dressing covers and contains drainage adequately
Enterocolitis	S		Use Contact Precautions for diapered or incontinent children for duration of illness
Multidrug-resistant (see multidrug-resistant			
Pneumonia	S		
Scalded skin syndrome	C	DI	Consider healthcare personnel as potential source of nursery, NICU outbreak [1095].
Toxic shock syndrome	S		
Streptobacillus moniliformis disease (rat-bite	S		Not transmitted from person to person
Streptococcal disease (group A streptococcus)			
Skin, wound, or burn			
Major	C,D	U 24 hrs	No dressing or dressing does not contain drainage adequately
Minor or limited	S		Dressing covers and contains drainage adequately
Endometritis (puerperal sepsis)	S		
Pharyngitis in infants and young children	D	U 24 hrs	
Pneumonia	D	U 24 hrs	
Scarlet fever in infants and young children	D	U 24 hrs	

(Continued).

Infection/Condition	Precautions		
	Type *	Duration †	Comments
Serious invasive disease	D	U24 hrs	Outbreaks of serious invasive disease have occurred secondary to transmission among patients and healthcare personnel [162, 972, 1096-1098] Contact Precautions for draining wound as above; follow rec. for antimicrobial prophylaxis in selected conditions [160].
Streptococcal disease (group B streptococcus),	S		
Streptococcal disease (not group A or B) unless	S		
Multidrug-resistant (see multidrug-resistant			
Strongyloidiasis	S		
Syphilis			
Latent (tertiary) and seropositivity without lesions	S		
Skin and mucous membrane, including congenital, primary, Secondary	S		
Tapeworm disease			
Hymenolepis nana	S		Not transmitted from person to person
Taenia solium (pork)	S		
Other	S		
Tetanus	S		Not transmitted from person to person
Tinea (e.g., dermatophytosis, dermatomycosis,	S		Rare episodes of person-to-person transmission
Toxoplasmosis	S		Transmission from person to person is rare; vertical transmission from mother to child, transmission through organs and blood transfusion rare
Toxic shock syndrome (staphylococcal disease, streptococcal disease)	S		Droplet Precautions for the first 24 hours after implementation of antibiotic therapy if Group A streptococcus is a likely etiology
Trachoma, acute	S		

Transmissible spongiform encephalopathy (see Creutzfeld-Jacob disease, CJD, vCJD)		
Trench mouth (Vincent's angina)	S	
Trichinosis	S	
Trichomoniasis	S	
Trichuriasis (whipworm disease)	S	
Tuberculosis (M. tuberculosis)		
Extrapulmonary, draining lesion	A,C	Discontinue precautions only when patient is improving clinically, and drainage has ceased or there are three consecutive negative cultures of continued drainage [1025, 1026]. Examine for evidence of active pulmonary tuberculosis.
Extrapulmonary, no draining lesion, meningitis	S	Examine for evidence of pulmonary tuberculosis. For infants and children, use Airborne Precautions until active pulmonary tuberculosis in visiting family members ruled out [42]
Pulmonary or laryngeal disease, confirmed	A	Discontinue precautions only when patient on effective therapy is improving clinically and has three consecutive sputum smears negative for acid-fast bacilli collected on separate days(MMWR 2005; 54: RR-17 http://www.cdc.gov/mmwr/preview/mmwrhtml/rr5417a1.htm?scid=rr5 417a1e) 12.
Skin-test positive with no evidence of current	S	Discontinue precautions only when the likelihood of infectious TB
Tularemia		
Draining lesion	S	Not transmitted from person to person
Pulmonary	S	Not transmitted from person to person

(Continued).

Infection/Condition	Precautions Type *	Duration †	Comments
Typhoid (*Salmonella typhi*) fever (see Typhus)			
Rickettsia pro wazekii (Epidemic or Louse-borne typhus)	S		Transmitted from person to person through close personal or clothing contact
Rickettsia typhi	S		Not transmitted from person to person
Urinary tract infection (including pyelonephritis), with or without urinary catheter	S		
Vaccinia (vaccination site, adverse events following vaccination) *			Only vaccinated HCWs have contact with active vaccination sites and care for persons with adverse vaccinia events; if unvaccinated, only HCWs without contraindications to vaccine may provide care.
Vaccination site care (including autoinoculated areas)	S		Vaccination recommended for vaccinators; for newly vaccinated HCWs: semi-permeable dressing over gauze until scab separates, with dressing change as fluid accumulates, ~3-5 days; gloves, hand hygiene for dressing change; vaccinated HCW or HCW without contraindication to vaccine for dressing changes [205, 221, 225].
Eczema vaccinatum	C	Until lesions dry and crusted, scabs separated	For contact with virus-containing lesions and exudative material
Fetal vaccinia	C		
Generalized vaccinia	C		
Progressive vaccinia	C		
Postvaccinia encephalitis	S		
Blepharitis or conjunctivitis	S/C		Use Contact Precautions if there is copious drainage

Iritis or keratitis	S		
Vaccinia-associated erythema multiforme (Stevens Johnson Syndrome)	S		Not an infectious condition
Secondary bacterial infection (e.g., S. aureus, group A beta hemolytic streptococcus	S/C		Follow organism-specific (strep, staph most frequent) recommendations and consider magnitude of drainage
Varicella Zoster	A,C	Until lesions dry and crusted	Susceptible HCWs should not enter room if immune caregivers are available; no recommendation for face protection of immune HCWs; no recommendation for type of protection, i.e. surgical mask or respirator for susceptible HCWs. In immunocompromised host with varicella pneumonia, prolong duration of precautions for duration of illness. Post-exposure prophylaxis: provide post-exposure vaccine ASAP but within 120 hours; for susceptible exposed persons for whom vaccine is contraindicated (immunocompromised persons, pregnant women, newborns whose mother's varicella onset is <5days before delivery or within 48 hrs after delivery) provide VZIG, when available, within 96 hours; if unavailable, use IVIG, Use Airborne Precautions for exposed susceptible persons and exclude exposed susceptible healthcare workers beginning 8 days after first exposure until 21 days after last exposure or 28 if received VZIG, regardless of postexposure vaccination. [1036].
Variola (see smallpox)			
Vibrio parahaemolyticus (see gastroenteritis)			
Vincent's angina (trench mouth)	S		

(Continued).

Infection/Condition	Precautions		Comments
	Type *	Duration †	
Viral hemorrhagic fevers due to Lassa, Ebola, Marburg, Crimean-Congo fever viruses	S, D, C	DI	Single-patient room preferred. Emphasize: 1) use of sharps safety devices and safe work practices; 2) hand hygiene; 3) barrier protection against blood and body fluids upon entry into room (single gloves and fluid-resistant or impermeable gown, face/eye protection with masks, goggles or face shields); and 4) appropriate waste handling. Use N95 or higher respirators when performing aerosol-generating procedures. Largest viral load in final stages of illness when hemorrhage may occur; additional PPE, including double gloves, leg and shoe coverings may be used, especially in resource-limited settings where options for cleaning and laundry are limited. Notify public health officials immediately if Ebola is suspected [212, 314, 740, 772] Also see Table 3 for Ebola as a bioterrorism agent
Viral respiratory diseases (not covered elsewhere)			
Adults	S		
Infants and young children (see respiratory infectious disease, acute)			
Whooping cough (see pertussis)			
Wound infections			
Major	C	DI	No dressing or dressing does not contain drainage adequately
Minor or limited	S		Dressing covers and contains drainage adequately
Yersinia enterocolitica gastroenteritis (see			
Zoster (varicella-zoster) (see herpes zoster)			
Zygomycosis (phycomycosis, mucormycosis)	S		Not transmitted person-to-person

1 Type of Precautions: A, Airborne Precautions; C, Contact; D, Droplet; S, Standard; when A, C, and D are specified, also use S.

† Duration of precautions: CN, until off antimicrobial treatment and culture-negative; DI, duration of illness (with wound lesions, DI means until wounds stop draining); DE, until environment completely decontaminated; U, until time specified in hours (hrs) after initiation of effective therapy; Unknown: criteria for establishing eradication of pathogen has not been determined.

Table 1. History of Guidelines for Isolation Precautions in Hospitals*

YEAR (Ref)	DOCUMENT ISSUED	COMMENT
1970 1099	Isolation Techniques for Use in Hospitals, 1st ed.	- Introduced seven isolation precaution categories with color-coded cards: Strict, Respiratory, Protective, Enteric, Wound and Skin, Discharge, and Blood
		- No user decision-making required
		- Simplicity a strength; over isolation prescribed for some infections
1975 1100	Isolation Techniques for Use in Hospitals, 2nd ed.	- Same conceptual framework as 1st edition
1983 1101	CDC Guideline for Isolation Precautions in Hospitals	- Provided two systems for isolation: category-specific and disease-specific
		- Protective Isolation eliminated; Blood Precautions expanded to include Body Fluids
		- Categories included Strict, Contact, Respiratory, AFB, Enteric, Drainage/Secretion, Blood and Body
		- Emphasized decision-making by users
1985-88	Universal Precautions	- Developed in response to HIV/AIDS epidemic

Table 1. (Continued)

YEAR (Ref)	DOCUMENT ISSUED	COMMENT
780, 896		- Dictated application of Blood and Body Fluid precautions to all patients, regardless of infection status
		- Did not apply to feces, nasal secretions, sputum, sweat, tears, urine, or vomitus unless contaminated by visible blood
		- Added personal protective equipment to protect HCWs from mucous membrane exposures
		- Handwashing recommended immediately after glove removal
		- Added specific recommendations for handling needles and other sharp devices; concept became integral to OSHA's 1991 rule on occupational exposure to blood-borne pathogens in healthcare settings
1987	Body Substance Isolation	- Emphasized avoiding contact with all moist and potentially infectious
YEAR (Ref)	DOCUMENT ISSUED	COMMENT
1102		body substances except sweat even if blood not present
		- Shared some features with Universal Precautions
		- Weak on infections transmitted by large droplets or by contact with dry surfaces
		- Did not emphasize need for special ventilation to contain airborne infections
		- Handwashing after glove removal not specified in the absence of visible soiling
1996	Guideline for Isolation Precautions	- Prepared by the Healthcare Infection Control Practices Advisory
1	Hospitals	Committee (HICPAC)
		- Melded major features of Universal Precautions and Body Substance Isolation into Standard Precautions to be used with all patients at all times
		- Included three transmission-based precaution categories: airborne, droplet, and contact
		- Listed clinical syndromes that should dictate use of empiric isolation until an etiological diagnosis is established

* Derived from Garner ICHE 1996.

Table 2. Clinical Syndromes or Conditions Warranting Empiric Transmission-Based Precautions in Addition to Standard Precautions Pending Confirmation of Diagnosis*

Clinical Syndrome or Condition†	Potential Pathogens‡	Empiric Precautions (Always includes Standard Precautions)
DIARRHEA		
Acute diarrhea with a likely infectious cause in an incontinent or diapered patient	Enteric pathogens§	Contact Precautions (pediatrics and adult)
MENINGITIS	Neisseria meningitidis Enteroviruses M. tuberculosis	Droplet Precautions for first 24 hrs of antimicrobial therapy; mask and face protection for intubation Contact Precautions for infants and children Airborne Precautions if pulmonary infiltrate Airborne Precautions plus Contact Precautions if potentially infectious draining body fluid present
RASH OR EXANTHEMS, GENERALIZED, ETIOLOGY UNKNOWN		
Petechial/ecchymotic with fever (general) - If positive history of travel to an area with an ongoing outbreak of VHF in the 10 days before onset of fever	Neisseria meningitidis Ebola, Lassa, Marburg viruses	Droplet Precautions for first 24 hrs of antimicrobial therapy Droplet Precautions plus Contact Precautions, with face/eye protection, emphasizing safety sharps and barrier precautions when blood exposure likely. Use N95 or higher respiratory protection when aerosol-generating procedure performed
Vesicular	Varicella-zoster, *herpes simplex*, variola (smallpox), vaccinia viruses Vaccinia virus	Airborne plus Contact Precautions; Contact Precautions only if *herpes simplex*, localized zoster in an immunocompetent host or vaccinia viruses most likely
Maculopapular with cough, coryza and fever	Rubeola (measles) virus	Airborne Precautions

Table 2. (Continued).

Clinical Syndrome or Condition†	Potential Pathogens‡	Empiric Precautions (Always includes Standard Precautions)
RESPIRATORY INFECTIONS		
Cough/fever/upper lobe pulmonary infiltrate in an HIV-negative patient or a patient at low risk for human immunodeficiency virus (HIV) infection	M. tuberculosis, Respiratory viruses, S. pneumoniae, S. aureus (MSSA or MRSA)	Airborne Precautions plus Contact precautions
Cough/fever/pulmonary infiltrate in any lung location in an HIV-infected patient or a patient at high risk for HIV infection	M. tuberculosis, Respiratory viruses, S. pneumoniae, S. aureus (MSSA or MRSA)	Airborne Precautions plus Contact Precautions Use eye/face protection if aerosol-generating procedure performed or contact with respiratory secretions anticipated. If tuberculosis is unlikely and there are no AIIRs and/or respirators available, use Droplet Precautions instead of Airborne Precautions Tuberculosis more likely in HIV-infected individual than in HIV negative individual
Cough/fever/pulmonary infiltrate in any lung location in a patient with a history of recent travel (10-21 days) to countries with active outbreaks of SARS, avian influenza	*M. tuberculosis*, severe acute respiratory syndrome virus (SARS- CoV), avian influenza	Airborne plus Contact Precautions plus eye protection. If SARS and tuberculosis unlikely, use Droplet Precautions instead of Airborne Precautions.

Respiratory infections, particularly bronchiolitis and pneumonia, in infants and young children	Respiratory syncytial virus, parainfluenza virus, adenovirus, influenza virus, Human metapneumovirus	Contact plus Droplet Precautions; Droplet Precautions may be discontinued when adenovirus and influenza have been ruled out
Skin or Wound Infection		
Abscess or draining wound that cannot be covered	*Staphylococcus aureus* (MSSA or MRSA), group A streptococcus	Contact Precautions Add Droplet Precautions for the first 24 hours of appropriate antimicrobial therapy if invasive Group A streptococcal disease is suspected

* Infection control professionals should modify or adapt this table according to local conditions. To ensure that appropriate empiric precautions are implemented always, hospitals must have systems in place to evaluate patients routinely according to these criteria as part of their preadmission and admission care.

† Patients with the syndromes or conditions listed below may present with atypical signs or symptoms (e.g.neonates and adults with pertussis may not have paroxysmal or severe cough). The clinician's index of suspicion should be guided by the prevalence of specific conditions in the community, as well as clinical judgment.

‡ The organisms listed under the column "Potential Pathogens" are not intended to represent the complete, or even most likely, diagnoses, but rather possible etiologic agents that require additional precautions beyond Standard Precautions until they can be ruled out.

§ These pathogens include enterohemorrhagic *Escherichia coli* O1 57:H7, *Shigella spp*, hepatitis A virus, noroviruses, rotavirus, *C. difficile*.

Table 3. Infection Control Considerations for High-Priority (CDC Category A) Diseases that May Result from Bioterrorist Attacks or Are Considered to Be Bioterrorist Threats (www.Bt.Cdc.Gov) A

Disease	Anthrax
Site(s) of Infection; Transmission Mode Cutaneous and inhalation disease have occurred in past bioterrorist incidents	Cutaneous (contact with spores);RT (inhalation of spores);GIT (ingestion of spores - rare) Comment: Spores can be inhaled into the lower respiratory tract. The infectious dose of *B. anthracis* in humans by any route is not precisely known. In primates, the LD50 (i.e., the dose required to kill 50% of animals) for an aerosol challenge with *B. anthracis* is estimated to be 8,000–50,000 spores; the infectious dose may be as low as 1-3 spores
Incubation Period	Cutaneous: 1 to12 days; RT: Usually 1 to 7 days but up to 43 days reported; GIT: 15-72 hours
Clinical Features	Cutaneous: Painless, reddish papule, which develops a central vesicle or bulla in 1-2 days; over next 3-7 days lesion becomes pustular, and then necrotic, with black eschar; extensive surrounding edema. RT: initial flu-like illness for 1-3 days with headache, fever, malaise, cough; by day 4 severe dyspnea and shock, and is usually fatal (85%-90% if untreated; meningitis in 50% of RT cases. GIT: : if intestinal form, necrotic, ulcerated edematous lesions develop in intestines with fever, nausea and vomiting, progression to hematemesis and bloody diarrhea; 25-60% fatal
Diagnosis	Cutaneous: Swabs of lesion (under eschar) for IHC, PCR and culture; punch biopsy for IHC, PCR and culture; vesicular fluid aspirate for Gram stain and culture; blood culture if systemic symptoms; acute and convalescent sera for ELISA serology RT: CXR or CT demonstrating wide mediastinal widening and/or pleural effusion, hilar abnormalities; blood for culture and PCR; pleural effusion for culture, PCR and IHC; CSF if meningeal signs present for IHC, PCR and culture; acute and convalescent sera for ELISA serology; pleural and/or bronchial biopsies IHC. GIT: blood and ascites fluid, stool samples, rectal swabs, and swabs of oropharyngeal lesions if present for culture, PCR and IHC
Infectivity	Cutaneous: Person-to-person transmission from contact with lesion of untreated patient possible, but extremely rare.
	RT and GIT: Person-to-person transmission does not occur.
	Aerosolized powder, environmental exposures: Highly infectious if aerosolized
Recommended	Cutaneous: Standard Precautions; Contact Precautions if uncontained copious drainage.

Precautions	RT and GIT: Standard Precautions.
	Aerosolized powder, environmental exposures: Respirator (N95 mask or PAPRs), protective clothing; decontamination of persons with powder on them
	(http://www.cdc.gov/mmwr/preview/mmwrhtml/mm5 1 35a3. htm)
	Hand hygiene: Handwashing for 30-60 seconds with soap and water or 2% chlorhexidene gluconate after spore contact (alcohol handrubs inactive against spores [Weber DJ JAMA 2003; 289:1274]).
	Post-exposure prophylaxis following environmental exposure: 60 days of antimicrobials (either doxycycline, ciprofloxacin, or levofloxacin) and post-exposure vaccine under IND
Site(s) of Infection; Transmission Mode	GIT: Ingestion of toxin-containing food, RT: Inhalation of toxin containing aerosol cause disease. Comment: Toxin ingested or potentially delivered by aerosol in bioterrorist incidents. LD_{50} for type A is 0.001 ig/ml/kg.
Incubation Period	1-5 days.
Clinical Features	Ptosis, generalized weakness, dizziness, dry mouth and throat, blurred vision, diplopia, dysarthria, dysphonia, and dysphagia followed by symmetrical descending paralysis and respiratory failure.
Diagnosis	Clinical diagnosis; identification of toxin in stool, serology unless toxin-containing material available for toxin neutralization bioassays.
Infectivity	Not transmitted from person to person. Exposure to toxin necessary for disease.
Recommended Precautions	Standard Precautions.
Site(s) of Infection; Transmission Mode	As a rule infection develops after exposure of mucous membranes or RT, or through broken skin or percutaneous injury.
Incubation Period	2-19 days, usually 5-10 days
Clinical Features	Febrile illnesses with malaise, myalgias, headache, vomiting and diarrhea that are rapidly complicated by hypotension, shock, and hemorrhagic features. Massive hemorrhage in < 50% pts.

Table 3. (Continued)

Disease	Anthrax
Diagnosis	Etiologic diagnosis can be made using RT-PCR, serologic detection of antibody and antigen, pathologic assessment with immunohistochemistry and viral culture with EM confirmation of morphology.
Infectivity	Person-to-person transmission primarily occurs through unprotected contact with blood and body fluids; percutaneous injuries (e.g., needlestick) associated with a high rate of transmission; transmission in healthcare settings has been reported but is prevented by use of barrier precautions.
Recommended Precautions	Hemorrhagic fever specific barrier precautions: If disease is believed to be related to intentional release of a bioweapon, epidemiology of transmission is unpredictable pending observation of disease transmission. Until the nature of the pathogen is understood and its transmission pattern confirmed, Standard, Contact and Airborne Precautions should be used. Once the pathogen is characterized, if the epidemiology of transmission is consistent with natural disease, Droplet Precautions can be substituted for Airborne Precautions. Emphasize: 1) use of sharps safety devices and safe work practices, 2) hand hygiene; 3) barrier protection against blood and body fluids upon entry into room (single gloves and fluid-resistant or impermeable gown, face/eye protection with masks, goggles or face shields); and 4) appropriate waste handling. Use N95 or higher respirators when performing aerosol-generating procedures. In settings where AIIRs are unavailable or the large numbers of patients cannot be accommodated by existing AIIRs, observe Droplet Precautions (plus Standard Precautions and Contact Precautions) and segregate patients from those not suspected of VHF infection. Limit blooddraws to those essential to care. See text for discussion and Appendix A for recommendations for naturally occurring VHFs.
Site(s) of Infection; Transmission Mode	RT: Inhalation of respiratory droplets. Comment: Pneumonic plague most likely to occur if used as a biological weapon, but some cases of bubonic and primary septicemia may also occur. Infective dose 100 to 500 bacteria
Incubation Period	1 to 6, usually 2 to 3 days.
Clinical Features	Pneumonic: fever, chills, headache, cough, dyspnea, rapid progression of weakness, and in a later stage hemoptysis, circulatory collapse, and bleeding diathesis
Diagnosis	Presumptive diagnosis from Gram stain or Wayson stain of sputum, blood, or lymph node aspirate; definitive diagnosis from cultures of same material, or paired acute/convalescent serology.

Infectivity	Person-to-person transmission occurs via respiratory droplets risk of transmission is low during first 20-24 hours of illness and requires close contact. Respiratory secretions probably are not infectious within a few hours after initiation of appropriate therapy.
Recommended Precautions	Standard Precautions, Droplet Precautions until patients have received 48 hours of appropriate therapy. Chemoprophylaxis: Consider antibiotic prophylaxis for HCWs with close contact exposure.
Site(s) of Infection; Transmission Mode	RT Inhalation of droplet or, rarely, aerosols; and skin lesions (contact with virus). Comment: If used as a biological weapon, natural disease, which has not occurred since 1977, will likely result.
Incubation Period	7 to 19 days (mean 12 days)
Clinical Features	Fever, malaise, backache, headache, and often vomiting for 2-3 days; then generalized papular or maculopapular rash (more on face and extremities), which becomes vesicular (on day 4 or 5) and then pustular; lesions all in same stage.
Diagnosis	Electron microscopy of vesicular fluid or culture of vesicular fluid by WHO approved laboratory (CDC); detection by PCR available only in select LRN labs, CDC and USAMRID
Infectivity	Secondary attack rates up to 50% in unvaccinated persons; infected persons may transmit disease from time rash appears until all lesions have crusted over (about 3 weeks); greatest infectivity during first 10 days of rash.
Recommended Precautions	Combined use of Standard, Contact, and Airborne Precautions[b] until all scabs have separated (3-4 weeks). Only immune HCWs to care for pts; post-exposure vaccine within 4 days. Vaccinia: HCWs cover vaccination site with gauze and semi-permeable dressing until scab separates (>21 days). Observe hand hygiene. Adverse events with virus-containing lesions: Standard plus Contact Precautions until all lesions crusted
Site(s) of Infection; Transmission Mode	RT: Inhalation of aerosolized bacteria. GIT: Ingestion of food or drink contaminated with aerosolized bacteria. Comment: Pneumonic or typhoidal disease likely to occur after bioterrorist event using aerosol delivery. Infective dose 10-50 bacteria
Incubation Period	2 to 10 days, usually 3 to 5 days

Table 3. (Continued).

Disease	Anthrax
Clinical Features	Pneumonic: malaise, cough, sputum production, dyspnea; Typhoidal: fever, prostration, weight loss and frequently an associated pneumonia.
Diagnosis	Diagnosis usually made with serology on acute and convalescent serum specimens; bacterium can be detected by PCR (LRN) or isolated from blood and other body fluids on cysteine-enriched media or mouse inoculation.
Infectivity	Person-to-person spread is rare. Laboratory workers who encounter/handle cultures of this organism are at high risk for disease if exposed.
Recommended Precautions	Standard Precautions

a Abbreviations used in this table: RT = respiratory tract; GIT = gastrointestinal tract; CXR = chest x-ray; CT = computerized axial tomography; CSF = cerebrospinal fluid; and LD50 = lethal dose for 50% of experimental animals; HCWs = healthcare worker; BSL = biosafety level; PAPR = powered air purifying respirator; PCR = polymerase chain reaction; IHC = immunohistochemistry.

2 Pneumonic plague is not as contagious as is often thought. Historical accounts and contemporary evidence indicate that persons with plague usually only transmit the infection when the disease is in the end stage. These persons cough copious amounts of bloody sputum that contains many plague bacteria. Patients in the early stage of primary pneumonic plague (approximately the first 20–24 h) apparently pose little risk [1, 2]. Antibiotic medication rapidly clears the sputum of plague bacilli, so that a patient generally is not infective within hours after initiation of effective antibiotic treatment [3]. This means that in modern times many patients will never reach a stage where they pose a significant risk to others. Even in the end stage of disease, transmission only occurs after close contact. Simple protective measures, such as wearing masks, good hygiene, and avoiding close contact, have been effective to interrupt transmission during many pneumonic plague outbreaks [2]. In the United States, the last known cases of person to person transmission of pneumonic plague occurred in 1925 [2]. Wu L-T. A treatise on pneumonic plague. Geneva: League of Nations, 1926. III. Health. Kool JL. Risk of person to person transmission of pneumonic plague. Clinical Infectious Diseases, 2005; 40 (8): 1166-1172 Butler TC. Plague and other Yersinia infections. In: Greenough WB, ed. Current topics in infectious disease. New York: Plenum Medical Book Company, 1983.

b Transmission by the airborne route is a rare event: Airborne Precautions is recommended when possible, but in the event of mass exposures, barrier precautions and containment within a designated area are most important 204, 212.

c Vaccinia adverse events with lesions containing infectious virus include inadvertent autoinoculation, ocular lesions (blepharitis, conjunctivitis), generalized vaccinia, progressive vaccinia, eczema vaccinatum; bacterial superinfection also requires addition of contact precautions if exudates cannot be contained 216, 217.

Table 4. Recommendations for Application of Standard Precautions for the Care of All Patients in All Healthcare Settings
(See Sections II.D.-II.J. and III.A.1)

COMPONENT	RECOMMENDATIONS
Hand hygiene	After touching blood, body fluids, secretions, excretions, contaminated items; immediately after removing gloves; between patient contacts.
Personal protective equipment (PPE)	
Gloves	For touching blood, body fluids, secretions, excretions, contaminated items; for touching mucous membranes and nonintact skin
Gown	During procedures and patient-care activities when contact of clothing/exposed skin with blood/body fluids, secretions, and excretions is anticipated.
Mask, eye protection (goggles), face shield*	During procedures and patient-care activities likely to generate splashes or sprays of blood, body fluids, secretions, especially suctioning, endotracheal intubation
Soiled patient-care equipment	Handle in a manner that prevents transfer of microorganisms to others and to the environment; wear gloves if visibly contaminated; perform hand hygiene.
Environmental control	Develop procedures for routine care, cleaning, and disinfection of environmental surfaces, especially frequently touched surfaces in patient-care areas.
Textiles and laundry	Handle in a manner that prevents transfer of microorganisms to others and to the environment
Needles and other sharps	Do not recap, bend, break, or hand-manipulate used needles; if recapping is required, use a one-handed scoop technique only; use safety features when available; place used sharps in puncture-resistant container
Patient resuscitation	Use mouthpiece, resuscitation bag, other ventilation devices to prevent contact with mouth and oral secretions

Table 4. (Continued).

COMPONENT	RECOMMENDATIONS
Patient placement	Prioritize for single-patient room if patient is at increased risk of transmission, is likely to contaminate the environment, does not maintain appropriate hygiene, or is at increased risk of acquiring infection or developing adverse outcome following infection.
Respiratory hygiene/cough etiquette (source containment of infectious respiratory secretions in symptomatic patients, beginning at initial point of encounter e.g., triage and reception areas in emergency departments and physician offices)	Instruct symptomatic persons to cover mouth/nose when sneezing/coughing; use tissues and dispose in no-touch receptacle; observe hand hygiene after soiling of hands with respiratory secretions; wear surgical mask if tolerated or maintain spatial separation, >3 feet if possible.

* * During aerosol-generating procedures on patients with suspected or proven infections transmitted by respiratory aerosols (e.g., SARS), wear a fit-tested N95 or higher respirator in addition to gloves, gown, and face/eye protection.

Table 5. Components of a Protective Environment (Adapted from MMWR 2003; 52 [RR-1 0])

I. Patients: allogeneic hematopoeitic stem cell transplant (HSCT) only

- Maintain in PE room except for required diagnostic or therapeutic procedures that cannot be performed in the room, e.g. radiology, operating room
- Respiratory protection e.g., N95 respirator, for the patient when leaving PE during periods of construction

II. Standard and Expanded Precautions
- Hand hygiene observed before and after patient contact
- Gown, gloves, mask NOT required for HCWs or visitors for routine entry into the room
- Use of gown, gloves, mask by HCWs and visitors according to Standard Precautions and as indicated for suspected or proven infections for which Transmission-Based Precautions are recommended

III. Engineering
- Central or point-of-use HEPA (99.97% efficiency) filters capable of removing particles 0.3 im in diameter for supply (incoming) air
- Well-sealed rooms

o Proper construction of windows, doors, and intake and exhaust ports o Ceilings: smooth, free of fissures, open joints, crevices
o Walls sealed above and below the ceiling
o If leakage detected, locate source and make necessary repairs

- Ventilation to maintain >12 ACH
- Directed air flow: air supply and exhaust grills located so that clean, filtered air enters from one side of the room, flows across the patient's bed, exits on opposite side of the room
- Positive room air pressure in relation to the corridor

o Pressure differential of >2.5 Pa [0.01" water gauge]

- Monitor and document results of air flow patterns daily using visual methods (e.g., flutter strips, smoke tubes) or a hand held pressure gauge
- Self-closing door on all room exits
- Maintain back-up ventilation equipment (e.g., portable units for fans or filters) for emergency provision of ventilation requirements for PE areas and take immediate steps to restore the fixed ventilation system
- For patients who require both a PE and Airborne Infection Isolation, use an anteroom to ensure proper air balance relationships and provide independent exhaust of contaminated air to the outside or place a HEPA filter in the exhaust duct. If an anteroom is not available, place patient in an AIIR and use portable ventilation units, industrial-grade HEPA filters to enhance filtration of spores.

Table 5. (Continued)

IV. Surfaces
- Daily wet-dusting of horizontal surfaces using cloths moistened with EPA- registered hospital disinfectant/detergent
- Avoid dusting methods that disperse dust
- No carpeting in patient rooms or hallways
- No upholstered furniture and furnishings

V. Other
- No flowers (fresh or dried) or potted plants in PE rooms or areas
- Use vacuum cleaner equipped with HEPA filters when vacuum cleaning is necessary

DONNING PPE

GOWN
- Fully cover torso from neck to knees, arms to end of wrist, and wrap around the back
- Fasten in back at neck and waist

MASK OR RESPIRATOR
- Secure ties or elastic band at middle of head and neck
- Fit flexible band to nose bridge
- Fit snug to face and below chin
- Fit-check respirator

GOGGLES/FACE SHIELD
- Put on face and adjust to fit

GLOVES
- Use non-sterile for isolation
- Select according to hand size
- Extend to cover wrist of isolation gown

SAFE WORK PRACTICES
- Keep hands away from face
- Work from clean to dirty
- Limit surfaces touched
- Change when torn or heavily contaminated
- Perform hand hygiene

Figure (Continued).

Guideline for Isolation Precautions

REMOVING PPE
Remove PPE at doorway before leaving patient room or in anteroom

GLOVES
- Outside of gloves are contaminated!
- Grasp outside of glove with opposite gloved hand; peel off
- Hold removed glove in gloved hand
- Slide fingers of ungloved hand under remaining glove at wrist

GOGGLES/FACE SHIELD
- Outside of goggles or face shield are contaminated!
- To remove, handle by "clean" head band or ear pieces
- Place in designated receptacle for reprocessing or in waste container

GOWN
- Gown front and sleeves are contaminated!
- Unfasten neck, then waist ties
- Remove gown using a peeling motion; pull gown from each shoulder toward the same hand
- Gown will turn inside out
- Hold removed gown away from body, roll into a bundle and discard into waste or linen receptacle

MASK OR RESPIRATOR
- Front of mask/respirator is contaminated – DO NOT TOUCH!
- Grasp ONLY bottom then top ties/elastics and remove
- Discard in waste container

HAND HYGIENE
Perform hand hygiene immediately after removing all PPE!

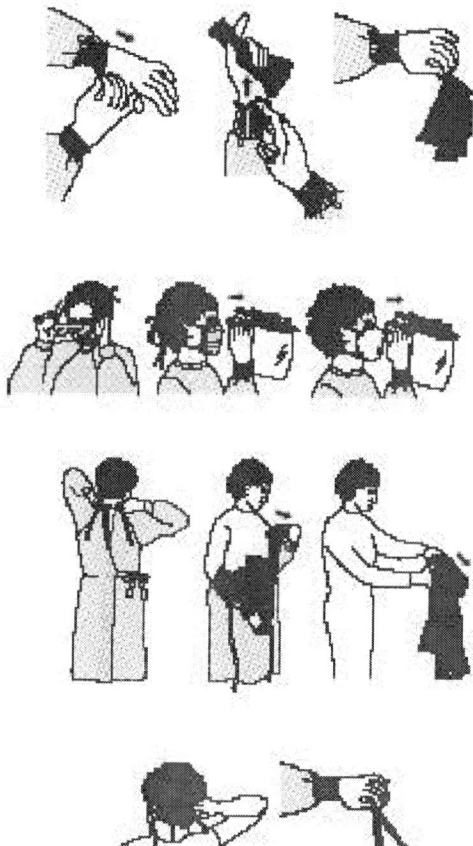

Figure. Example of Safe Donning and Removal of Personal Protective Equipment (PPE).

Additional information relevant to use of precautions was added in the comments column to assist the caregiver in decision-making. Citations were added as needed to support a change in or provide additional evidence for recommendations for a specific disease and for new infectious agents (e.g., SARS-CoV, avian influenza) that have been added to Appendix A. The reader may refer to more detailed discussion concerning modes of transmission and emerging pathogens in the background text and for MDRO control in Appendix B.

GLOSSARY

Airborne infection isolation room (AIIR). Formerly, negative pressure isolation room, an AIIR is a single-occupancy patient-care room used to isolate persons with a suspected or confirmed airborne infectious disease. Environmental factors are controlled in AIIRs to minimize the transmission of infectious agents that are usually transmitted from person to person by droplet nuclei associated with coughing or aerosolization of contaminated fluids. AIIRs should provide negative pressure in the room (so that air flows under the door gap into the room); **and** an air flow rate of 6-12 ACH (6 ACH for existing structures, 12 ACH for new construction or renovation); **and** direct exhaust of air from the room to the outside of the building or recirculation of air through a HEPA filter before retruning to circulation (MMWR 2005; 54 [RR-17]).

American Institute of Architects (AIA). A professional organization that develops standards for building ventilation, The "2001Guidelines for Design and Construction of Hospital and Health Care Facilities", the development of which was supported by the AIA, Academy of Architecture for Health, Facilities Guideline Institute, with assistance from the U.S. Department of Health and Human Services and the National Institutes of Health, is the primary source of guidance for creating airborne infection isolation rooms (AIIRs) and protective environments (www.aia.org/aah).

Ambulatory care settings. Facilities that provide health care to patients who do not remain overnight (e.g., hospital-based outpatient clinics, nonhospital-based clinics and physician offices, urgent care centers, surgicenters, free-standing dialysis centers, public health clinics, imaging centers, ambulatory behavioral health and substance abuse clinics, physical therapy and rehabilitation centers, and dental practices.

Bioaerosols. An airborne dispersion of particles containing whole or parts of biological entities, such as bacteria, viruses, dust mites, fungal hyphae, or fungal spores. Such aerosols usually consist of a mixture of mono-dispersed and aggregate cells, spores or viruses, carried by other materials, such as respiratory secretions and/or inert particles. Infectious bioaerosols (i.e., those that contain biological agents capable of causing an infectious disease) can be generated from human sources (e.g., expulsion from the respiratory tract during coughing, sneezing, talking or singing; during suctioning or wound irrigation), wet environmental sources (e.g. HVAC and cooling tower water with Legionella) or dry sources (e.g.,constuction dust with spores produced by *Aspergillus* spp.). Bioaerosols include large respiratory droplets and small droplet nuclei (Cole EC. AJIC 1998;26: 453-64).

Caregivers.. All persons who are not employees of an organization, are not paid, and provide or assist in providing healthcare to a patient (e.g., family member, friend) and acquire technical training as needed based on the tasks that must be performed.

Cohorting. In the context of this guideline, this term applies to the practice of grouping patients infected or colonized with the same infectious agent together to confine their care to one area and prevent contact with susceptible patients (cohorting patients). During outbreaks, healthcare personnel may be assigned to a cohort of patients to further limit opportunities for transmission (cohorting staff).

Colonization. Proliferation of microorganisms on or within body sites without detectable host immune response, cellular damage, or clinical expression. The presence of a microorganism within a host may occur with varying duration, but may become a source of potential transmission. In many instances, colonization and carriage are synonymous.

Droplet nuclei. Microscopic particles < 5 μm in size that are the residue of evaporated droplets and are produced when a person coughs, sneezes, shouts, or sings. These particles can remain suspended in the air for prolonged periods of time and can be carried on normal air currents in a room or beyond, to adjacent spaces or areas receiving exhaust air.

Engineering controls. Removal or isolation of a workplace hazard through technology. AIIRs, a Protective Environment, engineered sharps injury prevention devices and sharps containers are examples of engineering controls.

Epidemiologically important pathogens . Infectious agents that have one or more of the following characteristics: 1) are readily transmissible; 2) have a proclivity toward causing outbreaks; 3) may be associated with a severe outcome; or 4) are difficult to treat. Examples include *Acinetobacter sp.*, *Aspergillus* sp., *Burkholderia cepacia*, *Clostridium difficile*, *Klebsiella* or *Enterobacter* sp., extended-spectru m-beta-lactamase producing gram negative bacilli [ESB Ls], methici ll in-resistant *Staphylococcus aureus* [M RSA], *Pseudomonas aeruginosa,* vancomyci n-resistant enterococci [VRE], meth ici ll in resistant *Staphylococcus aureus* [MRSA], vancomycin resistant *Staphylococcus aureus* [VRSA] influenza virus, respiratory syncytial virus [RSV], rotavirus, SARSCoV, noroviruses and the hemorrhagic fever viruses).

Hand hygiene. A general term that applies to any one of the following: 1) handwashing with plain (nonantimicrobial) soap and water); 2) antiseptic handwash (soap containing antiseptic agents and water); 3) antiseptic handrub (waterless antiseptic product, most often alcohol-based, rubbed on all surfaces of hands); or 4) surgical hand antisepsis (antiseptic handwash or antiseptic handrub performed preoperatively by surgical personnel to eliminate transient hand flora and reduce resident hand flora) [559].

Healthcare-associated infection (HAI). An infection that develops in a patient who is cared for in any setting where healthcare is delivered (e.g., acute care hospital, chronic care facility, ambulatory clinic, dialysis center, surgicenter, home) and is related to receiving health care (i.e., was not incubating or present at the time healthcare was provided). In ambulatory and home settings, HAI would apply to any infection that is associated with a medical or surgical intervention. Since the geographic location of infection acquisition is often uncertain, the preferred term is considered to be healthcare-*associated* rather than healthcare-*acquired*.

Healthcare epidemiologist. A person whose primary training is medical (M.D., D.O.) and/or masters or doctorate-level epidemiology who has received advanced training in healthcare epidemiology. Typically these professionals direct or provide consultation to an infection control program in a hospital, long term care facility (LTCF), or healthcare delivery system (also see infection control professional).

Healthcare personnel, healthcare worker (HCW). All paid and unpaid persons who work in a healthcare setting (e.g. any person who has professional or technical training in a healthcare-related field and provides patient care in a healthcare setting or any person who provides services that support the delivery of healthcare such as dietary, housekeeping, engineering, maintenance personnel).

Hematopoietic stem cell transplantation (HSCT). Any transplantation of blood- or bone marrow-derived hematopoietic stem cells, regardless of donor type (e.g., allogeneic or autologous) or cell source (e.g., bone marrow, peripheral blood, or placental/umbilical cord blood); associated with periods of severe immunosuppression that vary with the source of the cells, the intensity of chemotherapy required, and the presence of graft versus host disease (MMWR 2000; 49: RR-10).

High-efficiency particulate air (HEPA) filter. An air filter that removes >99.97% of particles > 0.3µm (the most penetrating particle size) at a specified flow rate of air. HEPA filters may be integrated into the central air handling systems, installed at the point of use above the ceiling of a room, or used as portable units (MMWR 2003; 52: RR-10).

Home care. A wide-range of medical, nursing, rehabilitation, hospice and social services delivered to patients in their place of residence (e.g., private residence, senior living center, assisted living facility). Home health-care services include care provided by home health aides and skilled nurses, respiratory therapists, dieticians, physicians, chaplains, and volunteers; provision of durable medical equipment; home infusion therapy; and physical, speech, and occupational therapy.

Immunocompromised patients. Those patients whose immune mechanisms are deficient because of congenital or acquired immunologic disorders (e.g., human immunodeficiency virus [HIV] infection, congenital immune deficiency syndromes), chronic diseases such as diabetes mellitus, cancer, emphysema, or cardiac failure, ICU care, malnutrition, and immunosuppressive therapy of another disease process [e.g., radiation, cytotoxic chemotherapy, anti-graft-rejection medication, corticosteroids, monoclonal antibodies directed against a specific component of the immune system]). The type of infections for which an immunocompromised patient has increased susceptibility is determined by the severity of immunosuppression and the specific component(s) of the immune system that is affected. Patients undergoing allogeneic HSCT and those with chronic graft versus host disease are considered the most vulnerable to HAIs. Immunocompromised states also make it more difficult to diagnose certain infections (e.g., tuberculosis) and are associated with more severe clinical disease states than persons with the same infection and a normal immune system.

Infection. The transmission of microorganisms into a host after evading or overcoming defense mechanisms, resulting in the organism's proliferation and invasion within host tissue(s). Host responses to infection may include clinical symptoms or may be subclinical, with manifestations of disease mediated by direct organisms pathogenesis and/or a function of cell-mediated or antibody responses that result in the destruction of host tissues.

Infection control and prevention professional (ICP). A person whose primary training is in either nursing, medical technology, microbiology, or epidemiology and who has acquired special training in infection control. Responsibilities may include collection, analysis, and feedback of infection data and trends to healthcare providers; consultation on infection risk assessment, prevention and control strategies; performance of education and training activities; implementation of evidence-based infection control practices or those mandated by regulatory and licensing agencies; application of epidemiologic principles to improve patient outcomes; participation in planning renovation and construction projects (e.g., to ensure appropriate containment of construction dust); evaluation of new products or procedures on patient outcomes; oversight of employee health services related to infection prevention; implementation of preparedness plans; communication within the healthcare setting, with local and state health departments, and with the community at large concerning infection control issues; and participation in research. Certification in infection control (CIC) is available through the Certification Board of Infection Control and Epidemiology.

Infection control and prevention program. A multidisciplinary program that includes a group of activities to ensure that recommended practices for the prevention of healthcare-associated infections are implemented and followed by HCWs, making the healthcare setting safe from infection for patients and healthcare personnel. The Joint Commission on Accreditation of Healthcare Organizations (JCAHO) requires the following five components of an infection control program for accreditation: 1) *surveillance*: monitoring patients and healthcare personnel for acquisition of infection and/or colonization; 2) *investigation:* identification and analysis of infection problems or undesirable trends; 3) *prevention*: implementation of measures to prevent transmission of infectious agents and to reduce risks for device- and procedure-related infections; 4) *control*: evaluation and management of outbreaks; and 5) *reporting:* provision of information to external agencies as required by state and federal law and regulation (www.jcaho.org). The infection control program staff has the ultimate authority to determine infection control policies for a healthcare organization with the approval of the organization's governing body.

Long-term care facilities (LTCFs). An array of residential and outpatient facilities designed to meet the bio-psychosocial needs of persons with sustained self-care deficits. These include skilled nursing facilities, chronic disease hospitals, nursing homes, foster and group homes, institutions for the developmentally disabled, residential care facilities, assisted living facilities, retirement homes, adult day health care facilities, rehabilitation centers, and long-term psychiatric hospitals.

Mask. A term that applies collectively to items used to cover the nose and mouth and includes both procedure masks and surgical masks (www.fda.gov/cdrh/ode/guidance/094.html#4).

Multidrug-resistant organisms (MDROs). In general, bacteria that are resistant to one or more classes of antimicrobial agents and usually are resistant to all but one or two commercially available antimicrobial agents (e.g., MRSA, VRE, extended spectrum beta-lactamase [ESBL]-producing or intrinsically resistant gram-negative bacilli) [176].

Nosocomial infection. A term that is derived from two Greek words "nosos" (disease) and "komeion" (to take care of) and refers to any infection that develops during or as a result of an admission to an acute care facility (hospital) and was not incubating at the time of admission.

Personal protective equipment (PPE). A variety of barriers used alone or in combination to protect mucous membranes, skin, and clothing from contact with infectious agents. PPE includes gloves, masks, respirators, goggles, face shields, and gowns.

Procedure Mask. A covering for the nose and mouth that is intended for use in general patient care situations. These masks generally attach to the face with ear loops rather than ties or elastic. Unlike surgical masks, procedure masks are not regulated by the Food and Drug Administration.

Protective Environment. A specialized patient-care area, usually in a hospital, that has a positive air flow relative to the corridor (i.e., air flows from the room to the outside adjacent space). The combination of high-efficiency particulate air (HEPA) filtration, high numbers (>12) of air changes per hour (ACH), and minimal leakage of air into the room creates an environment that can safely accommodate patients with a severely compromised immune system (e.g., those who have received allogeneic hemopoietic stem-cell transplant [HSCT]) and decrease the risk of exposure to spores produced by environmental fungi. Other components include use of scrubbable surfaces instead of materials such as upholstery or carpeting, cleaning to prevent dust accumulation, and prohibition of fresh flowers or potted plants.

Quasi-experimental studies. Studies to evaluate interventions but do not use randomization as part of the study design. These studies are also referred to as nonrandomized, pre-post-intervention study designs. These studies aim to demonstrate causality between an intervention and an outcome but cannot achieve the level of confidence concerning attributable benefit obtained through a randomized, controlled trial. In hospitals and public health settings, randomized control trials often cannot be implemented due to ethical, practical and urgency reasons; therefore, quasi-experimental design studies are used commonly. However, even if an intervention appears to be effective statistically, the question can be raised as to the possibility of alternative explanations for the result.. Such study design is used when it is not logistically feasible or ethically possible to conduct a randomized, controlled trial, (e.g., during outbreaks). Within the classification of quasi-experimental study designs, there is a hierarchy of design features that may contribute to validity of results (Harris et al. CID 2004:38: 1586).

Residential care setting. A facility in which people live, minimal medical care is delivered, and the psychosocial needs of the residents are provided for.

Respirator. A personal protective device worn by healthcare personnel to protect them from inhalation exposure to airborne infectious agents that are < 5 im in size. These include infectious droplet nuclei from patients with *M. tuberculosis,* variola virus [smallpox], SARS-CoV), and dust particles that contain infectious particles, such as spores of environmental fungi (e.g., *Aspergillus* sp.). The CDC's National Institute for Occupational Safety and Health (NIOSH) certifies respirators used in healthcare settings (www.cdc.gov/niosh/topics/respirators/). The N95 disposable particulate, air purifying, respirator is the type used most commonly by healthcare personnel. Other respirators used include N-99 and N-100 particulate respirators, powered air-purifying respirators (PAPRS) with high efficiency filters; and non-powered full-facepiece elastomeric negative pressure respirators. A listing of NIOSH-approved respirators can be found at www.cdc.gov/niosh/npptl/respirators/disp part/particlist. html. Respirators must be used in conjunction with a complete Respiratory Protection Program, as required by the Occupational Safety and Health Administration (OSHA), that includes fit testing, training, proper selection of respirators, medical clearance and respirator maintenance.

Respiratory Hygiene/ Cough Etiquette. A combination of measures designed to minimize the transmission of respiratory pathogens via droplet or airborne routes in healthcare settings. The components of Respiratory Hygiene/Cough Etiquette are 1) covering the mouth and nose during coughing and sneezing, 2) using tissues to contain respiratory secretions with prompt disposal into a no- touch receptacle, 3) offering a surgical mask to persons who are coughing to decrease contamination of the surrounding environment, and 4) turning the head away from others and maintaining spatial separation, ideally >3 feet, when coughing. These measures are targeted to all patients with symptoms of respiratory infection and their accompanying family members or friends beginning at the point of initial encounter with a healthcare setting (e.g., reception/triage in emergency departments, ambulatory clinics, healthcare provider offices) [126] (Srinivasin A ICHE 2004; 25: 1020; www.cdc.gov/flu/professionals/infectioncontrol/resphygiene.htm).

Safety culture/climate. The shared perceptions of workers and management regarding the expectations of safety in the work environment. A hospital safety climate includes the following six organizational components: 1) senior management support for safety programs; 2) absence of workplace barriers to safe work practices; 3) cleanliness and orderliness of the worksite; 4) minimal conflict and good communication among staff members; 5) frequent safety- related feedback/training by supervisors; and 6) availability of PPE and engineering controls [620].

Source Control. The process of containing an infectious agent either at the portal of exit from the body or within a confined space. The term is applied most frequently to containment of infectious agents transmitted by the respiratory route but could apply to other routes of transmission, (e.g., a draining wound, vesicular or bullous skin lesions). Respiratory Hygiene/Cough Etiquette that encourages individuals to "cover your cough" and/or wear a mask is a source control measure. The use of enclosing devices for local exhaust ventilation (e.g., booths for sputum induction or administration of aerosolized medication) is another example of source control.

Standard Precautions. A group of infection prevention practices that apply to all patients, regardless of suspected or confirmed diagnosis or presumed infection status. Standard Precautions is a combination and expansion of Universal Precautions [780] and Body Substance Isolation [1102]. Standard Precautions is based on the principle that all blood, body fluids, secretions, excretions except sweat, nonintact skin, and mucous membranes may contain transmissible infectious agents. Standard Precautions includes hand hygiene, and depending on the anticipated exposure, use of gloves, gown, mask, eye protection, or face shield. Also, equipment or items in the patient environment likely to have been contaminated with infectious fluids must be handled in a manner to prevent transmission of infectious agents, (e.g. wear gloves for handling, contain heavily soiled equipment, properly clean and disinfect or sterilize reusable equipment before use on another patient).

Surgical mask. A device worn over the mouth and nose by operating room personnel during surgical procedures to protect both surgical patients and operating room personnel from transfer of microorganisms and body fluids. Surgical masks also are used to protect healthcare personnel from contact with large infectious droplets (>5 im in size). According to draft guidance issued by the Food and Drug Administration on May 15, 2003, surgical masks are evaluated using standardized testing procedures for fluid resistance, bacterial filtration efficiency, differential pressure (air exchange), and flammability in order to mitigate the risks to health associated with the use of surgical masks. These specifications apply to any masks that are labeled surgical, laser, isolation, or dental or medical procedure (www.fda.gov/cdrh/ode/guidance/094.html#4). Surgical masks do not protect against inhalation of small particles or droplet nuclei and should not be confused with particulate respirators that are recommended for protection against selected airborne infectious agents, (e.g., *Mycobacterium tuberculosis).*

REFERENCES

[1] Garner JS. Guideline for isolation precautions in hospitals. The Hospital Infection Control Practices Advisory Committee. *Infect. Control Hosp. Epidemiol.* 1996; 17(1):53-80.(s).

[2] Harris AD, Bradham DD, Baumgarten M, Zuckerman IH, Fink JC, Perencevich EN. The use and interpretation of quasi-experimental studies in infectious diseases. *Clin. Infect. Dis.* 2004;38(1 1):1586-91.

[3] Morton V, Torgerson DJ. Effect of regression to the mean on decision making in health care. *BMJ.* 2003;326(7398):1083-4.

[4] Pocock SJ, Elbourne DR. Randomized trials or observational tribulations? *N. Engl. J. Med.* 2000;342(25):1907-9.

[5] Ioannidis JP, Haidich AB, Pappa M, et al. Comparison of evidence of treatment effects in randomized and nonrandomized studies. *Jama.* 2001;286(7):821 -30.

[6] Bent S, Shojania KG, Saint S. The use of systematic reviews and meta-analyses in infection control and hospital epidemiology. *Am. J. Infect. Control.* 2004;32(4):246-54.

[7] Harris AD, Lautenbach E, Perencevich E. A systematic review of quasi-experimental study designs in the fields of infection control and antibiotic resistance. *Clin. Infect. Dis.* 2005;41(1):77-82.

[8] Evans R, Lloyd JF, Abouzelof RH, Taylor CW, Anderson VR, Samore MH. System-wide Surveillance for Clinical Encounters by Patients Previously Identified with MRSA and VRE. *Medinfo.* 2004;2004:212-6.

[9] Srinivasan A, McDonald LC, Jernigan D, et al. Foundations of the severe acute respiratory syndrome preparedness and response plan for healthcare facilities. Infect. *Control Hosp. Epidemiol.* 2004;25(12):1020-5.

[10] www.cdc.gov/flu/avian/professional/infect-control.htm

[11] CDC. Guidelines for Environmental Infection Control in Health-Care Facilities. Recommendations of CDC and the Healthcare Infection Control Practices Advisory Committee (HICPAC). *MMWR.* 2003;52(RR10);1-42.

[12] CDC. Guidelines for preventing the transmission of Mycobacterium tuberculosis in health-care settings, 2005. *MMWR Recomm. Rep.* 2005;54(17):1-141.

[13] AIA. Guidelines for Design and Construction of Hospital and Health Care Facilities. In: American Institute of Architects. Washington, DC: American Institute of Architects Press; 2006.

[14] CDC. Guidelines for Preventing Health-Care-Associated Pneumonia, 2003. Recommendations of CDC and the Healthcare Infection Control Practices Advisory Committee. *MMWR Recomm. Rep.* 2004;53(RR-3):140.

[15] CDC. Guidelines for preventing opportunistic infections among hematopoietic stem cell transplant recipients. Recommendations of CDC, the Infectious Disease Society of America, and the American Society of Blood and Marrow Transplantation. *MMWR - Morbidity & Mortality Weekly Report.* 2000;49(RR-10):1-125.

[16] Boyce JM, Pittet D. Guideline for Hand Hygiene in Health-Care Settings. Recommendations of the Healthcare Infection Control Practices Advisory Committee and the HICPAC/SHEA/APIC/IDSA Hand Hygiene Task Force. Society for Healthcare Epidemiology of America/Association for Professionals in Infection Control/Infectious Diseases Society of America. *MMWR Recomm. Rep.* 2002;51(RR-16):1-45, quiz CE1-4.

[17] Bolyard EA, Tablan OC, Williams WW, Pearson ML, Shapiro CN, Deitchmann SD. Guideline for infection control in healthcare personnel, 1998. Hospital Infection Control Practices Advisory Committee. *Infect. Control Hosp. Epidemiol.* 1998; 19(6) :407-63.

[18] CDC. Recommendations for Preventing Transmission of Infections Among Chronic Hemodialysis Patients. *MMWR.* 2001 ;50(RR05):1-43.

[19] Kohn WG, Collins AS, Cleveland JL, Harte JA, Eklund KJ, Malvitz DM. Guidelines for infection control in dental health-care settings--2003. *MMWR. Recomm. Rep.* 2003 ;52(RR- 17): 1-61.

[20] Saiman L, Siegel J. Infection control recommendations for patients with cystic fibrosis: microbiology, important pathogens, and infection control practices to prevent patient-to-patient transmission. *Infect. Control Hosp. Epidemiol.* 2003;24(5 Suppl):S6-52.

[21] Varia M, Wilson S, Sarwal S, et al. Investigation of a nosocomial outbreak of severe acute respiratory syndrome (SARS) in Toronto, Canada. *Cmaj.* 2003; 1 69(4):285-92.

[22] Haley RW, Cushion NB, Tenover FC, et al. Eradication of endemic methicillin-resistant Staphylococcus aureus infections from a neonatal intensive care unit. *J. Infect. Dis.* 1995;171(3):614-24.

[23] Bridges CB, Kuehnert MJ, Hall CB. Transmission of influenza: implications for control in health care settings. *Clin. Infect. Dis.* 2003;37(8): 1094-101.

[24] Hall CB. Nosocomial respiratory syncytial virus infections: the "Cold War" has not ended. *Clin. Infect. Dis.* 2000;31(2):590-6.

[25] Campbell JR, Zaccaria E, Mason EO, Jr., Baker CJ. Epidemiological analysis defining concurrent outbreaks of Serratia marcescens and methicillin-resistant Staphylococcus aureus in a neonatal intensive-care unit. *Infect. Control Hosp. Epidemiol.* 1998;19(12):924-8.

[26] Pena C, Pujol M, Ardanuy C, et al. Epidemiology and successful control of a large outbreak due to *Klebsiella pneumoniae* producing extended- spectrum beta-lactamases. *Antimicrob. Agents Chemother.* 1 998;42(1): 538.

[27] Bonten MJ, Slaughter S, Ambergen AW, et al. The role of "colonization pressure" in the spread of vancomycin-resistant enterococci: an important infection control variable. *Arch. Intern. Med.* 1998;158(10):1127-32.

[28] Jensenius M, Ringertz SH, Berild D, Bell H, Espinoza R, Grinde B. Prolonged nosocomial outbreak of hepatitis A arising from an alcoholic with pneumonia. *Scand. J. Infect. Dis.* 1998;30(2):1 19-23.

[29] Zawacki A, O'Rourke E, Potter-Bynoe G, Macone A, Harbarth S, Goldmann D. An outbreak of Pseudomonas aeruginosa pneumonia and bloodstream infection associated with intermittent otitis externa in a healthcare worker. *Infect. Control Hosp. Epidemiol.* 2004;25(12): 1083-9.

[30] Foca M, Jakob K, Whittier S, et al. Endemic Pseudomonas aeruginosa infection in a neonatal intensive care unit. *N. Engl. J. Med.* 2000;343(1 0):695-700.

[31] Gupta A, Della-Latta P, Todd B, et al. Outbreak of extended-spectrum beta-lactamase-producing Klebsiella pneumoniae in a neonatal intensive care unit linked to artificial nails. *Infect. Control Hosp. Epidemiol.* 2004;25(3):210-5.

[32] Boyce JM, Opal SM, Potter-Bynoe G, Medeiros AA. Spread of methicillin-resistant Staphylococcus aureus in a hospital after exposure to a health care worker with chronic sinusitis. *Clin. Infect. Dis.* 1993; 1 7(3):496-504.

[33] Fliegel PE, Weinstein WM. Rubella outbreak in a prenatal clinic: management and prevention. *Am. J. Infect. Control.* 1982;10(1):29-33.

[34] Atkinson WL, Markowitz LE, Adams NC, Seastrom GR. Transmission of measles in medical settings--United States, 1985-1989. *Am. J. Med.* 1991;91(3B):320S-4S.

[35] Carman WF, Elder AG, Wallace LA, et al. Effects of influenza vaccination of health-care workers on mortality of elderly people in longterm care: a randomised controlled trial. *Lancet.* 2000;355(9198):93-7.

[36] CDC. Outbreaks of pertussis associated with hospitals--Kentucky, Pennsylvania, and Oregon, 2003. *MMWR Morb. Mortal Wkly. Rep.* 2005 ;54(3): 67-7 1.

[37] Mermel LA, McKay M, Dempsey J, Parenteau S. Pseudomonas surgical- site infections linked to a healthcare worker with onychomycosis. *Infect. Control Hosp. Epidemiol.* 2003 ;24(10) :749-52.

[38] Barnes GL, Callaghan SL, Kirkwood CD, Bogdanovic-Sakran N, Johnston LJ, Bishop RF. Excretion of serotype G1 rotavirus strains by asymptomatic staff: a possible source of nosocomial infection. *J. Pediatr.* 2003; 142(6):722-5.

[39] Wang JT, Chang SC, Ko WJ, et al. A hospital-acquired outbreak of methicillin-resistant Staphylococcus aureus infection initiated by a surgeon carrier. *J. Hosp. Infect.* 2001;47(2):104-9.

[40] Valenti WM, Pincus PH, Messner MK. Nosocomial pertussis: possible spread by a hospital visitor. *Am. J. Dis. Child.* 1 980; 1 34(5):520-1.

[41] Christie CD, Glover AM, Willke MJ, Marx ML, Reising SF, Hutchinson NM. Containment of pertussis in the regional pediatric hospital during the Greater Cincinnati epidemic of 1993. *Infect. Control Hosp. Epidemiol.* 1995;16(10):556-63.

[42] Munoz FM, Ong LT, Seavy D, Medina D, Correa A, Starke JR. Tuberculosis among adult visitors of children with suspected tuberculosis and employees at a children's hospital. *Infect. Control Hosp. Epidemiol.* 2002;23(10):568-72.

[43] Garcia R, Raad I, Abi-Said D, et al. Nosocomial respiratory syncytial virus infections: prevention and control in bone marrow transplant patients. *Infect. Control Hosp. Epidemiol.* 1997; 18(6) :412-6.

[44] Whimbey E, Champlin RE, Couch RB, et al. Community respiratory virus infections among hospitalized adult bone marrow transplant recipients. *Clin. Infect. Dis.* 1996;22(5):778-82.

[45] Saiman L, O'keefe M, Graham PL, et al. Hospital transmission of community-acquired methicillin-resistant Staphylococcus aureus among postpartum women. *Clin. Infect. Dis.* 2003;37(10):1313-9.

[46] Bonten MJ, Slaughter S, Hayden MK, Nathan C, van Voorhis J, Weinstein RA. External sources of vancomycin-resistant enterococci for intensive care units. *Crit. Care Med.* 1998;26(12):2001-4.

[47] Flynn DM, Weinstein RA, Nathan C, Gaston MA, Kabins SA. Patients' endogenous flora as the source of "nosocomial" Enterobacter in cardiac surgery. *J. Infect. Dis.* 1987;156(2):363-8.

[48] Olson B, Weinstein RA, Nathan C, Chamberlin W, Kabins SA. Epidemiology of endemic Pseudomonas aeruginosa: why infection control efforts have failed. *J. Infect. Dis.* 1984;150(6):808-16.

[49] Perl TM, Cullen JJ, Wenzel RP, et al. Intranasal mupirocin to prevent postoperative Staphylococcus aureus infections. *N. Engl. J. Med.* 2002;346(24):1871-7.

[50] Toltzis P, Hoyen C, et al. Factors that predict preexisting colonization with antibiotic-resistant gram-negative bacilli in patients admitted to a pediatric intensive care unit. *Pediatrics.* 1999;103 (4 Pt1):719-23.

[51] Sarginson RE, Taylor N, Reilly N, Baines PB, Van Saene HK. Infection in prolonged pediatric critical illness: A prospective four-year study based on knowledge of the carrier state. *Crit. Care Med.* 2004;32(3):839-47.

[52] Silvestri L, Monti Bragadin C, Milanese M, et al. Are most ICU infections really nosocomial? A prospective observational cohort study in mechanically ventilated patients. *J. Hosp. Infect.* 1 999;42(2): 125-33.

[53] Heggers JP, Phillips LG, Boertman JA, et al. The epidemiology of methicillin-resistant Staphylococcus aureus in a burn center. *J. Burn Care Rehabil.* 1988;9(6):610-2.

[54] Donskey CJ. The role of the intestinal tract as a reservoir and source for transmission of nosocomial pathogens. *Clin. Infect. Dis.* 2004;39(2):219-26.

[55] Osterholm MT, Hedberg CW, Moore KA. The epidemiology of infectious diseases. . In: G.L. M, Jr DRG, J.E. B, eds. Principles and Practice of Infectious Diseases. 5th ed ed. Philadelphia: Churchill Livingstone; 2000: 161-3.

[56] Thomsen RW, Hundborg HH, Lervang HH, Johnsen SP, Schonheyder HC, Sorensen HT. Risk of community-acquired pneumococcal bacteremia in patients with diabetes: a population-based case-control study. *Diabetes Care.* 2004;27(5): 1143-7.

[57] Carton JA, Maradona JA, Nuno FJ, Fernandez-Alvarez R, Perez-Gonzalez F, Asensi V. Diabetes mellitus and bacteraemia: a comparative study between diabetic and non-diabetic patients. *Eur. J. Med.* 1992;1(5):281-7.

[58] Hirschtick RE, Glassroth J, Jordan MC, et al. Bacterial pneumonia in persons infected with the human immunodeficiency virus. Pulmonary Complications of HIV Infection Study Group. *N. Engl. J. Med.* 1995;333(13): 845-5 1.

[59] Rosenberg AL, Seneff MG, Atiyeh L, Wagner R, Bojanowski L, Zimmerman JE. The importance of bacterial sepsis in intensive care unit patients with acquired immunodeficiency syndrome: implications for future

care in the age of increasing antiretroviral resistance. *Crit. Care Med.* 2001;29(3):548-56.

[60] Malone JL, Ijaz K, Lambert L, et al. Investigation of healthcare-associated transmission of Mycobacterium tuberculosis among patients with malignancies at three hospitals and at a residential facility. *Cancer.* 2004; 101(12):2713-21.

[61] Fishman JA, Rubin RH. Infection in organ-transplant recipients. *N. Engl. J. Med.* 1998;338(24):1741-51.

[62] Safdar N, Kluger DM, Maki DG. A review of risk factors for catheter- related bloodstream infection caused by percutaneously inserted, noncuffed central venous catheters: implications for preventive strategies. *Medicine.* (Baltimore) 2002;81(6):466-79.

[63] Jarvis WR, Robles B. Nosocomial infections in pediatric patients. *Adv. Pediatr. Infect. Dis.* 1996;12:243-959(js).

[64] Yogaraj JS, Elward AM, Fraser VJ. Rate, risk factors, and outcomes of nosocomial primary bloodstream infection in pediatric intensive care unit patients. *Pediatrics.* 2002; 11 0(3):48 1-5.

[65] Donlan RM. Biofilms: microbial life on surfaces. *Emerg. Infect. Dis.* 2002;8(9):881 -90.

[66] Rosen HR. Acquisition of hepatitis C by a conjunctival splash. *Am. J. Infect. Control.* 1997;25(3):242-7.

[67] Beltrami EM, Kozak A, Williams IT, et al. Transmission of HIV and hepatitis C virus from a nursing home patient to a health care worker. *Am. J. Infect. Control.* 2003;31(3):168-75.

[68] Obasanjo OO, Wu P, Conlon M, et al. An outbreak of scabies in a teaching hospital: lessons learned. *Infect. Control Hosp. Epidemiol.* 2001;22(1):13-8.

[69] Andersen BM, Haugen H, Rasch M, Heldal Haugen A, Tageson A. Outbreak of scabies in Norwegian nursing homes and home care patients: control and prevention. *J. Hosp. Infect.* 2000;45(2):160-4.

[70] Avitzur Y, Amir J. Herpetic whitlow infection in a general pediatrician-- an occupational hazard. *Infection.* 2002;30(4):234-6.

[71] Adams G, Stover BH, Keenlyside RA, et al. Nosocomial herpetic infections in a pediatric intensive care unit. *Am. J. Epidemiol.* 1981;1 13(2):126-32.

[72] Bhalla A, Pultz NJ, Gries DM, et al. Acquisition of nosocomial pathogens on hands after contact with environmental surfaces near hospitalized patients. *Infect. Control Hosp. Epidemiol.* 2004;25 (2): 164-7.

[73] Duckro AN, Blom DW, Lyle EA, Weinstein RA, Hayden MK. Transfer of vancomycin-resistant enterococci via health care worker hands. *Arch. Intern. Med.* 2005;165(3):302-7.
[74] Brooks SE, Veal RO, Kramer M, Dore L, Schupf N, Adachi M. Reduction in the incidence of Clostridium difficile-associated diarrhea in an acute care hospital and a skilled nursing facility following replacement of electronic thermometers with single-use disposables. *Infect. Control Hosp. Epidemiol.* 1992;13(2):98-103.
[75] CDC. Nosocomial hepatitis B virus infection associated with reusable fingerstick blood sampling devices--Ohio and New York City, 1996. *MMWR Morb. Mortal Wkly. Rep.* 1997;46 (10):217-21.
[76] Desenclos JC, Bourdiol-Razes M, Rolin B, et al. Hepatitis C in a ward for cystic fibrosis and diabetic patients: possible transmission by spring-loaded finger-stick devices for self-monitoring of capillary blood glucose. *Infect. Control Hosp. Epidemiol.* 2001;22(1 1):701-7.
[77] CDC. Transmission of hepatitis B virus among persons undergoing blood glucose monitoring in long-term-care facilities--Mississippi, North Carolina, and Los Angeles County, California, 2003-2004. *MMWR Morb. Mortal Wkly. Rep.* 2005;54(9):220-3.
[78] Hall CB, Douglas RG, Jr. Modes of transmission of respiratory syncytial virus. *J. Pediatr.* 1981;99(1):100-3.
[79] Hall CB, Douglas RG, Jr., Geiman JM. Possible transmission by fomites of respiratory syncytial virus. *J. Infect. Dis.* 1980;141(1):98-102.
[80] Buttery JP, Alabaster SJ, Heine RG, et al. Multiresistant Pseudomonas aeruginosa outbreak in a pediatric oncology ward related to bath toys. *Pediatr. Infect. Dis. J.* 1998;17(6):509-13.
[81] Agerton T, Valway S, Gore B, et al. Transmission of a highly drug-resistant strain (strain W1) of Mycobacterium tuberculosis. Community outbreak and nosocomial transmission via a contaminated bronchoscope. *JAMA.* 1997;278(13):1073-7.
[82] Bronowicki JP, Venard V, Botte C, et al. Patient-to-patient transmission of hepatitis C virus during colonoscopy. *N. Engl. J. Med.* 1997;337(4):237-40.
[83] Michele TM, Cronin WA, Graham NM, et al. Transmission of Mycobacterium tuberculosis by a fiberoptic bronchoscope. Identification by DNA fingerprinting. *JAMA.* 1997;278(13):1093-5.
[84] Schelenz S, French G. An outbreak of multidrug-resistant Pseudomonas aeruginosa infection associated with contamination of bronchoscopes and an endoscope washer-disinfector. *J. Hosp. Infect.* 2000;46(1):23-30.

[85] Weber DJ, Rutala WA. Lessons from outbreaks associated with bronchoscopy. *Infect. Control Hosp. Epidemiol.* 2001 ;22(7):403-8.

[86] Kirschke DL, Jones TF, Craig AS, et al. Pseudomonas aeruginosa and Serratia marcescens contamination associated with a manufacturing defect in bronchoscopes. *N. Engl. J. Med.* 2003;348(3):214-20.

[87] Srinivasan A, Wolfenden LL, Song X, et al. An outbreak of Pseudomonas aeruginosa infections associated with flexible bronchoscopes. *N. Engl. J. Med.* 2003;348(3):221-7.

[88] Boyce JM, Potter-Bynoe G, Chenevert C, King T. Environmental contamination due to methicillin-resistant Staphylococcus aureus: possible infection control implications. *Infect. Control Hosp. Epidemiol.* 1997; 1 8(9):622-7.(mj).

[89] Zachary KC, Bayne PS, Morrison VJ, Ford DS, Silver LC, Hooper DC. Contamination of gowns, gloves, and stethoscopes with vancomycinresistant enterococci. *Infect. Control Hosp. Epidemiol.* 2001 ;22(9):560-4.

[90] Perry C, Marshall R, Jones E. Bacterial contamination of uniforms. *J. Hosp. Infect.* 2001 ;48(3):238-41.

[91] Papineni RS, Rosenthal FS. The size distribution of droplets in the exhaled breath of healthy human subjects. *J. Aerosol Med.* 1997;10(2):105-16.

[92] Wells WF. On airborne infection: Study II. Droplets and droplet nuclei. *Am. J. Hygiene.* 1934;20:61 1-18.

[93] Loeb M, McGeer A, Henry B, et al. SARS among critical care nurses, Toronto. *Emerg. Infect. Dis.* 2004;10(2):251-5.

[94] Fowler RA, Guest CB, Lapinsky SE, et al. Transmission of severe acute respiratory syndrome during intubation and mechanical ventilation. *Am. J. Respir. Crit. Care Med.* 2004;169(1 1):1 198-202.

[95] Gehanno JF, Kohen-Couderc L, Lemeland JF, Leroy J. Nosocomial meningococcemia in a physician. *Infect. Control Hosp. Epidemiol.* 1 999;20(8):564-5.

[96] Scales D, et al. Illness in intensive-care staff after brief exposure to severe acute respiratory syndrome. *Emerg. Infect. Dis.* 2003;9(10):1205-10.

[97] Ensor E, Humphreys H, Peckham D, Webster C, Knox AJ. Is Burkholderia (Pseudomonas) cepacia disseminated from cystic fibrosis patients during physiotherapy? *J. Hosp. Infect.* 1 996;32(1): 9-15.

[98] Christian MD, Loutfy M, McDonald LC, et al. Possible SARS coronavirus transmission during cardiopulmonary resuscitation. *Emerg. Infect Dis.* 2004; 1 0(2):287-93.

[99] Valenzuela TD, Hooton TM, Kaplan EL, Schlievert P. Transmission of 'toxic strep' syndrome from an infected child to a firefighter during CPR. *Ann. Emerg. Med.* 1991;20(1):90-2.

[100] Bassinet L, Matrat M, Njamkepo E, Aberrane S, Housset B, Guiso N. Nosocomial pertussis outbreak among adult patients and healthcare workers. *Infect. Control Hosp. Epidemiol.* 2004;25(11):995-7.

[101] Wong TW, Lee CK, Tam W, et al. Cluster of SARS among medical students exposed to single patient, Hong Kong. *Emerg. Infect. Dis.* 2004; 10(2):269-76.

[102] Pachucki CT, Pappas SA, Fuller GF, Krause SL, Lentino JR, Schaaff DM. Influenza A among hospital personnel and patients. Implications for recognition, prevention, and control. *Arch. Intern. Med.* 1989;149(1):77-80.

[103] Feigin RD, Baker CJ, Herwaldt LA, Lampe RM, Mason EO, Whitney SE. Epidemic meningococcal disease in an elementary-school classroom. *N. Engl. J. Med.* 1982;307(20):1255-7.

[104] Dick EC, Jennings LC, Mink KA, Wartgow CD, Inhorn SL. Aerosol transmission of rhinovirus colds. *J. Infect. Dis.* 1987;156(3):442-8.

[105] Duguid JP. The size and duration of air-carriage of respiratory droplets and droplet nucleii. *J. Hyg.* (Lond) 1946;44:471-9.

[106] Hall CB, Douglas RG, Jr., Schnabel KC, Geiman JM. Infectivity of respiratory syncytial virus by various routes of inoculation. *Infect. Immun.* 1981;33(3):779-83.

[107] Downie AW, Meiklejohn M, St Vincent L, Rao AR, Sundara Babu BV, Kempe CH. The recovery of smallpox virus from patients and their environment in a smallpox hospital. *Bull. World Health Organ.* 1965;33(5):615-22.

[108] Fenner F, Henderson DA, Arita I, Jezek Z, Ladnyi ID. The epidemiology of smallpox. In: Smallpox and its eradication. Switzerland: World Health Orginization; 1988.

[109] Cole EC, Cook CE. Characterization of infectious aerosols in health care facilities: an aid to effective engineering controls and preventive strategies. *Am. J. Infect. Control.* 1998;26(4):453-64.

[110] Christie C, Mazon D, Hierholzer W, Jr., Patterson JE. Molecular heterogeneity of Acinetobacter baumanii isolates during seasonal increase in prevalence. *Infect. Control Hosp. Epidemiol.* 1995;16(10):590-4.

[111] Musher DM. How contagious are common respiratory tract infections? *N. Engl. J. Med.* 2003;348(13):1256-66.

[112] Steinberg P, White RJ, Fuld SL, Gutekunst RR, Chanock RM, Senterfit LB. Ecology of Mycoplasma pneumoniae infections in marine recruits at Parris Island, South Carolina. *Am. J. Epidemiol.* 1969;89(1):62-73.

[113] Seto WH, Tsang D, Yung RW, et al. Effectiveness of precautions against droplets and contact in prevention of nosocomial transmission of severe acute respiratory syndrome (SARS). *Lancet.* 2003 ;3 61(9368): 1519-20.

[114] Hamburger M, Robertson OH. Expulsion of group A haemolytic streptocicci in droplets and droplet nuclei by sneezing, coughing and talking. *Am. J. Med.* 1948;4:690.

[115] CDC. Nosocomial meningococcemia. *MMWR Morb. Mortal Wkly. Rep.* 1978;27:358.

[116] LeClair JM, Freeman J, Sullivan BF, Crowley CM, Goldmann DA. Prevention of nosocomial respiratory syncytial virus infections through compliance with glove and gown isolation precautions. *N. Engl. J. Med.* 1987;3 17(6):329-34.

[117] Madge P, Paton JY, McColl JH, Mackie PL. Prospective controlled study of four infection-control procedures to prevent nosocomial infection with respiratory syncytial virus. *Lancet.* 1 992;340(8827):1079-83.

[118] Bassetti S, Bischoff WE, Walter M, et al. Dispersal of Staphylococcus aureus Into the Air Associated With a Rhinovirus Infection. *Infec. Control Hosp. Epidemiol.* 2005;26(2):196-203.

[119] Eichenwald HF, Kotsevalov O, Fasso LA. The "cloud baby": an example of bacterial-viral interaction. *Am. J. Dis. Child.* 1960;100:161-73.

[120] Sheretz RJ, Reagan DR, Hampton KD, et al. A cloud adult: the Staphylococcus aureus-virus interaction revisited. *Ann. Intern. Med.* 1996; 124(6):539-47.

[121] Coronado VG, Beck-Sague CM, Hutton MD, et al. Transmission of multidrug-resistant Mycobacterium tuberculosis among persons with human immunodeficiency virus infection in an urban hospital: epidemiologic and restriction fragment length polymorphism analysis. *J. Infect. Dis.* 1993;168(4):1052-5.

[122] Bloch AB, Orenstein WA, Ewing WM, et al. Measles outbreak in a pediatric practice: airborne transmission in an office setting. *Pediatrics.* 1985;75(4):676-83.

[123] LeClair JM, Zaia JA, Levin MJ, Congdon RG, Goldmann DA. Airborne transmission of chickenpox in a hospital. *N. Engl. J. Med.* 1980;302(8):450-3.

[124] Riley RL, Mills CC, Nyka W, et al. Aerial dissemination of pulmonary tuberculosis. A two-year study of contagion in a tuberculosis ward. 1959. *Am. J. Hyg.* 1959;70:185-96.

[125] Beck-Sague C, Dooley SW, Hutton MD, et al. Hospital outbreak of multidrug-resistant Mycobacterium tuberculosis infections. Factors in

transmission to staff and HIV-infected patients. *JAMA.* 1 992;268(10): 1280-6.

[126] CDC. Guidelines for preventing the transmission of Mycobacterium tuberculosis in health-care facilities, 1994. Centers for Disease Control and Prevention. *MMWR Recomm. Rep.* 1994;43(RR-13):1-132.

[127] Haley CE, McDonald RC, Rossi L, Jones WD, Jr., Haley RW, Luby JP. Tuberculosis epidemic among hospital personnel. *Infect. Control Hosp. Epidemiol.* 1989;10(5):204-10.

[128] Wehrle PF, Posch J, Richter KH, Henderson DA. An airborne outbreak of smallpox in a German hospital and its significance with respect to other recent outbreaks in Europe. *Bull. World Health Organ.* 1970;43(5):669-79.

[129] Gelfand HM, Posch J. The recent outbreak of smallpox in Meschede, West Germany. *Am. J. Epidemiol.* 1971;93(4):234-7.

[130] Moser MR, Bender TR, Margolis HS, Noble GR, Kendal AP, Ritter DG. An outbreak of influenza aboard a commercial airliner. *Am. J. Epidemiol.* 1979;1 10(1):1-6.

[131] Alford RH, Kasel JA, Gerone PJ, Knight V. Human influenza resulting from aerosol inhalation. *Proc. Soc. Exp. Biol. Med.* 1966;122(3):800-4.

[132] Chadwick PR, McCann R. Transmission of a small round structured virus by vomiting during a hospital outbreak of gastroenteritis. *J. Hosp. Infect.* 1 994;26(4):25 1-9.

[133] Prince DS, Astry C, Vonderfecht S, Jakab G, Shen FM, Yolken RH. Aerosol transmission of experimental rotavirus infection. *Pediatr. Infect. Dis.* 1986;5(2):218-22. www.cdc.gov/ncidod/sars.

[134] Peiris JS, Yuen KY, Osterhaus AD, Stohr K. The severe acute respiratory syndrome. *N. Engl. J. Med.* 2003;349(25):2431-41.

[135] Olsen SJ, Chang HL, Cheung TY, et al. Transmission of the severe acute respiratory syndrome on aircraft. *N. Engl. J. Med.* 2003;349(25):2416-22.

[136] Wilder-Smith A, Leong HN, Villacian JS. In-flight transmission of Severe Acute Respiratory Syndrome (SARS): A Case Report. *J. Travel Med.* 2003; 1 0(5):299-300.

[137] Booth TF, Kournikakis B, Bastien N, et al. Detection of airborne severe acute respiratory syndrome (SARS) coronavirus and environmental contamination in SARS outbreak units. *J. Infect. Dis.* 2005;191(9):1472-7.

[138] Yu IT, Li Y, Wong TW, et al. Evidence of airborne transmission of the severe acute respiratory syndrome virus. *N. Engl. J. Med.* 2004;350(17): 1731-9.

[139] CDC. Update: Outbreak of severe acute respiratory syndrome--worldwide. *MMWR Morb. Mortal Wkly. Rep.* 2003;52 (12):241-6, 8.

[140] CDC. Cluster of severe acute respiratory syndrome cases among protected health-care workers--Toronto, Canada, April 2003. *MMWR Morb. Mortal Wkly. Rep.* 2003 ;52(19):433-6.
[141] Sawyer LA, Murphy JJ, Kaplan JE, et al. 25- to 30-nm virus particle associated with a hospital outbreak of acute gastroenteritis with evidence for airborne transmission. *Am. J. Epidemiol.* 1988;127(6):1261-71.
[142] Marks PJ, Vipond IB, Carlisle D, Deakin D, Fey RE, Caul EO. Evidence for airborne transmission of Norwalk-like virus (NLV) in a hotel restaurant. *Epidemiol. Infec.* 2000; 1 24(3):48 1-7.
[143] Salgado CD, Farr BM, Hall KK, Hayden FG. Influenza in the acute hospital setting. *Lancet Infect. Dis.* 2002;2(3): 145-55.
[144] Riley RL. Airborne infection. *Am. J. Med.* 1974;57(3):466-75.
[145] McLean R. General discussion. . *Am. Rev. Respir. Dis.* 1961;83 36–8.
[146] Cheesbrough JS, Green J, Gallimore CI, Wright PA, Brown DW. Widespread environmental contamination with Norwalk-like viruses (NLV) detected in a prolonged hotel outbreak of gastroenteritis. *Epidemiol. Infect.* 2000;125(1):93-8.
[147] Marks PJ, Vipond IB, Regan FM, Wedgwood K, Fey RE, Caul EO. A school outbreak of Norwalk-like virus: evidence for airborne transmission. *Epidemiol. Infect.* 2003; 131(1):727-36.
[148] Roy CJ, Milton DK. Airborne transmission of communicable infection-- the elusive pathway. *N. Engl. J. Med.* 2004;350(17):1710-2.
[149] Dull PM, Wilson KE, Kournikakis B, et al. Bacillus anthracis aerosolization associated with a contaminated mail sorting machine. *Emerg. Infect. Dis.* 2002; 8(10): 1044-7.
[150] Weis CP, Intrepido AJ, Miller AK, et al. Secondary aerosolization of viable Bacillus anthracis spores in a contaminated US Senate Office. *JAMA.* 2002;288(22):2853-8.
[151] Patterson JE, Zidouh A, Miniter P, Andriole VT, Patterson TF. Hospital epidemiologic surveillance for invasive aspergillosis: patient demographics and the utility of antigen detection. *Infect. Control Hosp. Epidemiol.* 1997;1 8(2): 104-8.
[152] Arnow PM, Andersen RL, Mainous PD, Smith EJ. Pumonary aspergillosis during hospital renovation. *Am. Rev. Respir. Dis.* 1978;1 18(1):49-53.
[153] Pegues DA, Lasker BA, McNeil MM, Hamm PM, Lundal JL, Kubak BM. Cluster of cases of invasive aspergillosis in a transplant intensive care unit:

evidence of person-to-person airborne transmission. *Clin. Infect. Dis.* 2002;34(3):41 2-6.

[154] Buffington J, Reporter R, Lasker BA, et al. Investigation of an epidemic of invasive aspergillosis: utility of molecular typing with the use of random amplified polymorphic DNA probes. *Pediatr. Infect. Dis. J.* 1994;13(5):38693.

[155] Krasinski K, Holzman RS, Hanna B, Greco MA, Graff M, Bhogal M. Nosocomial fungal infection during hospital renovation. *Infect. Control.* 1985;6(7):278-82.

[156] Humphreys H. Positive-pressure isolation and the prevention of invasive aspergillosis. What is the evidence? *J. Hosp. Infect.* 2004;56(2):93-100.

[157] Thio CL, Smith D, Merz WG, et al. Refinements of environmental assessment during an outbreak investigation of invasive aspergillosis in a leukemia and bone marrow transplant unit. *Infect. Control Hosp. Epidemiol.* 2000;21(1):18-23.

[158] Anaissie EJ, Stratton SL, Dignani MC, et al. Pathogenic Aspergillus species recovered from a hospital water system: a 3-year prospective study. *Clin. Infect. Dis.* 2002;34(6):780-9.

[159] CDC. Prevention of invasive group A streptococcal disease among household contacts of case patients and among postpartum and postsurgical patients: recommendations from the Centers for Disease Control and Prevention. *Clin. Infect. Dis.* 2002;35 (8):950-9.

[160] Gruteke P, van Belkum A, Schouls LM, et al. Outbreak of group A streptococci in a burn center: use of pheno- and genotypic procedures for strain tracking. *J. Clin. Microbiol.* 1996;34(1):1 14-8.

[161] Greene CM, Van Beneden CA, Javadi M, et al. Cluster of deaths from group A streptococcus in a long-term care facility--Georgia, 2001. *Am. J. Infect. Control.* 2005;33(2): 108-13.

[162] Sabria M, Campins M. Legionnaires' disease: update on epidemiology and management options. *Am. J. Respir. Med.* 2003 ;2(3):235-43.

[163] Bille J, Marchetti O, Calandra T. Changing face of health-care associated fungal infections. *Curr. Opin. Infect. Dis.* 2005;18(4):314-9.

[164] Hall IC, O'Toole E. Intestinal flora in newborn infants with a description of a new pathogenic anaerobe, Bacillus difficilis. *Am. J. Dis. Child.* 1935;49:390-402.

[165] George WL, Sutter VL, Finegold SM. Antimicrobial agent-induced diarrhea--a bacterial disease. *J. Infect. Dis.* 1977;136(6):822-8.

[166] McFarland LV, Mulligan ME, Kwok RY, Stamm WE. Nosocomial acquisition of Clostridium difficile infection. *N. Engl. J. Med.* 1 989;320(4):204-10.

[167] Pepin J, Valiquette L, Alary ME, et al. Clostridium difficile-associated diarrhea in a region of Quebec from 1991 to 2003: a changing pattern of disease severity. *Cmaj.* 2004; 171(5) :466-72.
[168] 169. Agency HP. Outbreak of Clostridium difficile infection in a hospital in south east England. *Communicable Disease Report Weekly.* 2005;3 1(24).
[169] Koopmans M, Wilbrink B, Conyn M, et al. Transmission of H7N7 avian influenza A virus to human beings during a large outbreak in commercial poultry farms in the Netherlands. *Lancet.* 2004;363(9409):587-93.
[170] McDonald LC, Killgore GE, Thompson A, et al. An epidemic, toxin gene-variant strain of Clostridium difficile. *N. Engl. J. Med.* 2005;353(23):2433-41.
[171] Loo VG, Poirier L, Miller MA, et al. A predominantly clonal multi-institutional outbreak of Clostridium difficile-associated diarrhea with high morbidity and mortality. *N. Engl. J. Med.* 2005;353(23):2442-9.
[172] Warny M, Pepin J, Fang A, et al. Toxin production by an emerging strain of Clostridium difficile associated with outbreaks of severe disease in North America and Europe. 2005;366(9491):1079-84.
[173] Layton BA ML, Gerding DN, Liedtke LA, Strausbaugh LJ. Perceived increases in the incidence and severity of Clostridium difficile disease: an emerging threat that continues to unfold. In: 15th Annual Scientific Meeting of the Society for Healthcare Epidemiology of America;. Los Angeles, CA.; 2005.
[174] Sohn S, Climo M, Diekema D, et al. Varying rates of Clostridium difficile-associated diarrhea at prevention epicenter hospitals. *Infect. Control Hosp. Epidemiol.* 2005 ;26(8): 676-9.
[175] IOM. Antimicrobial Resistance: Issues and Options. Workshop report. In: Harrison PF, Lederberg J, eds. Washington, DC: National Academy Press; 1998:8-74.
[176] Shlaes DM, Gerding DN, John JF, Jr., et al. Society for Healthcare Epidemiology of America and Infectious Diseases Society of America Joint Committee on the Prevention of Antimicrobial Resistance: guidelines for the prevention of antimicrobial resistance in hospitals. *Infect.Control Hosp. Epidemiol.* 1997; 18(4) :275-91.
[177] Whitener CJ, Park SY, Browne FA, et al. Vancomycin-resistant Staphylococcus aureus in the absence of vancomycin exposure. *Clin. Infect. Dis.* 2004;38(8): 1049-55.
[178] CDC. Staphylococcus aureus with reduced susceptibility to vancomycin-United States. *MMWR. Morb. Mortal. Wkly. Rep.* 1997;46 (33):765-6.

[179] CDC. Staphylococcus aureus resistant to vancomycin--United States, 2002. *MMWR. Morb. Mortal. Wkly. Rep.* 2002;51 (26):565-7.
[180] CDC. Public Health Dispatch: Vancomycin-Resistant Staphylococcus aureus --- Pennsylvania, 2002. *MMWR - Morbidity & Mortality Weekly Report.* 2002;5 1 (40):902.
[181] CDC. Vancomycin-resistant Staphylococcus aureus--New York, 2004. *MMWR. Morb. Mortal Wkly. Rep.* 2004;53(15):322-3.
[182] Chang S, Sievert DM, Hageman JC, et al. Infection with vancomycinresistant Staphylococcus aureus containing the vanA resistance gene. *N. Engl. J. Med.* 2003;348(14):1342-7.
[183] Fridkin SK, Hageman J, McDougal LK, et al. Epidemiological and microbiological characterization of infections caused by Staphylococcus aureus with reduced susceptibility to vancomycin, United States, 19972001. *Clin. Infect. Dis.* 2003;36(4):429-39.
[184] Gold HS, Moellering RC, Jr. Antimicrobial-drug resistance. *N. Engl. J. Med.* 1 996;335(1 9): 1445-53.
[185] Hageman JC, Pegues DA, Jepson C, et al. Vancomycin-intermediate Staphylococcus aureus in a home health-care patient. *Emerg. Infect. Dis.* 2001 ;7(6): 1023-5.
[186] Harwell JI, Brown RB. The drug-resistant pneumococcus: clinical relevance, therapy, and prevention. *Chest.* 2000;1 17(2):530-41.
[187] Jones RN. Resistance patterns among nosocomial pathogens: trends over the past few years. *Chest.* 2001;119(2 Suppl):397S-404S.
[188] Murray BE. Vancomycin-resistant enterococcal infections. *N. Engl. J. Med.* 2000;342(10):710-21.
[189] Neuhauser MM, Weinstein RA, Rydman R, Danziger LH, Karam G, Quinn JP. Antibiotic resistance among gram-negative bacilli in US
[190] intensive care units: implications for fluoroquinolone use. *JAMA.* 2003;289(7):885-8.
[191] Pitout JD, Sanders CC, Sanders WE, Jr. Antimicrobial resistance with focus on beta-lactam resistance in gram- negative bacilli. *Am. J. Med.* 1997;103(1):51-9.
[192] Rotun SS, McMath V, Schoonmaker DJ, et al. Staphylococcus aureus with reduced susceptibility to vancomycin isolated from a patient with fatal bacteremia. *Emerg. Infect. Dis.* 1999;5(1):147-9.
[193] Smith TL, Pearson ML, Wilcox KR, et al. Emergence of vancomycin resistance in Staphylococcus aureus. Glycopeptide-Intermediate Staphylococcus aureus Working Group. *N. Engl. J. Med.* 1999;340(7):49350 1.

[194] Srinivasan A, Dick JD, Perl TM. Vancomycin resistance in staphylococci. *Clin. Microbiol. Rev.* 2002; 1 5(3):430-8.
[195] Hyle EP, Lipworth AD, Zaoutis TE, et al. Risk Factors for Increasing Multidrug Resistance among Extended-Spectrum ß-lactamase-Lactamase-Producing *Escheria coli* and *Klebsiella* species. *Clin. Infect. Dis.* 2005;40(9): 1317-24.
[196] Gleich S, Morad Y, Echague R, et al. Streptococcus pneumoniae serotype 4 outbreak in a home for the aged: report and review of recent outbreaks. *Infect. Control. Hosp. Epidemiol.* 2000;21 :711.
[197] Fry AM, Udeagu CC, Soriano-Gabarro M, et al. Persistence of fluoroquinolone-resistant, multidrug-resistant Streptococcus pneumoniae in a long-term-care facility: efforts to reduce intrafacility transmission. *Infect. Control. Hosp. Epidemiol.* 2005;26(3):239-47.
[198] Carter RJ, Sorenson G, Heffernan R, et al. Failure to control an outbreak of multidrug-resistant Streptococcus pneumoniae in a long-term-care facility: emergence and ongoing transmission of a fluoroquinoloneresistant strain. *Infect. Control. Hosp. Epidemiol.* 2005;26(3):248-55.
[199] Blok HE, Troelstra A, Kamp-Hopmans TE, et al. Role of healthcare workers in outbreaks of methicillin-resistant Staphylococcus aureus: a 10- year evaluation from a Dutch university hospital. *Infect. Control Hosp. Epidemiol.* 2003 ;24(9):679-85.
[200] Muto CA, Jernigan JA, Ostrowsky BE, et al. SHEA guideline for preventing nosocomial transmission of multidrug-resistant strains of Staphylococcus aureus and enterococcus. *Infect. Control Hosp. Epidemiol.* 2003 ;24(5):362-86.
[201] Tammelin A, Klotz F, Hambraeus A, Stahle E, Ransjo U. Nasal and hand carriage of Staphylococcus aureus in staff at a Department for Thoracic and Cardiovascular Surgery: endogenous or exogenous source? *Infect. Control Hosp. Epidemiol.* 2003;24(9):686-9.
[202] CDC. Biological and chemical terrorism: strategic plan for preparedness and response. Recommendations of the CDC Strategic Planning Workgroup. *MMWR. Recomm. Rep.* 2000;49(RR-4):1-14.
[203] Inglesby TV, O'Toole T, Henderson DA, et al. Anthrax as a biological weapon, 2002: updated recommendations for management. *JAMA.* 2002;287(1 7):2236-52.
[204] Henderson DA, Inglesby TV, Bartlett JG, et al. Smallpox as a biological weapon: medical and public health management. Working Group on Civilian Biodefense. *JAMA.* 1 999;28 1 (22):2 127-37.
[205] www.bt.cdc.gov/agent/smallpox/

[206] www.who.int/csr/disease/smallpox/en/
[207] Kool JL. Risk of person-to-person transmission of pneumonic plague. *Clin. Infect. Dis.* 2005;40(8):1 166-72.
[208] Inglesby TV, Dennis DT, Henderson DA, et al. Plague as a biological weapon: medical and public health management. Working Group on Civilian Biodefense. *JAMA.* 2000;283 (1 7):228 1-90.
[209] Arnon SS, Schechter R, Inglesby TV, et al. Botulinum toxin as a biological weapon: medical and public health management. *JAMA.* 2001 ;285(8): 1059-70.
[210] Dennis DT, Inglesby TV, Henderson DA, et al. Tularemia as a biological weapon: medical and public health management. *JAMA.* 2001;285(21):2763-73.
[211] CDC. Notice to Readers Update: Management of Patients with Suspected Viral Hemorrhagic Fever -- United States. *MMWR Recomm. Rep.* 1995;44(25):475-9.
[212] Borio L, Inglesby T, Peters CJ, et al. Hemorrhagic fever viruses as biological weapons: medical and public health management. *JAMA.* 2002;287(1 8):2391-405.
[213] Neff JM, Lane JM, Fulginiti VA, Henderson DA. Contact vaccinia-transmission of vaccinia from smallpox vaccination. *JAMA.* 2002;288(1 5): 1901-5.
[214] Sepkowitz KA. How contagious is vaccinia? *N. Engl. J. Med.* 2003 ;348(5):439-46.
[215] Lane JM, Fulginiti VA. Transmission of vaccinia virus and rationale for measures for prevention. *Clin. Infect. Dis.* 2003;37(2):281-4.
[216] CDC. Smallpox Vaccination and Adverse Reactions: Guidance for Clinicians. *MMWR - Morbidity & Mortality Weekly Report.* 2003;52(RR04): 1-28.
[217] Fulginiti VA, Papier A, Lane JM, Neff JM, Henderson DA. Smallpox vaccination: a review, part II. Adverse events. *Clin. Infect. Dis.* 2003;37(2):25 1-71.
[218] www.smallpox.mil./event/SPSafetySum.asp
[219] CDC. Update: adverse events following civilian smallpox vaccination--United States, 2003. *MMWR Morb. Mortal Wkly. Rep.* 2003;52(18):41920.
[220] CDC. Secondary and tertiary transfer of vaccinia virus among U.U. military personnel--United States and worldwide, 2002-2004. *MMWR Morb. Mortal Wkly Rep.* 2004;53(5):103-5.
[221] Talbot TR, Ziel E, Doersam JK, LaFleur B, Tollefson S, Edwards KM. Risk of vaccinia transfer to the hands of vaccinated persons after smallpox immunization. *Clin. Infect. Dis.* 2004;3 8(4): 536-41.

[222] Hepburn MJ, Dooley DP, Murray CK, et al. Frequency of vaccinia virus isolation on semipermeable versus nonocclusive dressings covering smallpox vaccination sites in hospital personnel. *Am. J. Infect. Control.* 2004;32(3): 126-30.

[223] Waibel KH, Ager EP, Topolski RL, Walsh DS. Randomized trial comparing vaccinia on the external surfaces of 3 conventional bandages applied to smallpox vaccination sites in primary vaccinees. *Clin. Infect. Dis.* 2004;39(7): 1004-7.

[224] Tenorio AR, Peeples M, Patri M, et al. Quantitative Vaccinia Cultures and Evolution of Vaccinia-Specific CD8+ Cytotoxic T-lymphocytes (CTL) Responses in Revaccinees. Abstract #823, 41st Annual Meeting IDSA, October 2003, San Diego 2003.

[225] Wharton M, Strikas RA, Harpaz R, et al. Recommendations for using smallpox vaccine in a pre-event vaccination program. Supplemental recommendations of the Advisory Committee on Immunization Practices (ACIP) and the Healthcare Infection Control Practices Advisory Committee (HICPAC). *MMWR Recomm. Rep.* 2003;52(RR-7):1-16.

[226] CDC. Surveillance for Creutzfeldt-Jakob Disease -- United States. *MMWR.* 1996;45(31):665-8.

[227] Johnson RT, Gibbs CJ, Jr. Creutzfeldt-Jakob disease and related transmissible spongiform encephalopathies. *N. Engl. J. Med.* 1998;339(27): 1994-2004.

[228] Brown P, Gajdusek DC, Gibbs CJ, Jr., Asher DM. Potential epidemic of Creutzfeldt-Jakob disease from human growth hormone therapy. *N. Engl. J. Med.* 1985;313(12):728-31.

[229] Frasier SD, Foley TP, Jr. Clinical review 58: Creutzfeldt-Jakob disease in recipients of pituitary hormones. *J. Clin. Endocrinol. Metab.* 1 994;78(6): 1277-9.

[230] CDC. Update: Creutzfeldt-Jakob disease associated with cadaveric dura mater grafts--Japan, 1979-2003. *MMWR Morb Mortal Wkly. Rep.* 2003;52(48):1 179-81.

[231] Lang CJ, Heckmann JG, Neundorfer B. Creutzfeldt-Jakob disease via dural and corneal transplants. *J. Neurol. Sci.*1998;160(2):128-39.

[232] el Hachimi KH, Chaunu MP, Cervenakova L, Brown P, Foncin JF. Putative neurosurgical transmission of Creutzfeldt-Jakob disease with analysis of donor and recipient: agent strains. *C R Acad. Sci.* III 1 997;320(4):3 19-28.

[233] Will RG, Matthews WB. Evidence for case-to-case transmission of Creutzfeldt-Jakob disease. *J. Neurol. Neurosurg. Psychiatry.* 1 982;45(3):2358.

[234] Bernoulli C, Siegfried J, Baumgartner G, et al. Danger of accidental person-to-person transmission of Creutzfeldt-Jakob disease by surgery. *Lancet.* 1977;1(8009):478-9.
[235] Rutala WA, Weber DJ. Creutzfeldt-Jakob disease: recommendations for disinfection and sterilization. *Clin. Infect. Dis.* 2001;32(9): 1348-56.
[236] Belay ED, Maddox RA, Williams ES, Miller MW, Gambetti P, Schonberger LB. Chronic wasting disease and potential transmission to humans. *Emerg. Infect. Dis.* 2004;10(6):977-84.
[237] Collinge J, Sidle KC, Meads J, Ironside J, Hill AF. Molecular analysis of prion strain variation and the aetiology of 'new variant' CJD. *Nature.* 1 996;3 83(6602):685-90.
[238] Belay ED, Schonberger LB. The public health impact of prion diseases. *Annu. Rev. Public Health.* 2005;26:191-212.
[239] Belay ED, Schonberger LB. Variant Creutzfeldt-Jakob disease and bovine spongiform encephalopathy. *Clin. Lab. Med.* 2002;22(4):849-62, v-vi.
[240] Hill AF, Butterworth RJ, Joiner S, et al. Investigation of variant Creutzfeldt-Jakob disease and other human prion diseases with tonsil biopsy samples. *Lancet.*1 999;3 53(9148): 183-9.
[241] Evatt B. Creutzfeldt-Jakob disease and haemophilia: assessment of risk. *Haemophilia.* 2000;6 Suppl 1:94-9.
[242] Chamberland ME. Emerging infectious agents: do they pose a risk to the safety of transfused blood and blood products? *Clin. Infect. Dis.* 2002;34(6):797-805.
[243] www.fda.gov/cber/gdlns/cjdvcjd.htm
[244] Llewelyn CA, Hewitt PE, Knight RS, et al. Possible transmission of variant Creutzfeldt-Jakob disease by blood transfusion. *Lancet.* 2004;363(9407):417-21.
[245] Peden AH, Head MW, Ritchie DL, Bell JE, Ironside JW. Preclinical vCJD after blood transfusion in a PRNP codon 129 heterozygous patient. *Lancet.* 2004;364(9433):527-9.
[246] Brown P. Guidelines for high risk autopsy cases: special precautions for Creutzfeldt-Jakob Disease. In: Hutchins G, ed. Autopsy Performance and Reporting, Northfield, Ill.:. *College of American Pathologists.* 1990:68-74.
[247] Drosten C, Gunther S, Preiser W, et al. Identification of a novel coronavirus in patients with severe acute respiratory syndrome. *N. Engl. J. Med.* 2003;348(20): 1967-76.
[248] Ksiazek TG, Erdman D, Goldsmith CS, et al. A novel coronavirus associated with severe acute respiratory syndrome. *N. Engl. J. Med.* 2003;348(20): 1953-66.

[249] Chan WM, Kwan YW, Wan HS, Leung CW, Chiu MC. Epidemiologic linkage and public health implication of a cluster of severe acute respiratory syndrome in an extended family. *Pediatr. Infect. Dis. J.* 2004;23(12):1 156-9.

[250] Leung CW, Kwan YW, Ko PW, et al. Severe acute respiratory syndrome among children. *Pediatrics.* 2004;1 13(6):e535-43.

[251] Bitnun A, Allen U, Heurter H, et al. Children hospitalized with severe acute respiratory syndrome-related illness in Toronto. *Pediatrics.* 2003;1 12(4):e261.

[252] Chow KY, Lee CE, Ling ML, Heng DM, Yap SG. Outbreak of severe acute respiratory syndrome in a tertiary hospital in Singapore, linked to an index patient with atypical presentation: epidemiological study. *Bmj.* 2004;328(7433): 195.

[253] Shen Z, Ning F, Zhou W, et al. Superspreading SARS events, Beijing, 2003. *Emerg. Infect. Dis.* 2004;10(2):256-60.

[254] Chen Y-C, Huang L-M, Chan C-C, et al. SARS in Hospital Emergency Room. *Emerg. Infect. Dis.* 2004;10:782-8.

[255] Chung Y-C, Huang L-M, Chan C-C, et al. SARS in Hospital Emergency Room. *Emerg. Infect. Dis.* 2004;10:782-8.

[256] Gamage B, Moore D, Copes R, Yassi A, Bryce E. Protecting health care workers from SARS and other respiratory pathogens: a review of the infection control literature. *Am. J. Infect. Control.* 2005 ;3 3(2): 114-21.

[257] Moore D, Gamage B, Bryce E, Copes R, Yassi A. Protecting health care workers from SARS and other respiratory pathogens: organizational and individual factors that affect adherence to infection control guidelines. *Am. J. Infect. Control.* 2005;33(2):88-96.

[258] Dowell SF, Simmerman JM, Erdman DD, et al. Severe acute respiratory syndrome coronavirus on hospital surfaces. *Clin. Infect. Dis.* 2004;39(5):652-7.

[259] Public Health Guidance for Community-Level Preparedness and Response to Severe Acute Respiratory Syndrome (SARS). 2004. (Accessed at http://www.cdc.gov/ncidod/sars/guidance/I/occupational.htm.)

[260] Le DH, Bloom SA, Nguyen QH, et al. Lack of SARS transmission among public hospital workers, *Vietnam. Emerg. Infect. Dis.* 2004;10(2):265-8.

[261] Lim PL, Kurup A, Gopalakrishna G, et al. Laboratory-acquired severe acute respiratory syndrome. *N. Engl. J. Med.* 2004;350(17):1740-5.

[262] CDC. www.cdc.gov/ncidod/sars. 2003.

[263] Reed KD, Melski JW, Graham MB, et al. The detection of monkeypox in humans in the Western Hemisphere. *N. Engl. J. Med.* 2004;350(4):342-50.

[264] Anderson MG, Frenkel LD, Homann S, Guffey J. A case of severe monkeypox virus disease in an American child: emerging infections and changing professional values. *Pediatr. Infect. Dis. J.* 2003;22:1093-6.

[265] Jezek Z, Fenner F. Human monkey pox. In: Melnick JL ed. Monographs in virology. Vol. 17. Basel, Switzerland: S Karger AG. 1988:81-102.

[266] Marennikova SS, Jezek Z, Szczeniowski M, Mbudi PM, Vernette M. [Contagiousness of monkey pox for humans: results of an investigation of 2 outbreaks of the infection in Zaire]. *Zh. Mikrobiol. Epidemiol. Immunobiol.* 1985(8):38-43.

[267] Jezek Z, Arita I, Mutombo M, Dunn C, Nakano JH, Szczeniowski M. Four generations of probable person-to-person transmission of human monkeypox. *Am. J. Epidemiol.* 1986;123(6):1004-12.

[268] Learned LA, Reynolds MG, Wassa DW, et al. Extended interhuman transmission of monkeypox in a hospital community in the Republic of the Congo, 2003. *Am. J. Trop. Med. Hyg.* 2005;73(2):428-34.

[269] Fleischauer AT, Kile JC, Davidson M, et al. Evaluation of human-tohuman transmission of monkeypox from infected patients to health care workers. *Clin. Infect. Dis.* 2005 ;40(5):689-94.

[270] Likos AM, Sammons SA, Olson VA, et al. A tale of two clades: monkeypox viruses. *J. Gen. Virol.* 2005;86(Pt 10):2661-72.

[271] Fine PE, Jezek Z, Grab B, Dixon H. The transmission potential of monkeypox virus in human populations. *Int. J. Epidemiol.* 1988;17(3):64350.

[272] Jezek Z, Grab B, Paluku KM, Szczeniowski MV. Human monkeypox: disease pattern, incidence and attack rates in a rural area of northern Zaire. *Trop. Geogr. Med.* 1988;40(2):73-83.

[273] CDC. "Norwalk-Like Viruses":Public Health Consequences and Outbreak Management. *MMWR - Morbidity & Mortality Weekly Report.* 2001 ;50 (RR-09)(June): 1-18.

[274] Evans MR, Meldrum R, Lane W, et al. An outbreak of viral gastroenteritis following environmental contamination at a concert hall. *Epidemiol. Infect.* 2002; 129(2):355-60.

[275] Wu HM, Fornek M, Kellogg JS, et al. A Norovirus Outbreak at a LongTerm-Care Facility: The Role of Environmental Surface Contamination. *Infect. Control Hosp. Epidemiol.* 2005;26(10):802-10.

[276] Duizer E, Schwab KJ, Neill FH, Atmar RL, Koopmans MP, Estes MK. Laboratory efforts to cultivate noroviruses. *J. Gen. Virol.* 2004;85(Pt 1):7987.

[277] Zingg W, Colombo C, Jucker T, Bossart W, Ruef C. Impact of an outbreak of norovirus infection on hospital resources. *Infect. Control Hosp. Epidemiol.* 2005;26:263-7.
[278] Calderon-Margalit R, Sheffer R, Halperin T, Orr N, Cohen D, Shohat T. A large-scale gastroenteritis outbreak associated with Norovirus in nursing homes. *Epidemiol. Infect* .2005; 133(1): 35-40.
[279] Marx A, Shay DK, Noel JS, et al. An outbreak of acute gastroenteritis in a geriatric long-term-care facility: combined application of epidemiological and molecular diagnostic methods. *Infect. Control Hosp. Epidemiol.* 1999;20(5):306-1 1.
[280] Gellert GA, Waterman SH, Ewert D, et al. An outbreak of acute gastroenteritis caused by a small round structured virus in a geriatric convalescent facility. *Infect. Control Hosp. Epidemiol.* 1990; 11 (9):459-64.
[281] Cooper E, Blamey S. A Norovirus Gastroenteritis Epidemic in a Long-Term-Care Facility. *Infect. Control Hosp. Epidemiol.* 2005;26(3):256.
[282] Navarro G, Sala RM, Segura F, et al. An Outbreak of Norovirus Infection in a Long-Term-Care. *Infect. Control Hosp. Epidemiol.* 2005;26(3):259.
[283] Green KY, Belliot G, Taylor JL, et al. A predominant role for Norwalk- like viruses as agents of epidemic gastroenteritis in Maryland nursing homes for the elderly. *J. Infect. Dis.* 2002;185(2):133-46.
[284] Widdowson MA, Cramer EH, Hadley L, et al. Outbreaks of acute gastroenteritis on cruise ships and on land: identification of a predominant circulating strain of norovirus--United States, 2002. *J. Infect. Dis.* 2004; 1 90(1):27-36.
[285] CDC. Outbreaks of gastroenteritis associated with noroviruses on cruise ships-- United States, 2002. *MMWR Morb. Mortal. Wkly. Rep.* 2002;51(49):1 112-5.
[286] CDC. Norovirus outbreak among evacuees from hurricane Katrina-- Houston, Texas, September 2005. *MMWR. Morb. Mortal. Wkly. Rep.* 2005;54(40): 1016-8.
[287] Mattner F, Mattner L, Borck HU, Gastmeier P. Evaluation of the Impact of the Source (Patient Versus Staff) on Nosocomial Norovirus Outbreak Severity. *Infect. Control Hosp. Epidemiol.* 2005;26(3):268-72.
[288] Isakbaeva ET, Bulens SN, Beard RS, et al. Norovirus and child care: challenges in outbreak control. *Pediatr. Infect. Dis. J.* 2005;24(6):561-3.
[289] Kapikian AZ, Estes MK, Chanock RM. Norwalk group of viruses. In: Fields BN, Knipe DM, Howley PM, eds. Fields virology. 3rd ed. Philadelphia, PA: Lippincott-Raven. 1996:783-810.

[290] Duizer E, Bijkerk P, Rockx B, De Groot A, Twisk F, Koopmans M. Inactivation of caliciviruses. *Appl. Environ. Microbiol.* 2004;70(8):453 8-43.
[291] Doultree JC, Druce JD, Birch CJ, Bowden DS, Marshall JA. Inactivation of feline calicivirus, a Norwalk virus surrogate. *J. Hosp. Infect.* 1999;41(1):51-7.
[292] Barker J, Vipond IB, Bloomfield SF. Effects of cleaning and disinfection in reducing the spread of Norovirus contamination via environmental surfaces. *J. Hosp. Infect.* 2004;58(1):42-9.
[293] Gulati BR, Allwood PB, Hedberg CW, Goyal SM. Efficacy of commonly used disinfectants for the inactivation of calicivirus on strawberry, lettuce, and a food-contact surface. *J. Food Prot.* 2001;64(9): 1430-4.
[294] Gehrke C, Steinmann J, Goroncy-Bermes P. Inactivation of feline calicivirus, a surrogate of norovirus (formerly Norwalk-like viruses), by different types of alcohol in vitro and in vivo. *J. Hosp. Infect.* 2004;56(1):49-55.
[295] Hutson AM, Atmar RL, Graham DY, Estes MK. Norwalk virus infection and disease is associated with ABO histo-blood group type. *J. Infect. Dis.* 2002; 185(9): 1335-7.
[296] National Center for Infectious Diseases - Division of Viral and Rickettsial Diseases. (www.cdc.gov/ncidod/dvrd/index.htm
[297] LeDuc JW. Epidemiology of hemorrhagic fever viruses. *Rev. Infect. Dis.* 1989;11 Suppl 4:S730-5.
[298] Roels TH, Bloom AS, Buffington J, et al. Ebola hemorrhagic fever, Kikwit, Democratic Republic of the Congo, 1995: risk factors for patients without a reported exposure. *J. Infect. Dis.* 1999 Feb;179 Suppl. 1:S92-7.
[299] Suleiman MN, Muscat-Baron JM, Harries JR, et al. Congo/Crimean haemorrhagic fever in Dubai. An outbreak at the Rashid Hospital. *Lancet.* 1 980;2(8201):939-41.
[300] Monath TP, Mertens PE, Patton R, et al. A hospital epidemic of Lassa fever in Zorzor, Liberia, March-April 1972. *Am. J. Trop. Med. Hyg.* 1973 ;22(6):773-9.
[301] Dowell SF, Mukunu R, Ksiazek TG, Khan AS, Rollin PE, Peters CJ. Transmission of Ebola hemorrhagic fever: a study of risk factors in family members, Kikwit, Democratic Republic of the Congo, 1995. *J. Infect. Dis.* 1999 Feb;179 Suppl 1:S87-91.
[302] Peters CJ. Marburg and Ebola--arming ourselves against the deadly filoviruses. *N. Engl. J. Med.* 2005;352(25):2571-3.

[303] Ebola haemorrhagic fever in Zaire, 1976. *Bull. World Health. Organ.* 1978;56(2):271-93.
[304] Emond RT, Evans B, Bowen ET, Lloyd G. A case of Ebola virus infection. *Br. Med. J.* 1977;2(6086):541-4.
[305] Zaki SR, Shieh WJ, Greer PW, et al. A novel immunohistochemical assay for the detection of Ebola virus in skin: implications for diagnosis, spread, and surveillance of Ebola hemorrhagic fever. Commission de Lutte contre les Epidemies a Kikwit. *J. Infect. Dis.* 1999;179 Suppl 1:S36-47.
[306] Khan AS, Tshioko FK, Heymann DL, et al. The reemergence of Ebola hemorrhagic fever, Democratic Republic of the Congo, 1995. Commission de Lutte contre les Epidemies a Kikwit. *J. Infect. Dis.* 1999;179 Suppl 1:S76-86.
[307] Muyembe-Tamfum JJ, Kipasa M, Kiyungu C, Colebunders R. Ebola outbreak in Kikwit, Democratic Republic of the Congo: discovery and control measures. *J. Infect. Dis.* 1999;179 Suppl. 1:S259-62.
[308] Haas WH, Breuer T, Pfaff G, et al. Imported Lassa fever in Germany: surveillance and management of contact persons. *Clin. Infect. Dis.* 2003;36(10): 1254-8.
[309] Simpson DI. Marburg agent disease: in monkeys. *Trans. R. Soc. Trop. Med. Hyg.* 1969;63(3):303-9.
[310] Jaax NK, Davis KJ, Geisbert TJ, et al. Lethal experimental infection of rhesus monkeys with Ebola-Zaire (Mayinga) virus by the oral and conjunctival route of exposure. *Arch. Pathol. Lab. Med.* 1996;120(2):140-55.
[311] Stephenson EH, Larson EW, Dominik JW. Effect of environmental factors on aerosol-induced Lassa virus infection. *J. Med. Virol.* 1984;14(4):295303.
[312] Johnson E, Jaax N, White J, Jahrling P. Lethal experimental infections of rhesus monkeys by aerosolized Ebola virus. *Int. J. Exp. Pathol.* 1 995;76(4):227-36.
[313] Jaax N, Jahrling P, Geisbert T, et al. Transmission of Ebola virus (Zaire strain) to uninfected control monkeys in a biocontainment laboratory. *Lancet.* 1 995;346(899 1-8992): 1669-71.
[314] www.bt.cdc.gov/agent/vhf/.
[315] Nguyen GT, Proctor SE, Sinkowitz-Cochran RL, Garrett DO, Jarvis WR. Status of infection surveillance and control programs in the United States, 1992-1996. Association for Professionals in Infection Control and Epidemiology, Inc. *Am. J. Infect. Control.* 2000;28(6):392-400.
[316] Richards C, Emori TG, Edwards J, Fridkin S, Tolson J, Gaynes R. Characteristics of hospitals and infection control professionals participating

in the National Nosocomial Infections Surveillance System 1999. *Am. J. Infect. Control.* 2001;29(6):400-3.

[317] Wenzel RP, Thompson RL, Landry SM, et al. Hospital-acquired infections in intensive care unit patients: an overview with emphasis on epidemics. *Infect. Control.* 1983;4(5):371-5.

[318] Wenzel RP, Gennings C. Bloodstream infections due to Candida species in the intensive care unit: identifying especially high-risk patients to determine prevention strategies. *Clin. Infect. Dis.* 2005 ;4 1 Suppl 6:S389-93.

[319] San Miguel LG, Cobo J, Otheo E, Sanchez-Sousa A, Abraira V, Moreno S. Secular trends of candidemia in a large tertiary-care hospital from 1988 to 2000: emergence of Candida parapsilosis. *Infect. Control Hosp. Epidemiol.* 2005;26(6):548-52.

[320] NNIS. National Nosocomial Infections Surveillance (NNIS) System Report, data summary from January 1992 through June 2004, issued October 2004. *Am. J. Infect. Control.* 2004;32(8):470-85.

[321] Richards MJ, Edwards JR, Culver DH, Gaynes RP. Nosocomial infections in medical intensive care units in the United States. National Nosocomial Infections Surveillance System. *Crit. Care Med.* 1999;27(5):887-92.

[322] Richards MJ, Edwards JR, Culver DH, Gaynes RP. Nosocomial infections in combined medical-surgical intensive care units in the United States. *Infect. Control Hosp. Epidemiol.* 2000;21(8):510-5.

[323] Hugonnet S, Eggimann P, Borst F, Maricot P, Chevrolet JC, Pittet D. Impact of ventilator-associated pneumonia on resource utilization and patient outcome. *Infect. Control Hosp. Epidemiol.* 2004;25(12): 1090-6.

[324] O'Neill JM, Schutze GE, Heulitt MJ, Simpson PM, Taylor BJ. Nosocomial infections during extracorporeal membrane oxygenation. *Intensive Care Med.* 2001 ;27(8): 1247-53.

[325] Villegas MV, Hartstein AI. Acinetobacter Outbreaks, 1977–2000. *Infect. Control Hosp. Epidemiol.* 2003;24(4):284-95.

[326] Gordon SM, Schmitt SK, Jacobs M, et al. Nosocomial bloodstream infections in patients with implantable left ventricular assist devices. *Ann. Thorac. Surg.* 2001;72(3):725-30.

[327] Giamarellou H. Nosocomial cardiac infections. *J. Hosp. Infect.* 2002;50(2):91 - 105.

[328] Fridkin SK. Increasing prevalence of antimicrobial resistance in intensive care units. *Crit. Care Med.* 2001 ;29(4 Suppl):N64-8.

[329] Kollef MH, Fraser VJ. Antibiotic resistance in the intensive care unit. *Ann. Intern. Med.* 2001;134(4):298-314.

[330] Fridkin SK, Edwards JR, Courval JM, et al. The effect of vancomycin and third-generation cephalosporins on prevalence of vancomycin-resistant enterococci in 126 U.S. adult intensive care units. *Ann. Intern. Med.* 2001;135(3):175-83.

[331] Crnich CJ, Safdar N, Maki DG. The role of the intensive care unit environment in the pathogenesis and prevention of ventilator-associated pneumonia. *Respir. Care.* 2005 ;50(6):813-36; discussion 36-8.

[332] Knaus WA, Wagner DP, Zimmerman JE, Draper EA. Variations in mortality and length of stay in intensive care units. *Ann. Intern. Med.* 1993;1 18(10):753-61.

[333] Villarino ME, Stevens LE, Schable B, et al. Risk factors for epidemic Xanthomonas maltophilia infection/colonization in intensive care unit patients. *Infect. Control Hosp. Epidemiol.* 1992;13(4):201-6.

[334] Sanchez V, Vazquez JA, Barth-Jones D, Dembry L, Sobel JD, Zervos MJ. Nosocomial acquisition of Candida parapsilosis: an epidemiologic study. *Am. J. Med.* 1993;94(6):577-82.

[335] Husni RN, Goldstein LS, Arroliga AC, et al. Risk factors for an outbreak of multi-drug-resistant Acinetobacter nosocomial pneumonia among intubated patients. *Chest.* 1999;1 15(5):1378-82.

[336] McDonald LC, Walker M, Carson L, et al. Outbreak of Acinetobacter spp. bloodstream infections in a nursery associated with contaminated aerosols and air conditioners. *Pediatr. Infect. Dis. J.* 1998;17(8):716-22.

[337] Trick WE, Kioski CM, Howard KM, et al. Outbreak of Pseudomonas aeruginosa ventriculitis among patients in a neurosurgical intensive care unit. *Infect. Control Hosp. Epidemiol.* 2000;21(3):204-8.

[338] Guidry GG, Black-Payne CA, Payne DK, Jamison RM, George RB, Bocchini JA, Jr. Respiratory syncytial virus infection among intubated adults in a university medical intensive care unit. *Chest.* 1991;100(5):137784.

[339] Wurtz R, Karajovic M, Dacumos E, Jovanovic B, Hanumadass M. Nosocomial infections in a burn intensive care unit. *Burns.* 1995;21(3):181-4.

[340] Rodgers GL, Mortensen J, Fisher MC, Lo A, Cresswell A, Long SS. Predictors of infectious complications after burn injuries in children. *Pediatr. Infect. Dis. J.* 2000;19(10):990-5.

[341] Pruitt BA, Jr., McManus AT, Kim SH, Goodwin CW. Burn wound infections: current status. *World J. Surg.* 1998;22(2):135-45.

[342] Weber J, ed. Epidemiology of Infections and Strategies for Control in Burn Care and Therapy. St. Louis: Mosby, Inc.; 1998.

[343] Heggers JP, McCoy L, Reisner B, Smith M, Edgar P, Ramirez RJ. Alternate antimicrobial therapy for vancomycin-resistant enterococci burn wound infections. *J. Burn. Care Rehabil.* 1998;19(5):399-403.

[344] Sheridan RL, Weber J, Benjamin J, Pasternack MS, Tompkins RG. Control of methicillin-resistant Staphylococcus aureus in a pediatric burn unit. *Am. J. Infect. Control.* 1994;22(6):340-5.

[345] Matsumura H, Yoshizawa N, Narumi A, Harunari N, Sugamata A, Watanabe K. Effective control of methicillin-resistant Staphylococcus aureus in a burn unit. *Burns.* 1996;22(4):283-6.

[346] McGregor JC. Profile of the first four years of the Regional Burn Unit based at St. John's Hospital, West Lothian (1992-1996). *J. R. Coll. Surg. Edinb.* 1998;43(1):45-8.

[347] Desai MH, Rutan RL, Heggers JP, Herndon DN. Candida infection with and without nystatin prophylaxis. A 11-year experience with patients with burn injury. *Arch. Surg.* 1992;127(2):159-62.

[348] Ekenna O, Sherertz RJ, Bingham H. Natural history of bloodstream infections in a burn patient population: the importance of candidemia. *Am. J. Infect. Control.* 1993 ;2 1(4): 189-95.

[349] Bowser-Wallace BH, Graves DB, Caldwell FT. An epidemiological profile and trend analysis of wound flora in burned children: 7 years' experience. *Burns. Incl. Therm. Inj.* 1984;11(1):16-25.

[350] Tredget EE, Shankowsky HA, Rennie R, Burrell RE, Logsetty S. Pseudomonas infections in the thermally injured patient. *Burns.* 2004;30(1):3-26.

[351] Edgar P, Mlcak R, Desai M, Linares HA, Phillips LG, Heggers JP. Containment of a multiresistant Serratia marcescens outbreak. *Burns.* 1997;23(1):15-8.

[352] Embil JM, McLeod JA, Al-Barrak AM, et al. An outbreak of methicillin resistant *Staphylococcus aureus* on a burn unit: potential role of contaminated hydrotherapy equipment. *Burns.* 2001 ;27(7) :681-8.

[353] Meier PA, Carter CD, Wallace SE, Hollis RJ, Pfaller MA, Herwaldt LA. A prolonged outbreak of methicillin-resistant Staphylococcus aureus in the burn unit of a tertiary medical center. *Infect. Control Hosp. Epidemiol.* 1996; 17(12):798-802.

[354] Snyder LL, Wiebelhaus P, Boon SE, Morin RA, Goering R. Methicillin-resistant Staphylococcus aureus eradication in a burn center. *J. Burn Care Rehabil.* 1993;14(2 Pt 1):164-8.

[355] May AK, Melton SM, McGwin G, Cross JM, Moser SA, Rue LW. Reduction of vancomycin-resistant enterococcal infections by limitation of

broad-spectrum cephalosporin use in a trauma and burn intensive care unit. *Shock.* 2000;14(3):259-64.

[356] Sheridan RL, Weber JM, Budkevich LG, Tompkins RG. Candidemia in the pediatric patient with burns. *J. Burn Care Rehabil.* 1995;16(4):440-3.

[357] Mayhall CG. The epidemiology of burn wound infections: then and now. *Clin. Infect. Dis.* 2003 ;37(4) :543-50.

[358] McManus AT, Mason AD, Jr., McManus WF, Pruitt BA, Jr. A decade of reduced gram-negative infections and mortality associated with improved isolation of burned patients. *Arch. Surg.* 1994; 129(12): 1306-9.

[359] Bryce EA, Walker M, Scharf S, et al. An outbreak of cutaneous aspergillosis in a tertiary-care hospital. *Infect. Control Hosp. Epidemiol.* 1996; 17(3): 170-2.

[360] Levenson C, Wohlford P, Djou J, Evans S, Zawacki B. Preventing postoperative burn wound aspergillosis. *J. Burn Care Rehabil.* 1991; 12(2): 132-5.

[361] Tredget EE, Shankowsky HA, Joffe AM, et al. Epidemiology of infections with Pseudomonas aeruginosa in burn patients: the role of hydrotherapy. *Clin. Infect. Dis.* 1992;15(6):941-9.

[362] Wisplinghoff H, Perbix W, Seifert H. Risk factors for nosocomial bloodstream infections due to Acinetobacter baumannii: a case-control study of adult burn patients. *Clin. Infect. Dis.* 1999;28(1):59-66.

[363] Weber JM, Sheridan RL, Schulz JT, Tompkins RG, Ryan CM. Effectiveness of bacteria-controlled nursing units in preventing cross-colonization with resistant bacteria in severely burned children. *Infect. Control. Hosp. Epidemiol.* 2002;23 (9): 549-51.

[364] Bayat A, Shaaban H, Dodgson A, Dunn KW. Implications for Burns Unit design following outbreak of multi-resistant Acinetobacter infection in ICU and Burns Unit. *Burns.* 2003;29(4):303-6.

[365] Lee JJ, Marvin JA, Heimbach DM, Grube BJ, Engrav LH. Infection control in a burn center. *J. Burn. Care Rehabil.* 1990;11(6):575-80.

[366] Raymond J, Aujard Y. Nosocomial infections in pediatric patients: a European, multicenter prospective study. European Study Group. *Infect. Control Hosp. Epidemiol.* 2000;2 1 (4):260-3.

[367] Campins M, Vaque J, Rossello J, et al. Nosocomial infections in pediatric patients: a prevalence study in Spanish hospitals. EPINE Working Group. *Am. J. Infect. Control.* 1993;21(2):58-63.

[368] Allen U, Ford-Jones EL. Nosocomial infections in the pediatric patient: an update. *Am. J. Infect Control.* 1990;18(3):176-93.

[369] Grohskopf LA, Sinkowitz-Cochran RL, Garrett DO, et al. A national point-prevalence survey of pediatric intensive care unit-acquired infections in the United States. *J. Pediatr.* 2002;140(4):432-8.

[370] Sohn AH, Garrett DO, Sinkowitz-Cochran RL, et al. Prevalence of nosocomial infections in neonatal intensive care unit patients: Results from the first national point-prevalence survey. *J. Pediatr.* 2001;139(6):8217.

[371] Gaynes RP, Edwards JR, Jarvis WR, Culver DH, Tolson JS, Martone WJ. Nosocomial infections among neonates in high-risk nurseries in the United States. National Nosocomial Infections Surveillance System. *Pediatrics.* 1996;98(3 Pt 1):357-61.

[372] Richards MJ, Edwards JR, Culver DH, Gaynes RP. Nosocomial infections in pediatric intensive care units in the United States. National Nosocomial Infections Surveillance System. *Pediatrics.* 1999; 103 (4):e39.

[373] Maltezou HC, Drancourt M. Nosocomial influenza in children. *J. Hosp. Infect.* 2003;55(2):83-91.

[374] Moisiuk SE, Robson D, Klass L, et al. Outbreak of parainfluenza virus type 3 in an intermediate care neonatal nursery. *Pediatr. Infect. Dis. J.* 1998; 17(1):49-53.(mj).

[375] Mullins JA, Erdman DD, Weinberg GA, et al. Human metapneumovirus infection among children hospitalized with acute respiratory illness. *Emerg. Infect. Dis.* 2004;10(4):700-5.

[376] Hatherill M, Levin M, Lawrenson J, Hsiao NY, Reynolds L, Argent A. Evolution of an adenovirus outbreak in a multidisciplinary children's hospital. *J. Paediatr. Child Health.* 2004;40(8):449-54.

[377] Langley JM, Hanakowski M. Variation in risk for nosocomial chickenpox after inadvertent exposure. *J. Hosp. Infect.* 2000;44(3):224-6.

[378] Ratner AJ, Neu N, Jakob K, et al. Nosocomial rotavirus in a pediatric hospital. *Infect. Control Hosp. Epidemiol.* 2001 ;22(5):299-301.

[379] Avila-Aguero ML, German G, Paris MM, Herrera JF. Toys in a pediatric hospital: are they a bacterial source? *Am. J. Infect. Control.* 2004;32(5):28790.

[380] Nyqvist KH, Lutes LM. Co-bedding twins: a developmentally supportive care strategy. *J. Obstet. Gynecol. Neonatal Nurs.* 1998;27(4):450-6.

[381] Feldman R, Eidelman AI, Sirota L, Weller A. Comparison of skin-to-skin (kangaroo) and traditional care: parenting outcomes and preterm infant development. *Pediatrics.* 2002;1 10(1 Pt 1):16-26.

[382] Conde-Agudelo A, Diaz-Rossello JL, Belizan JM. Kangaroo mother care to reduce morbidity and mortality in low birthweight infants. *Cochrane Database Syst. Rev.* 2003(2):CD002771.

[383] Adcock PM, Pastor P, Medley F, Patterson JE, Murphy TV. Methicillinresistant Staphylococcus aureus in two child care centers. *J. Infect. Dis.* 1998; 178(2):577-80.

[384] Shahin R, Johnson IL, Jamieson F, McGeer A, Tolkin J, Ford-Jones EL. Methicillin-resistant Staphylococcus aureus carriage in a child care center following a case of disease. Toronto Child Care Center Study Group. *Arch. Pediatr. Adolesc. Med.* 1999; 153(8): 864-8.

[385] Stover BH, Duff A, Adams G, Buck G, Hancock G, Rabalais G. Emergence and control of methicillin-resistant Staphylococcus aureus in a children's hospital and pediatric long-term care facility. *Am. J. Infect. Control.* 1992;20(5):248-55.

[386] Herold BC, Immergluck LC, Maranan MC, et al. Community-acquired methicillin-resistant Staphylococcus aureus in children with no identified predisposing risk. *JAMA.* 1998;279(8):593-8.

[387] CDC. Four pediatric deaths from community-acquired methicillinresistant Staphylococcus aureus--Minnesota and North Dakota, 19971999. *MMWR - Morbidity & Mortality Weekly Report.* 1999;48:707-10.

[388] Abi-Hanna P, Frank AL, Quinn JP, et al. Clonal features of community-acquired methicillin-resistant Staphylococcus aureus in children. *Clin. Infect. Dis.* 2000;30(3):630-1.

[389] Fergie JE, Purcell K. Community-acquired methicillin-resistant Staphylococcus aureus infections in south Texas children. *Pediatr. Infect. Dis. J.* 2001;20(9):860-3.

[390] Sattler CA, Mason EO, Jr., Kaplan SL. Prospective comparison of risk factors and demographic and clinical characteristics of community- acquired, methicillin-resistant versus methicillin-susceptible Staphylococcus aureus infection in children. *Pediatr. Infect. Dis. J.* 2002;21(10):910-7.

[391] Kaplan SL, Hulten KG, Gonzalez BE, et al. Three-year surveillance of community-acquired Staphylococcus aureus infections in children. *Clin. Infect. Dis.* 2005;40(12):1785-91.

[392] Jarvis WR. Infection control and changing health-care delivery systems. *Emerg. Infect. Dis.* 2001;7(2): 170-3.

[393] Garibaldi RA. Residential care and the elderly: the burden of infection. *J. Hosp. Infect.* 1999;43 Suppl:S9-18.

[394] 394. Hsu K, Harris JA. Control of infections in nonacute care pediatric settings. *Seminars Pedi. Infect. Dis.* 2001;12(2):92-9.

[395] Strausbaugh LJ, Joseph CL. The burden of infection in long-term care. *Infect. Control Hosp. Epidemiol.* 2000;21(10):674-9.

[396] Centers for Medicare and Medicaid Services. Healthcare Industry Market Update. http://wwwcmshhsgov/reports/hcimu/hcimu_05202003pdf May 2003.
[397] Lee YL, Thrupp LD, Friis RH, Fine M, Maleki P, Cesario TC. Nosocomial infection and antibiotic utilization in geriatric patients: a pilot prospective surveillance program in skilled nursing facilities. *Gerontology.* 1 992;38(4):223-32.
[398] Stevenson KB. Regional data set of infection rates for long-term care facilities: description of a valuable benchmarking tool. *Am. J. Infect. Control.* 1999;27(1):20-6.
[399] Jackson MM, Fierer J, Barrett-Connor E, et al. Intensive surveillance for infections in a three-year study of nursing home patients. *Am. J. Epidemiol.* 1992; 1 35(6):685-96.
[400] Darnowski SB, Gordon M, Simor AE. Two years of infection surveillance in a geriatric long-term care facility. *Am. J. Infect. Control.* 1991; 19(4): 18590.
[401] Hoffman N, Jenkins R, Putney K. Nosocomial infection rates during a one-year period in a nursing home care unit of a Veterans Administration hospital. *Am. J. Infect. Control.* 1990;18(2):55-63.
[402] Tsan L, Hojlo C, Kearns MA, et al. Infection surveillance and control programs in the Department of Veterans Affairs nursing home care units: a preliminary assessment. *Am. J. Infect. Control.* 2006;34(2):80-3.
[403] Kane RA, Caplan AL, Urv-Wong EK, Freeman IC, Aroskar MA, Finch M. Everyday matters in the lives of nursing home residents: wish for and perception of choice and control. *J. Am. Geriatr. Soc.* 1997;45:1086-93.
[404] Libow LS, Starer P. Care of the nursing home patient. *N. Engl. J. Med.* 1989;321 (2):93-6.
[405] Perls TT, Herget M. Higher respiratory infection rates on an Alzheimer's special care unit and successful intervention. *J. Am. Geriatr. Soc.* 1995;43(12):1341-4.
[406] Bradley SF. Issues in the management of resistant bacteria in long-term- care facilities. Infect. *Control Hosp. Epidemiol.* 1999;20(5):362-6.
[407] Crossley K. Vancomycin-resistant enterococci in long-term-care facilities. *Infect. Control. Hosp. Epidemiol.* 1998; 19(7): 521-5.
[408] Strausbaugh LJ, Crossley KB, Nurse BA, Thrupp LD. Antimicrobial resistance in long-term-care facilities. *Infect. Control Hosp. Epidemiol.* 1996; 17(2): 129-40.
[409] Richards CL. Infections in Long-Term-Care Facilities: Screen or Clean? *Infect. Control Hosp. Epidemiol.* 2005;26(10):800-01.

[410] Drinka PJ, Krause P, Nest L, Goodman BM, Gravenstein S. Risk of acquiring influenza A in a nursing home from a culture-positive roommate. *Infect. Control Hosp. Epidemiol.* 2003 ;24(1 1):872-4.
[411] Falsey AR, Treanor JJ, Betts RF, Walsh EE. Viral respiratory infections in the institutionalized elderly: clinical and epidemiologic findings. *J. Am. Geriatr. Soc.* 1992;40(2):115-9.
[412] Ellis SE, Coffey CS, Mitchel EF, Jr., Dittus RS, Griffin MR. Influenza- and respiratory syncytial virus-associated morbidity and mortality in the nursing home population. *J. Am. Geriatr. Soc.* 2003;51(6):761-7.
[413] Louie JK, Yagi S, Nelson FA, et al. Rhinovirus outbreak in a long term care facility for elderly persons associated with unusually high mortality. *Clin. Infect. Dis.* 2005;41(2):262-5.
[414] Piednoir E, Bureau-Chalot F, Merle C, Gotzamanis A, Wuibout J, Bajolet O. Direct costs associated with a nosocomial outbreak of adenoviral conjunctivitis infection in a long-term care institution. *Am. J. Infect. Control.* 2002;30(7):407- 10.
[415] Addiss DG, Davis JP, Meade BD, et al. A pertussis outbreak in a Wisconsin nursing home. *J. Infect. Dis.* 1991;164(4):704-10.
[416] Gaynes R, Rimland D, Killum E, et al. Outbreak of Clostridium difficile infection in a long-term care facility: association with gatifloxacin use. *Clin. Infect. Dis.* 2004;38(5):640-5.
[417] High KP, Bradley S, Loeb M, Palmer R, Quagliarello V, Yoshikawa T. A new paradigm for clinical investigation of infectious syndromes in older adults: assessment of functional status as a risk factor and outcome measure. *Clin. Infect. Dis.* 2005;40(1):1 14-22.
[418] Loeb MB, Craven S, McGeer AJ, et al. Risk factors for resistance to antimicrobial agents among nursing home residents. *Am. J. Epidemiol.* 2003; 1 57(1):40-7.
[419] Vergis EN, Brennen C, Wagener M, Muder RR. Pneumonia in long-term care: a prospective case-control study of risk factors and impact on survival. *Arch. Intern. Med.* 2001;161(19):2378-81.
[420] Loeb M, McGeer A, McArthur M, Walter S, Simor AE. Risk factors for pneumonia and other lower respiratory tract infections in elderly residents of long-term care facilities. *Arch. Intern. Med.* 1999; 159(1 7):205 8-64.
[421] Brandeis GH, Ooi WL, Hossain M, Morris JN, Lipsitz LA. A longitudinal study of risk factors associated with the formation of pressure ulcers in nursing homes. *J. Am. Geriatr. Soc.* 1994;42(4):388-93.

[422] Allard JP, Aghdassi E, McArthur M, et al. Nutrition risk factors for survival in the elderly living in Canadian long-term care facilities. *J. Am. Geriatr. Soc.* 2004;52(1):59-65.
[423] Pick N, McDonald A, Bennett N, et al. Pulmonary aspiration in a longterm care setting: clinical and laboratory observations and an analysis of risk factors. *J. Am. Geriatr. Soc.* 1996;44(7):763-8.
[424] Nicolle LE. The chronic indwelling catheter and urinary infection in longterm-care facility residents. *Infect. Control Hosp. Epidemiol.* 2001;22(5):316-21.
[425] Pien EC, Hume KE, Pien FD. Gastrostomy tube infections in a community hospital. *Am. J. Infect. Control.* 1996;24(5):353-8.
[426] Gomes GF, Pisani JC, Macedo ED, Campos AC. The nasogastric feeding tube as a risk factor for aspiration and aspiration pneumonia. *Curr. Opin. Clin. Nutr. Metab. Care.* 2003;6(3):327-33.
[427] Bula CJ, Ghilardi G, Wietlisbach V, Petignat C, Francioli P. Infections and functional impairment in nursing home residents: a reciprocal relationship. *J. Am. Geriatr. Soc.* 2004;52(5):700-6.
[428] Bradley SF, Terpenning MS, Ramsey MA, et al. Methicillin-resistant Staphylococcus aureus: colonization and infection in a long-term care facility. *Ann. Intern. Med.* 1991;115(6):417-22.
[429] Washio M, Nishisaka S, Kishikawa K, et al. Incidence of methicillin-resistant Staphylococcus aureus (MRSA) isolation in a skilled nursing home: a third report on the risk factors for the occurrence of MRSA infection in the elderly. *J. Epidemiol.* 1996;6(2):69-73.
[430] Trick WE, Weinstein RA, DeMarais PL, et al. Colonization of skilled-care facility residents with antimicrobial-resistant pathogens. *J. Am. Geriatr. Soc.* 2001;49(3):270-6.
[431] Nicolle LE, Garibaldi RA. Infection control in long-term-care facilities. *Infect. Control Hosp. Epidemiol.* 1995; 16(6): 348-53 .(s).
[432] Crossley K. Long-term care facilities as sources of antibiotic-resistant nosocomial pathogens. *Curr. Opin. Infect. Dis.* 2001;14(4):455-9.
[433] Smith PW, Rusnak PG. Infection prevention and control in the long-term-care facility. SHEA Long-Term-Care Committee and APIC Guidelines Committee. *Infect. Control Hosp. Epidemiol.* 1997; 18(12): 831-49. (s).
[434] Friedman C, Barnette M, Buck AS, et al. Requirements for infrastructure and essential activities of infection control and epidemiology in out-ofhospital settings: a consensus panel report. Association for Professionals in Infection Control and Epidemiology and Society for Healthcare Epidemiology of America. *Infect. Control Hosp. Epidemiol.* 1999;20(10):695-705.

[435] Nicolle LE. Infection control in long-term care facilities. *Clin. Infect. Dis.* 2000;3 1 (3):752-6.
[436] Bradley SF. Methicillin-resistant Staphylococcus aureus: long-term care concerns. *Am. J. Med.* 1999;106(5A):2S-10S; discussion 48S-52S.
[437] www.cms.hhs.gov/manuals/Downloads/som107ap_pp_guidelines_ltcf
[438] Mylotte JM, Goodnough S, Tayara A. Antibiotic-resistant organisms among long-term care facility residents on admission to an inpatient geriatrics unit: Retrospective and prospective surveillance. *Am. J. Infect. Control.* 2001 ;29(3): 139-44.
[439] Strausbaugh LJ, Jacobson C, Yost T. Methicillin-resistant Staphylococcus aureus in a nursing home and affiliated hospital: a four-year perspective. *Infect. Control. Hosp. Epidemiol.* 1993; 14(6): 331-6.
[440] Wiener J, Quinn JP, Bradford PA, et al. Multiple antibiotic-resistant Klebsiella and Escherichia coli in nursing homes. *Jama.* 1999;281(6):51723.
[441] Pop-Vicas AE, D'Agata EM. The rising influx of multidrug-resistant gram-negative bacilli into a tertiary care hospital. *Clin. Infect. Dis.* 2005;40(12): 1792-8.
[442] Ly N, McCaig LF. National Hospital Ambulatory Medical Care Survey: 2000 outpatient department summary. *Adv. Data.* 2002(3 27): 1-27.
[443] Cherry DK, Woodwell DA. National Ambulatory Medical Care Survey: 2000 summary. *Adv. Data.* 2002(328):1-32.
[444] Finelli L, Miller JT, Tokars JI, Alter MJ, Arduino MJ. National surveillance of dialysis-associated diseases in the United States, 2002. *Semin. Dial.* 2005;18(1):52-61.
[445] D'Agata EM. Antimicrobial-resistant, Gram-positive bacteria among patients undergoing chronic hemodialysis. *Clin. Infect. Dis.* 2002;35(10): 12 12-8.
[446] Goodman RA, Solomon SL. Transmission of infectious diseases in outpatient health care settings. *JAMA.* 1991;265(18):2377-81.
[447] Nafziger DA, Lundstrom T, Chandra S, Massanari RM. Infection control in ambulatory care. *Infect. Dis. Clin. North Am.* 1997;1 1(2):279-96.
[448] Herwaldt LA, Smith SD, Carter CD. Infection control in the outpatient setting. *Infect. Control Hosp. Epidemiol.* 1998;19(1):41-74.
[449] Hlady WG, Hopkins RS, Ogilby TE, Allen ST. Patient-to-patient transmission of hepatitis B in a dermatology practice. *Am. J. Public Health.* 1993;83(12): 1689-93.
[450] Birnie GG, Quigley EM, Clements GB, Follet EA, Watkinson G. Endoscopic transmission of hepatitis B virus. *Gut.* 1983;24(2):171-4.

[451] Chant K, Lowe D, Rubin G, et al. Patient-to-patient transmission of HIV in private surgical consulting rooms. *Lancet.* 1993;342(8886-8887):1548-9.

[452] Chant K, Kociuba K, Munro R, et al. Investigation of Possible Patient-toPatient Transmission of Hepatitis C in a Hospital. *NSW Public Health Bull.* 1994;5(5):47-51.

[453] CDC. Transmission of hepatitis B and C viruses in outpatient settings-- New York, Oklahoma, and Nebraska, 2000-2002. *MMWR. Morb. Mortal Wkly. Rep.* 2003 ;52(3 8):901-6.

[454] Williams IT, Perz JF, Bell BP. Viral hepatitis transmission in ambulatory health care settings. *Clin. Infect. Dis.* 2004;38(11):1592-8.

[455] Couldwell DL, Dore GJ, Harkness JL, et al. Nosocomial outbreak of tuberculosis in an outpatient HIV treatment room. *Aids.* 1996;10(5):521-5.

[456] CDC. Mycobacterium tuberculosis Transmission in a Health Clinic -- Florida. *MMWR.* 1989;38(15):256-8; 63-64.

[457] Calder RA, Duclos P, Wilder MH, Pryor VL, Scheel WJ. Mycobacterium tuberculosis transmission in a health clinic. *Bull. Int. Union Tuberc. Lung Dis.* 1991;66(2-3):103-6.

[458] Istre GR, McKee PA, West GR, et al. Measles spread in medical settings: an important focus of disease transmission? *Pediatrics.* 1987;79(3):356-8.

[459] Dawson C, Darrell R. Infections due to adenovirus type 8 in the United States. I. An outbreak of epidemic keratoconjunctivitis originating in a physician's office. *N. Engl. J. Med.* 1963;268:1031-4.

[460] Montessori V, Scharf S, Holland S, Werker DH, Roberts FJ, Bryce E. Epidemic keratoconjunctivitis outbreak at a tertiary referral eye care clinic. *Am. J. Infect. Control.* 1998;26(4):399-405.

[461] Jernigan JA, Lowry BS, Hayden FG, et al. Adenovirus type 8 epidemic keratoconjunctivitis in an eye clinic: risk factors and control. *J. Infect. Dis.* 1993;167(6):1307-13.

[462] Buehler JW, Finton RJ, Goodman RA, et al. Epidemic keratoconjunctivitis: report of an outbreak in an ophthalmology practice and recommendations for prevention. *Infect. Control.* 1984;5(8):390-4.

[463] Johnston CP, Cooper L, Ruby W, Teeter T, al. E. Community-associated methicillin resistant *Staphyloccoccus aureus* skin infections among outpatient healthcare workers and its isolation in the clinic environment. Presented at the 15th Annual Scientific Meeting of the Society for Healthcare Epidemiology of America (SHEA), Los Angeles, California, 4/10/05. Abstract #132 2005.

[464] Biddick R, Spilker T, Martin A, LiPuma JJ. Evidence of transmission of Burkholderia cepacia, Burkholderia multivorans and Burkholderia dolosa among persons with cystic fibrosis. *FEMS Microbiol. Lett.* 2003 ;228(1):5762.

[465] Griffiths AL, Jamsen K, Carlin JB, et al. Effects of segregation on an epidemic Pseudomonas aeruginosa strain in a cystic fibrosis clinic. *Am. J. Respir. Crit. Care Med.* 2005;171(9):1020-5.

[466] Danzig LE, Short LJ, Collins K, et al. Bloodstream infections associated with a needleless intravenous infusion system in patients receiving home infusion therapy. *JAMA.* 1995;273(23):1862-4.

[467] Kellerman S, Shay DK, Howard J, et al. Bloodstream infections in home infusion patients: the influence of race and needleless intravascular access devices. *J. Pediatr*.1996;129(5):71 1-7.

[468] Do AN, Ray BJ, Banerjee SN, et al. Bloodstream infection associated with needleless device use and the importance of infection-control practices in the home health care setting. *J. Infect. Dis.* 1999;179(2):442-8.

[469] Tokars JI, Cookson ST, McArthur MA, Boyer CL, McGeer AJ, Jarvis WR. Prospective evaluation of risk factors for bloodstream infection in patients receiving home infusion therapy. *Ann. Intern. Med.* 1999; 131 (5):340-7.

[470] Manangan LP, Pearson ML, Tokars JI, Miller E, Jarvis WR. Feasibility of national surveillance of health-care-associated infections in home-care settings. *Emerg. Infect. Dis.* 2002;8(3):233-6.

[471] Shah SS, Manning ML, Leahy E, Magnusson M, Rheingold SR, Bell LM. Central venous catheter-associated bloodstream infections in pediatric oncology home care. *Infect. Control Hosp. Epidemiol.* 2002;23(2):99-101.

[472] Gorski LA. Central venous access device outcomes in a homecare agency: a 7-year study. *J. Infus. Nurs.* 2004;27(2):104-1 1.

[473] Rosenheimer L, Embry FC, Sanford J, Silver SR. Infection surveillance in home care: device-related incidence rates. *Am. J. Infect. Control.* 1998;26(3):359-63.

[474] White MC, Ragland KE. Surveillance of intravenous catheter-related infections among home care clients. *Am. J. Infect. Control.* 1 994;22(4):23 15.

[475] Beltrami EM, McArthur MA, McGeer A, et al. The nature and frequency of blood contacts among home healthcare workers. *Infect. Control Hosp. Epidemiol.* 2000;21(12):765-70.

[476] Embry FC, Chinnes LF. Draft definitions for surveillance of infections in home health care. *Am. J. Infect. Control.* 2000;28(6):449-53.

[477] Fraser TG, Stosor V, Wang Q, Allen A, Zembower TR. Vancomycin and home health care. *Emerg. Infect. Dis.* 2005;1 1(10):1558-64.

[478] Carrico RM, Niner S. Multidrug resistant organisms--VRE and MRSA: practical home care tips. *Home Healthc. Nurse.* 2002;20(1):23-8; quiz 8-9.
[479] Friedman MM, Rhinehart E. Improving infection control in home care: from ritual to science-based practice. *Home Healthc. Nurse.* 2000; 1 8(2):99105; quiz 6.
[480] Friedman MM, Rhinehart E. Putting infection control principles into practice in home care. *Nurs Clin. North Am.* 1999;34(2):463-82.
[481] Davis PL, Madigan EA. Evidence-based practice and the home care nurse's bag. *Home Healthc Nurse.* 1999;17(5):295-9.
[482] Sitzman KL, Pett MA, Bloswick DS. An exploratory study of nurse bag use by home visiting nurses. *Home Healthc Nurse.* 2002;20(4):237-43.
[483] Anderson MA, Madigan EA, Helms LB. Nursing research in home health care: endangered species? *Home Care Provid.* 2001 ;6(6):200-4.
[484] White MC. Identifying infectious diseases in prisons: surveillance, protection, and intervention. *West J. Med.* 1999;170(3):177.
[485] Puisis M. Update on public health in correctional facilities. *West J. Med.* 1998; 1 69(6):374.
[486] Levy MH, Lerwitworapong J. Issues facing TB control (3.1). Tuberculosis in prisons. *Scott. Med. J.* 2000;45(5 Suppl):30-2; discussion 3.
[487] Parece MS, Herrera GA, Voigt RF, Middlekauff SL, Irwin KL. STD testing policies and practices in U.S. city and county jails. *Sex Transm. Dis.* 1 999;26(8):43 1-7.
[488] Cieslak PR, Curtis MB, Coulombier DM, Hathcock AL, Bean NH, Tauxe RV. Preventable disease in correctional facilities. Desmoteric foodborne outbreaks in the United States, 1974-1991. *Arch. Intern. Med.* 1996;156(16): 1883-8.
[489] CDC. Public health dispatch: tuberculosis outbreak in a homeless population--Portland, Maine, 2002-2003. *MMWR Morb. Mortal Wkly. Rep.* 2003;52(48): 1184.
[490] CDC. Public health dispatch: tuberculosis outbreak among homeless persons--King County, Washington, 2002-2003. *MMWR Morb. Mortal Wkly Rep.* 2003;52(49):1209-10.
[491] CDC. Tuberculosis transmission in a homeless shelter population--New York, 2000-2003. *MMWR Morb. Mortal Wkly. Rep.* 2005;54(6):149-52.
[492] Baillargeon J, Kelley MF, Leach CT, Baillargeon G, Pollock BH. Methicillin-resistant Staphylococcus aureus infection in the Texas prison system. *Clin. Infect. Dis.* 2004;38(9):e92-5.
[493] Young DM, Harris HW, Charlebois ED, et al. An epidemic of methicillinresistant Staphylococcus aureus soft tissue infections among

medically underserved patients. *Arch. Surg.* 2004;139(9):947-51; discussion 51-3.

[494] Pan ES, Diep BA, Carleton HA, et al. Increasing prevalence of methicillin-resistant Staphylococcus aureus infection in California jails. *Clin. Infect. Dis.* 2003;37(10):1384-8.

[495] CDC. Drug-susceptible tuberculosis outbreak in a state correctional facility housing HIV-infected inmates--South Carolina, 1999-2000. *MMWR Morb. Mortal Wkly. Rep.* 2000;49(46):1041-4.

[496] CDC. Methicillin-resistant Staphylococcus aureus skin or soft tissue infections in a state prison--Mississippi, 2000. *MMWR Morb. Mortal Wkly. Rep.* 2001;50(42):919-22.

[497] Mohle-Boetani JC, Miguelino V, Dewsnup DH, et al. Tuberculosis outbreak in a housing unit for human immunodeficiency virus-infected patients in a correctional facility: transmission risk factors and effective outbreak control. *Clin. Infect. Dis.* 2002;34(5):668-76.

[498] CDC. Prevention and Control of Tuberculosis in Correctional Facilities. Recommendations of the Advisory Council for the Elimination of Tuberculosis. *MMWR Recomm. Rep.* 1 996;45(RR-8):1-37.

[499] Whimbey E, Englund JA, Couch RB. Community respiratory virus infections in immunocompromised patients with cancer. *Am. J. Med.* 1997; 1 02(3A): 10-8; *discussion.* 25-6.

[500] Zambon M, Bull T, Sadler CJ, Goldman JM, Ward KN. Molecular epidemiology of two consecutive outbreaks of parainfluenza 3 in a bone marrow transplant unit. *J. Clin. Microbiol.* 1998;36(8):2289-93.

[501] Gamis AS, Howells WB, DeSwarte-Wallace J, Feusner JH, Buckley JD, Woods WG. Alpha hemolytic streptococcal infection during intensive treatment for acute myeloid leukemia: a report from the Children's cancer group study CCG-2891. *J. Clin. Oncol.* 2000;18(9):1845-55.

[502] Ek T, Mellander L, Andersson B, Abrahamsson J. Immune reconstitution after childhood acute lymphoblastic leukemia is most severely affected in the high risk group. *Pediatr. Blood Cancer.* 2005;44(5):461-8.

[503] Pascual V, Allantaz F, Arce E, Punaro M, Banchereau J. Role of interleukin- 1 (IL-1) in the pathogenesis of systemic onset juvenile idiopathic arthritis and clinical response to IL-1 blockade. *J. Exp. Med.* 2005;201 (9): 1479-86.

[504] Marchesoni A, Puttini PS, Gorla R, et al. Cyclosporine in addition to infliximab and methotrexate in refractory rheumatoid arthritis. *Clin. Exp. Rheumatol.* 2005;23(6):91 6-7.

[505] Isaacs KL, Lewis JD, Sandborn WJ, Sands BE, Targan SR. State of the art: IBD therapy and clinical trials in IBD. *Inflamm. Bowel Dis.* 2005;1 1 Suppl 1:S3-12.
[506] CDC. Guidelines for preventing opportunitic infections among HIV-infected persons. *MMWR Morb. Mortal Wkly Rep.* 2002;51 (RR-8):1-52.
[507] Kusne S, and Krystofak S. Infection control issues after solid organ transplantation in transplant infections (Second Edition), ed. Bowden RA, Ljungman P, Paya CV. Lippincott, Williams and Wilkins. Philadelphia; 2003.
[508] Anderson D, DeFor T, Burns L, et al. A comparison of related donor peripheral blood and bone marrow transplants: importance of late-onset chronic graft-versus-host disease and infections. *Biol. Blood Marrow Transplant.* 2003;9(1):52-9.
[509] Pitchford KC, Corey M, Highsmith AK, et al. Pseudomonas species contamination of cystic fibrosis patients' home inhalation equipment. *J. Pediatr.* 1987;1 1 1(2):212-6.
[510] Hamill RJ, Houston ED, Georghiou PR, et al. An outbreak of Burkholderia (formerly Pseudomonas) cepacia respiratory tract colonization and infection associated with nebulized albuterol therapy. *Ann. Intern. Med.* 1995;122(10):762-6.
[511] Hutchinson GR, Parker S, Pryor JA, et al. Home-use nebulizers: a potential primary source of Burkholderia cepacia and other colistinresistant, gram-negative bacteria in patients with cystic fibrosis. *J. Clin. Microbiol.* 1996;34(3):584-7.
[512] Jakobsson BM, Onnered AB, Hjelte L, Nystrom B. Low bacterial contamination of nebulizers in home treatment of cystic fibrosis patients. *J. Hosp. Infect.* 1997;36(3):201-7.
[513] Rosenfeld M, Joy P, Nguyen CD, Krzewinski J, Burns JL. Cleaning home nebulizers used by patients with cystic fibrosis: is rinsing with tap water enough? *J. Hosp. Infect.* 2001;49(3):229-30.
[514] Govan JR. Infection control in cystic fibrosis: methicillin-resistant Staphylococcus aureus, Pseudomonas aeruginosa and the Burkholderia cepacia complex. *J. R. Soc. Med.* 2000;93(Suppl 38):40-5.
[515] Frederiksen B, Koch C, Hoiby N. Changing epidemiology of Pseudomonas aeruginosa infection in Danish cystic fibrosis patients (1974-1995). *Pediatr. Pulmonol.* 1999;28(3):159-66.
[516] Isles A, Maclusky I, Corey M, et al. Pseudomonas cepacia infection in cystic fibrosis: an emerging problem. *J. Pediatr.* 1984;104(2):206-10.

[517] LiPuma JJ. Burkholderia cepacia. Management issues and new insights. *Clin. Chest Med.* 1998;19(3):473-86, vi.

[518] Tablan OC, Chorba TL, Schidlow DV, et al. Pseudomonas cepacia colonization in patients with cystic fibrosis: risk factors and clinical outcome. *J. Pediatr.* 1985;107(3):382-7.

[519] Hudson VL, Wielinski CL, Regelmann WE. Prognostic implications of initial oropharyngeal bacterial flora in patients with cystic fibrosis diagnosed before the age of two years. *J. Pediatr.* 1993;122(6):854-60.

[520] Farrell PM, Li Z, Kosorok MR, et al. Bronchopulmonary disease in children with cystic fibrosis after early or delayed diagnosis. *Am. J. Respir. Crit. Care Med.* 2003;168(9):1100-8.

[521] Smith DL, Gumery LB, Smith EG, Stableforth DE, Kaufmann ME, Pitt TL. Epidemic of Pseudomonas cepacia in an adult cystic fibrosis unit: evidence of person-to-person transmission. *J. Clin. Microbiol.* 1993;31(11):3017-22.js.

[522] Pegues DA, Schidlow DV, Tablan OC, Carson LA, Clark NC, Jarvis WR. Possible nosocomial transmission of Pseudomonas cepacia in patients with cystic fibrosis. *Arch. Pediatr. Adolesc. Med.* 1994;148(8):805-12.

[523] Govan JR, Brown PH, Maddison J, et al. Evidence for transmission of Pseudomonas cepacia by social contact in cystic fibrosis. *Lancet.* 1993;342(8862):15-9.

[524] Pegues DA, Carson LA, Tablan OC, et al. Acquisition of Pseudomonas cepacia at summer camps for patients with cystic fibrosis. Summer Camp Study Group. *J. Pediatr.* 1994;124(5 Pt 1):694-702.

[525] Tablan OC, Martone WJ, Doershuk CF, et al. Colonization of the respiratory tract with Pseudomonas cepacia in cystic fibrosis. Risk factors and outcomes. *Chest.* 1987;91(4):527-32.

[526] Thomassen MJ, Demko CA, Doershuk CF, Stern RC, Klinger JD. Pseudomonas cepacia: decrease in colonization in patients with cystic fibrosis. *Am. Rev. Respir. Dis.* 1986;134(4):669-71.js.

[527] Weber DJ, Rutala WA. Gene therapy: a new challenge for infection control. *Infect. Control. Hosp. Epidemiol.* 1999;20(8):530-2.

[528] Evans ME, Lesnaw JA. Infection control for gene therapy: a busy physician's primer. *Clin. Infect. Dis.* 2002;35(5):597-605.

[529] Strausbaugh LJ. Gene therapy and infection control: more light on the way. *Infect. Control Hosp. Epidemiol.* 2000;21(10):630-2.

[530] CDC. West Nile virus infections in organ transplant recipients--New York and Pennsylvania, August-September, 2005. *MMWR Morb. Mortal Wkly. Rep.* 2005;54(40):1021-3.

[531] Lawson CA. Cytomegalovirus after kidney transplantation: a case review. *Prog. Transplant.* 2005;15(2):157-60.
[532] Tugwell BD, Patel PR, Williams IT, et al. Transmission of hepatitis C virus to several organ and tissue recipients from an antibody-negative donor. *Ann. Intern. Med.* 2005;143(9):648-54.
[533] Kainer MA, Linden JV, Whaley DN, et al. Clostridium infections associated with musculoskeletal-tissue allografts. *N. Engl. J. Med.* 2004;350(25):2564-71.
[534] CDC. Invasive Streptococcus pyogenes after allograft implantation-- Colorado, 2003. *MMWR Morb. Mortal Wkly. Rep.* 2003;52(48):1 174-6.
[535] Mungai M, Tegtmeier G, Chamberland M, Parise M. Transfusion-transmitted malaria in the United States from 1963 through 1999. *N. Engl. J. Med.* 2001;344(26):1973-8.
[536] Lux JZ, Weiss D, Linden JV, et al. Transfusion-associated babesiosis after heart transplant. *Emerg. Infect. Dis.* 2003;9(1):1 16-9.
[537] CDC. Chagas Disease After Organ Transplantation --- United States, 2001. *MMWR.* 2002;51(10):210-2.
[538] CDC. Lymphocytic choriomeningitis virus infection in organ transplant recipients--Massachusetts, Rhode Island, 2005. *MMWR Morb. Mortal Wkly. Rep.* 2005;54(21):537-9.
[539] Srinivasan A, Burton EC, Kuehnert MJ, et al. Transmission of rabies virus from an organ donor to four transplant recipients. *N. Engl. J. Med.* 2005;352(1 1):1 103-11.
[540] Gottesdiener KM. Transplanted infections: donor-to-host transmission with the allograft. *Ann. Intern. Med.* 1989;1 10(12):1001-16.
[541] Borie DC, Cramer DV, Phan-Thanh L, et al. Microbiological hazards related to xenotransplantation of porcine organs into man. *Infect. Control Hosp. Epidemiol.* 1998;19(5):355-65.
[542] CDC. U.S. Public Health Service Guideline on Infectious Disease Issues in Xenotransplantation. Centers for Disease Control and Prevention. MMWR - Morbidity & Mortality Weekly Report 2001 ;50 (RR- 1 5)(August): 1-46.
[543] IOM. Institute of Medicine. To err is human: building a safer health system. Washington DC National Academy Press; 1 999;http://www.iom.edu/report.asp?id=5575.
[544] Gerberding JL. Hospital-onset infections: a patient safety issue. *Ann. Intern. Med.* 2002;137(8):665-70.
[545] Leape LL, Berwick DM, Bates DW. What practices will most improve safety? Evidence-based medicine meets patient safety. *JAMA.* 2002;288(4):501 -7.

[546] Burke JP. Patient safety: infection control - a problem for patient safety. *N. Engl. J. Med.* 2003;348(7):651-6.
[547] Shulman L, Ost D. Managing infection in the critical care unit: how can infection control make the ICU safe? *Crit.Care Clin.* 2005;21(1):1 11-28, ix.
[548] Goldmann DA, Weinstein RA, Wenzel RP, et al. Strategies to Prevent and Control the Emergence and Spread of Antimicrobial-Resistant Microorganisms in Hospitals. A challenge to hospital leadership. *JAMA.* 1 996;275(3):234-40.
[549] Scheckler WE, Brimhall D, Buck AS, et al. Requirements for infrastructure and essential activities of infection control and epidemiology in hospitals: a consensus panel report. Society for Healthcare Epidemiology of America. *Infect. Control Hosp. Epidemiol.* 1998;19(2):1 14-24.
[550] www.jointcommission.org/PatientSafety/NationalPatientSafetyGoals/
[551] Jackson M, Chiarello LA, Gaynes RP, Gerberding JL. Nurse staffing and health care-associated infections: Proceedings from a working group meeting. *Am. J. Infect. Control.* 2002;30(4): 199-206.
[552] O'Boyle C, Jackson M, Henly SJ. Staffing requirements for infection control programs in US health care facilities: *Delphi project. Am. J. Infect. Control.* 2002;30(6):321-33.
[553] Peterson LR, Hamilton JD, Baron EJ, et al. Role of clinical microbiology laboratories in the management and control of infectious diseases and the delivery of health care. *Clin. Infect. Dis.* 2001;32(4):605-1 1.
[554] McGowan JE, Jr., Tenover FC. Confronting bacterial resistance in healthcare settings: a crucial role for microbiologists. *Nat. Rev. Microbiol.* 2004;2(3):25 1-8.
[555] (Accessed at
[556] Curtis JR, Cook DJ, Wall RJ, et al. Intensive care unit quality improvement: a "how-to" guide for the interdisciplinary team. *Crit. Care Med.* 2006;34(1):21 1-8.
[557] Pronovost PJ, Nolan T, Zeger S, Miller M, Rubin H. How can clinicians measure safety and quality in acute care? *Lancet.* 2004;363(9414):1061-7.
[558] Goldrick BA, Dingle DA, Gilmore GK, Curchoe RM, Plackner CL, Fabrey LJ. Practice analysis for infection control and epidemiology in the new millennium. *Am. J. Infect. Control.* 2002;30(8):437-48.
[559] CDC. Guideline for Hand Hygiene in Health-Care Settings: Recommendations of the Healthcare Infection Control Practices Advisory Committee and the HICPAC/SHEA/APIC/IDSA Hand Hygiene Task Force. *MMWR.* 2002;5 1(1 6)(RR-1 6): 1-44.

[560] Bonomo RA, Rice LB. Emerging issues in antibiotic resistant infections in long-term care facilities. *J. Gerontol. A Biol. Sci. Med. Sci.* 1999;54(6):B2607.

[561] Larson EL, Early E, Cloonan P, Sugrue S, Parides M. An organizational climate intervention associated with increased handwashing and decreased nosocomial infections. *Behav. Med.* 2000;26(1):14-22.

[562] Pittet D, Hugonnet S, Harbarth S, et al. Effectiveness of a hospital-wide programme to improve compliance with hand hygiene. Infection Control Programme. *Lancet.* 2000;356(923 8): 1307-12.

[563] Murthy R. Implementation of strategies to control antimicrobial resistance. *Chest.* 2001;1 19(2 Suppl):405S-1 1S.

[564] Rondeau KV, Wagar TH. Organizational learning and continuous quality improvement: examining the impact on nursing home performance. *Healthc Manage Forum.* 2002; 15(2): 17-23.

[565] Stelfox HT, Bates DW, Redelmeier DA. Safety of patients isolated for infection control. *JAMA.* 2003 ;290(14): 1899-905.

[566] Haley RW, Culver DH, White JW, et al. The efficacy of infection surveillance and control programs in preventing nosocomial infections in US hospitals. *Am. J. Epidemiol.* 1985;121(2):182-205.

[567] McArthur BJ, Pugliese G, Weinstein S, et al. A national task analysis of infection control practitioners, 1982. Part One: methodology and demography. *Am. J. Infect. Control.* 1984;12(2):88-95.

[568] Shannon R, McArthur BJ, Weinstein S, et al. A national task analysis of infection control practitioners, 1982. Part Two: Tasks, knowledge, and abilities for practice. *Am. J. Infect. Control.* 1984;12(3):187-96.

[569] Pugliese G, McArthur BJ, Weinstein S, et al. A national task analysis of infection control practitioners, 1982. Part Three: The relationship between hospital size and tasks performed. *Am. J. Infect. Control.* 1984;12(4):221-7.

[570] Larson E, Eisenberg R, Soule BM. Validating the certification process for infection control practice. *Am. J. Infect. Control.* 1988;16(5):198-205.

[571] Bjerke NB, Fabrey LJ, Johnson CB, et al. Job analysis 1992: infection control practitioner. *Am. J. Infect. Control.* 1993;21(2):51-7.

[572] Turner JG, Kolenc KM, Docken L. Job analysis 1996: Infection control professional. Certification Board in Infection Control and Epidemiology, Inc, 1996 Job Analysis Committee. *Am. J. Infect. Control.* 1999;27(2):14557.

[573] Health Canada. Nosocomial and Occupational Infections Section. Development of a resource model for infection prevention and control programs in acute, long term, and home care settings: conference proceedings of the Infection Prevention and Control Alliance. *AJIC.* 2004;32:2-6.

[574] Lee TH, Meyer GS, Brennan TA. A middle ground on public accountability. *N. Engl. J. Med.* 2004;350(23):2409-12.

[575] Stevenson KB, Murphy CL, Samore MH, et al. Assessing the status of infection control programs in small rural hospitals in the western United States. *Am. J. Infect. Control.* 2004;32(5):255-61.

[576] Simonds DN, Horan TC, Kelley R, Jarvis WR. Detecting pediatric nosocomial infections: how do infection control and quality assurance personnel compare? *Am. J. Infect. Control.* 1997;25(3):202-8.

[577] Dawson SJ. The role of the infection control link nurse. *J. Hosp. Infect.* 2003;54(4):251-7; quiz 320.

[578] Wright J, Stover BH, Wilkerson S, Bratcher D. Expanding the infection control team: development of the infection control liaison position for the neonatal intensive care unit. *Am. J. Infect. Control.* 2002;30(3):174-8.

[579] Teare EL, Peacock A. The development of an infection control link-nurse programme in a district general hospital. *J. Hosp. Infect.* 1996;34(4):267-78.

[580] Ching TY, Seto WH. Evaluating the efficacy of the infection control liaison nurse in the hospital. *J. Adv. Nurs.* 1990;15(10):1 128-31.

[581] Amundsen J, Drennan DP. An infection control nurse-advisor program. *Am. J. Infect. Control.* 1983;1 1(1):20-3.

[582] Ross KA. A program for infection surveillance utilizing an infection control liaison nurse. *Am. J. Infect. Control.* 1982;10(1):24-8.

[583] Needleman J, Buerhaus P, Mattke S, Stewart M, Zelevinsky K. Nurse- staffing levels and the quality of care in hospitals. *N. Engl. J. Med.* 2002;346(22): 1715-22.

[584] Dimick JB, Swoboda SM, Pronovost PJ, Lipsett PA. Effect of nurse-topatient ratio in the intensive care unit on pulmonary complications and resource use after hepatectomy. *Am. J. Crit. Care.* 2001;10(6):376-82.

[585] Mayhall CG, Lamb VA, Gayle WE, Jr., Haynes BW, Jr. *Enterobacter cloacae* septicemia in a burn center: epidemiology and control of an outbreak. *J. Infect. Dis.* 1979;139(2):166-71.

[586] Goldmann DA, Durbin WA, Jr., Freeman J. Nosocomial infections in a neonatal intensive care unit. *J. Infect. Dis.* 1981;144(5):449-59.(mj).

[587] Arnow P, Allyn PA, Nichols EM, Hill DL, Pezzlo M, Bartlett RH. Control of methicillin-resistant Staphylococcus aureus in a burn unit: role of nurse staffing. *J. Trauma.* 1982;22(1 1):954-9.

[588] Haley RW, Bregman DA. The role of understaffing and overcrowding in recurrent outbreaks of staphylococcal infection in a neonatal special-care unit. *J. Infect. Dis.* 1982;145(6):875-85.

[589] Fridkin SK, Pear SM, Williamson TH, Galgiani JN, Jarvis WR. The role of understaffing in central venous catheter-associated bloodstream infections. *Infect. Control Hosp. Epidemiol.* 1996; 17(3): 150-8.

[590] Robert J, Fridkin SK, Blumberg HM, et al. The influence of the composition of the nursing staff on primary bloodstream infection rates in a surgical intensive care unit. *Infect. Control Hosp. Epidemiol.* 2000;21(1): 12-7.(mj).

[591] Li J, Birkhead GS, Strogatz DS, Coles FB. Impact of institution size, staffing patterns, and infection control practices on communicable disease outbreaks in New York State nursing homes. *Am. J. Epidemiol.* 1996; 143(10): 1042-9.

[592] Archibald LK, Manning ML, Bell LM, Banerjee S, Jarvis WR. Patient density, nurse-to-patient ratio and nosocomial infection risk in a pediatric cardiac intensive care unit. *Pediatr. Infect. Dis. J.* 1997;16(1 1):1045-8.

[593] Harbarth S, Sudre P, Dharan S, Cadenas M, Pittet D. Outbreak of Enterobacter cloacae related to understaffing, overcrowding, and poor hygiene practices. *Infect. Control Hosp. Epidemiol.* 1999;20(9):598-603.

[594] Vicca AF. Nursing staff workload as a determinant of methicillin-resistant Staphylococcus aureus spread in an adult intensive therapy unit. *J. Hosp. Infect.* 1999;43(2):109-13.

[595] Stegenga J, Bell E, Matlow A. The role of nurse understaffing in nosocomial viral gastrointestinal infections on a general pediatrics ward. *Infect. Control Hosp. Epidemiol.* 2002;23(3):133-6.

[596] Alonso-Echanove J, Edwards JR, Richards MJ, et al. Effect of nurse staffing and antimicrobial-impregnated central venous catheters on the risk for bloodstream infections in intensive care units. *Infect. Control Hosp. Epidemiol.* 2003;24(12):91 6-25.

[597] Petrosillo N, Gilli P, Serraino D, et al. Prevalence of infected patients and understaffing have a role in hepatitis C virus transmission in dialysis. *Am. J. Kidney Dis.* 2001;37(5):1004-10.

[598] Pfaller MA, Herwaldt LA. The clinical microbiology laboratory and infection control: emerging pathogens, antimicrobial resistance, and new technology. *Clin. Infect. Dis.* 1 997;25(4):858-70.

[599] Simor AE. The role of the laboratory in infection prevention and control programs in long-term-care facilities for the elderly. *Infect. Control Hosp. Epidemiol.* 2001 ;22(7):459-63.

[600] Weinstein RA, Mallison GF. The role of the microbiology laboratory in surveillance and control of nosocomial infections. *Am. J. Clin. Pathol.* 1978;69(2): 130-6.

[601] Kolmos HJ. Interaction between the microbiology laboratory and clinician: what the microbiologist can provide. *J. Hosp. Infect.* 1999;43 Suppl:S285-91.
[602] Clinical and Laboratory Standards Institute. www.clsi.org/
[603] Ginocchio CC. Role of NCCLS in antimicrobial susceptibility testing and monitoring. *Am. J. Health Syst. Pharm.* 2002;59(8 Suppl 3):S7-1 1.
[604] National Committee for Clinical Laboratory Standards. Performance standards for antimicrobial susceptibility testing; twelfth informational supplement. Document M100-S12. NCCLS, Wayne (PA) 2002.
[605] NCCLS. (2002). Analysis and Presentation of Cumulative Antimicrobial Susceptibility Test Data. Approved Guideline. NCCLS document M39-A (ISBN 1-56238-422-9). Wayne: PA, NCCLS. 2002.
[606] Halstead DC, Gomez N, McCarter YS. Reality of developing a community-wide antibiogram. *J. Clin. Microbiol.* 2004;42(1):1-6.
[607] Ernst EJ, Diekema DJ, BootsMiller BJ, et al. Are United States hospitals following national guidelines for the analysis and presentation of cumulative antimicrobial susceptibility data? *Diagn. Microbiol. Infect. Dis.* 2004;49(2): 141-5.
[608] Bergeron MG, Ouellette M. Preventing antibiotic resistance through rapid genotypic identification of bacteria and of their antibiotic resistance genes in the clinical microbiology laboratory. *J. Clin. Microbiol.* 1998;3 6(8):2 16972.
[609] Hacek DM, Suriano T, Noskin GA, Kruszynski J, Reisberg B, Peterson LR. Medical and economic benefit of a comprehensive infection control program that includes routine determination of microbial clonality. *Am. J. Clin. Pathol.* 1999;1 1 1(5):647-54.
[610] Rodriguez WJ, Schwartz RH, Thorne MM. Evaluation of diagnostic tests for influenza in a pediatric practice. *Pediatr. Infect. Dis. J.* 2002;2 1(3): 193-6.
[611] CDC. Prevention and control of influenza. Recommendations of the Advisory Committee on Immunization Practices (ACIP). *MMWR Recomm. Rep.* 2005;54(RR-8):1-40.
[612] Uyeki TM. Influenza diagnosis and treatment in children: a review of studies on clinically useful tests and antiviral treatment for influenza. *Pediatr. Infect. Dis. J.* 2003;22(2):164-77.
[613] Chan EL, Antonishyn N, McDonald R, et al. The use of TaqMan PCR assay for detection of Bordetella pertussis infection from clinical specimens. *Arch. Pathol. Lab. Med.* 2002;126(2):173-6.

[614] Barenfanger J, Drake C, Kacich G. Clinical and financial benefits of rapid bacterial identification and antimicrobial susceptibility testing. *J. Clin. Microbiol.* 1999;37(5): 1415-8.

[615] Barenfanger J, Drake C, Leon N, Mueller T, Troutt T. Clinical and financial benefits of rapid detection of respiratory viruses: an outcomes study. *J. Clin. Microbiol.* 2000;38(8):2824-8.

[616] Ramers C, Billman G, Hartin M, Ho S, Sawyer MH. Impact of a diagnostic cerebrospinal fluid enterovirus polymerase chain reaction test on patient management. *JAMA.* 2000;283(20):2680-5.

[617] Mackie PL, Joannidis PA, Beattie J. Evaluation of an acute point-of-care system screening for respiratory syncytial virus infection. *J. Hosp. Infect.* 2001;48(1):66-71.

[618] Guillemot D, Courvalin P. Better control of antibiotic resistance. *Clin. Infect. Dis.* 2001;33(4):542-7.

[619] Paterson DL. The role of antimicrobial management programs in optimizing antibiotic prescribing within hospitals. *Clin. Infect. Dis.* 2006;42 Suppl 2:S90-5.

[620] Lundstrom T, Pugliese G, Bartley J, Cox J, Guither C. Organizational and environmental factors that affect worker health and safety and patient outcomes. *Am. J. Infect. Control.* 2002;30(2):93-106.

[621] www.patientsafety.com/vision.html

[622] Pronovost PJ, Jenckes MW, Dorman T, et al. Organizational characteristics of intensive care units related to outcomes of abdominal aortic surgery. *JAMA.* 1999;281(14):1310-7.

[623] Pronovost PJ, Angus DC, Dorman T, Robinson KA, Dremsizov TT, Young TL. Physician staffing patterns and clinical outcomes in critically ill patients: a systematic review. *JAMA.* 2002;288(17):2151-62.

[624] Pronovost PJ, Weast B, Holzmueller CG, et al. Evaluation of the culture of safety: survey of clinicians and managers in an academic medical center. *Qual. Saf. Health Care.* 2003; 12(6) :405-10.

[625] Nieva VF, Sorra J. Safety culture assessment: a tool for improving patient safety in healthcare organizations. *Qual. Saf. Health Care.* 2003;12 Suppl 2:ii17-23.

[626] Clarke SP, Rockett JL, Sloane DM, Aiken LH. Organizational climate, staffing, and safety equipment as predictors of needlestick injuries and near-misses in hospital nurses. *Am. J. Infect. Control.* 2002;30(4):207-16.

[627] Rivers DL, Aday LA, Frankowski RF, Felknor S, White D, Nichols B. Predictors of nurses' acceptance of an intravenous catheter safety device. *Nurs. Res.* 2003;52(4):249-55.

[628] Gershon RR, Karkashian CD, Grosch JW, et al. Hospital safety climate and its relationship with safe work practices and workplace exposure incidents. *Am. J. Infect. Control.* 2000;28(3):211-21.

[629] Gershon RR, Vlahov D, Felknor SA, et al. Compliance with universal precautions among health care workers at three regional hospitals. *Am. J. Infect. Control.* 1995;23(4):225-36.

[630] Michalsen A, Delclos GL, Felknor SA, et al. Compliance with universal precautions among physicians. *J. Occup. Environ. Med.* 1997;39(2):130-7.

[631] Vaughn TE, McCoy KD, Beekmann SE, Woolson RE, Torner JC, Doebbeling BN. Factors promoting consistent adherence to safe needle precautions among hospital workers. *Infect. Control Hosp. Epidemiol.* 2004;25(7):548-55.

[632] Grosch JW, Gershon RR, Murphy LR, DeJoy DM. Safety climate dimensions associated with occupational exposure to blood-borne pathogens in nurses. *Am. J. Ind. Med.* 1999;Suppl 1:122-4.

[633] Piotrowski MM, Hinshaw DB. The safety checklist program: creating a culture of safety in intensive care units. *Jt. Comm. J. Qual. Improv.* 2002;28(6):306-1 5.

[634] Weeks WB, Bagian JP. Developing a culture of safety in the Veterans Health Administration. *Eff. Clin. Pract.* 2000;3(6):270-6.

[635] Bagian JP, Gosbee JW. Developing a culture of patient safety at the VA. *Ambul. Outreach.* 2000:25-9.

[636] Tokars JI, McKinley GF, Otten J, et al. Use and efficacy of tuberculosis infection control practices at hospitals with previous outbreaks of multidrug-resistant tuberculosis. *Infect. Control Hosp. Epidemiol.* 2001;22(7):449-55.

[637] Maloney SA, Pearson ML, Gordon MT, Del Castillo R, Boyle JF, Jarvis WR. Efficacy of control measures in preventing nosocomial transmission of multidrug-resistant tuberculosis to patients and health care workers. *Ann. Intern. Med.* 1995;122(2):90-5.

[638] Montecalvo MA, Jarvis WR, Uman J, et al. Infection-control measures reduce transmission of vancomycin-resistant enterococci in an endemic setting. *Ann. Intern. Med.* 1999;131(4):269-72.

[639] Sherertz RJ, Ely EW, Westbrook DM, et al. Education of physicians-in-training can decrease the risk for vascular catheter infection. *Ann. Intern. Med.* 2000;132(8):641-8.

[640] Lynch P, Cummings MJ, Roberts PL, Herriott MJ, Yates B, Stamm WE. Implementing and evaluating a system of generic infection precautions: body substance isolation. *Am. J. Infect. Control.* 1990;18(1):1-12.

[641] Kelen GD, DiGiovanna TA, Celentano DD, et al. Adherence to Universal (barrier) Precautions during interventions on critically ill and injured emergency department patients. *J. Acquir. Immune Defic. Syndr.* 1990;3(10):987-94.

[642] Courington KR, Patterson SL, Howard RJ. Universal precautions are not universally followed. *Arch. Surg.* 1991;126(1):93-6.

[643] Kaczmarek RG, Moore RM, Jr., McCrohan J, et al. Glove use by health care workers: results of a tristate investigation. *Am. J. Infect. Control.* 1991;19(5):228-32.

[644] Freeman SW, Chambers CV. Compliance with universal precautions in a medical practice with a high rate of HIV infection. *J. Am. Board Fam. Pract.* 1992;5(3):313-8.

[645] Friedland LR, Joffe M, Wiley JF, 2nd, Schapire A, Moore DF. Effect of educational program on compliance with glove use in a pediatric emergency department. *Am. J. Dis. Child.* 1992;146(11):1355-8.

[646] Henry K, Campbell S, Maki M. A comparison of observed and self-reported compliance with universal precautions among emergency department personnel at a Minnesota public teaching hospital: implications for assessing infection control programs. *Ann. Emerg. Med.* 1992;21(8):940-6.

[647] Henry K, Campbell S, Collier P, Williams CO. Compliance with universal precautions and needle handling and disposal practices among emergency department staff at two community hospitals. *Am. J. Infect. Control.* 1994;22(3):129-37.

[648] Eustis TC, Wright SW, Wrenn KD, Fowlie EJ, Slovis CM. Compliance with recommendations for universal precautions among prehospital providers. *Ann. Emerg. Med.* 1995;25(4):512-5.

[649] DiGiacomo JC, Hoff WS, Rotondo MF, et al. Barrier precautions in trauma resuscitation: real-time analysis utilizing videotape review. *Am. J. Emerg. Med.* 1997;15(1):34-9.

[650] Thompson BL, Dwyer DM, Ussery XT, Denman S, Vacek P, Schwartz B. Handwashing and glove use in a long-term-care facility. *Infect. Control Hosp. Epidemiol.* 1997;18(2):97-103.(s).

[651] Helfgott AW, Taylor-Burton J, Garcini FJ, Eriksen NL, Grimes R. Compliance with universal precautions: knowledge and behavior of residents and students in a department of obstetrics and gynecology. *Infect. Dis. Obstet. Gynecol.* 1998;6(3):123-8.

[652] Moore S, Goodwin H, Grossberg R, Toltzis P. Compliance with universal precautions among pediatric residents. *Arch. Pediatr. Adolesc. Med.* 1998;152(6):554-7.

[653] Akduman D, Kim LE, Parks RL, et al. Use of personal protective equipment and operating room behaviors in four surgical subspecialties: personal protective equipment and behaviors in surgery. *Infect. Control Hosp. Epidemiol.* 1999;20(2):110-4.

[654] Brooks AJ, Phipson M, Potgieter A, Koertzen H, Boffard KD. Education of the trauma team: video evaluation of the compliance with universal barrier precautions in resuscitation. *Eur. J. Surg.* 1999;165(12):1 125-8.

[655] Kidd F, Heitkemper P, Kressel AB. A comprehensive educational approach to improving patient isolation practice. *Clin. Perform. Qual. Health Care.* 1999;7(2):74-6.

[656] Madan AK, Rentz DE, Wahle MJ, Flint LM. Noncompliance of health care workers with universal precautions during trauma resuscitations. *South Med. J.* 2001;94(3):277-80.

[657] Madan AK, Raafat A, Hunt JP, Rentz D, Wahle MJ, Flint LM. Barrier precautions in trauma: is knowledge enough? *J. Trauma.* 2002;52(3):540-3.

[658] Jeffe DB, Mutha S, Kim LE, Evanoff BA, Fraser VJ. Evaluation of a preclinical, educational and skills-training program to improve students' use of blood and body fluid precautions: one-year follow-up. *Prev. Med.* 1999;29(5):365-73.

[659] Williams CO, Campbell S, Henry K, Collier P. Variables influencing worker compliance with universal precautions in the emergency department. *Am. J. Infect. Control.* 1994;22(3):138-48.

[660] Larson E, McGeer A, Quraishi ZA, et al. Effect of an automated sink on handwashing practices and attitudes in high-risk units. *Infect. Control Hosp. Epidemiol.* 1991;12(7):422-8.

[661] Swoboda SM, Earsing K, Strauss K, Lane S, Lipsett PA. Electronic monitoring and voice prompts improve hand hygiene and decrease nosocomial infections in an intermediate care unit. *Crit. Care Med.* 2004;32(2):358-63.

[662] Kretzer EK, Larson EL. Behavioral interventions to improve infection control practices. *Am. J. Infect. Control.* 1998;26(3):245-53.

[663] CDC. Updated Guidelines for Evaluating Public Health Surveillance Systems. Recommendations from the Guidelines Working Group. *MMWR. Recomm. Rep.* 2001;50(RR-13):1-35.

[664] Semmelweiss IP. Die aetiologie, der begriff und die prophylaxis des kindbettfiebers. Pest, Wein, und Leipzig:. CA Harleben's VerlagsExpedition 1861.

[665] Bratzler DW, Houck PM. Antimicrobial prophylaxis for surgery: an advisory statement from the National Surgical Infection Prevention Project. *Clin. Infect. Dis.* 2004 Jun 15;38:1706-15.

[666] Bloom BT, Craddock A, Delmore PM, et al. Reducing acquired infections in the NICU: observing and implementing meaningful differences in process between high and low acquired infection rate centers. *J. Perinatol.* 2003 ;23 :489-92.

[667] Braun BI, Kritchevsky SB, Wong ES, et al. Preventing central venous catheter-associated primary bloodstream infections: characteristics of practices among hospitals participating in the Evaluation of Processes and Indicators in Infection Control (EPIC) study. *Infect. Control Hosp. Epidemiol.* 2003 ;24(1 2):926-35.

[668] Baker OG. Process surveillance: an epidemiologic challenge for all health care organizations. *AJIC.* 1997;25:96-101.

[669] Loeb M, McGeer A, McArthur M, Peeling RW, Petric M, Simor AE. Surveillance for outbreaks of respiratory tract infections in nursing homes. *Cmaj.* 2000;162(8):1133-7.

[670] Nicolle LE. Preventing infections in non-hospital settings: long-term care. *Emerg. Infect. Dis.* 2001 ;7(2):205-7.

[671] Pottinger JM, Herwaldt LA, Perl TM. Basics of surveillance--an overview. *Infect. Control Hosp. Epidemiol.* 1997; 18(7): 513-27.

[672] Lee TB, Baker OG, Lee JT, Scheckler WE, Steele L, Laxton CE. Recommended practices for surveillance. Association for Professionals in Infection Control and Epidemiology, Inc. Surveillance Initiative working Group. *Am. J. Infect. Control.* 1998;26(3):277-88.

[673] Haley RW. The scientific basis for using surveillance and risk factor data to reduce nosocomial infection rates. *J. Hosp. Infect.* 1995;30 Suppl:3-14.

[674] Benneyan JC, Lloyd RC, Plsek PE. Statistical process control as a tool for research and healthcare improvement. *Qual. Saf. Health Care.* 2003; 1 2(6):458-64.

[675] Lemmen SW, Zolldann D, Gastmeier P, Lutticken R. Implementing and evaluating a rotating surveillance system and infection control guidelines in 4 intensive care units. *Am. J. Infect. Control.* 2001;29(2):89-93.

[676] Gaynes R, Richards C, Edwards J, et al. Feeding back surveillance data to prevent hospital-acquired infections. *Emerg. Infect. Dis.* 2001 ;7(2):295-8.

[677] Tokars JI, Richards C, Andrus M, et al. The changing face of surveillance for health care-associated infections. *Clin. Infect. Dis.* 2004;39: 1347-52.

[678] Sands KE, Yokoe DS, Hooper DC, et al. Detection of postoperative surgical-site infections: comparison of health plan-based surveillance with hospital-based programs. *Infect. Control Hosp. Epidemiol.* 2003 ;24(10):741 -3.

[679] Jodra VM, Rodela AR, Martinez EM, Fresnena NL. Standardized infection ratios for three general surgery procedures: a comparison between Spanish hospitals and U.S. centers participating in the National Nosocomial Infections Surveillance System. *Infect. Control Hosp. Epidemiol.* 2003 ;24(1 0):744-8.

[680] McKibben L, Horan T, Tokars JI, et al. Guidance on public reporting of healthcare-associated infections: recommendations of the Healthcare Infection Control Practices Advisory Committee. *Am. J. Infect. Control.* 2005;33(4):217-26.

[681] Gould D, Chamberlain A. The use of a ward-based educational teaching package to enhance nurses' compliance with infection control procedures. *J. Clin. Nurs.* 1997;6(1):55-67.

[682] Calabro K, Weltge A, Parnell S, Kouzekanani K, Ramirez E. Intervention for medical students: effective infection control. *Am. J. Infect. Control.* 1998;26(4):43 1-6.

[683] Haiduven DJ, Hench CP, Simpkins SM, Stevens DA. Standardized management of patients and employees exposed to pertussis. *Infect. Control Hosp. Epidemiol.* 1998;19(1 1):861-4.

[684] Macartney KK, Gorelick MH, Manning ML, Hodinka RL, Bell LM. Nosocomial respiratory syncytial virus infections: the cost- effectiveness and cost-benefit of infection control. *Pediatrics.* 2000; 106(3): 520-6.

[685] Beekmann SE, Vaughn TE, McCoy KD, et al. Hospital bloodborne pathogens programs: program characteristics and blood and body fluid exposure rates. *Infect. Control Hosp. Epidemiol.* 2001 ;22(2):73-82.

[686] Sokas RK, Simmens S, Scott J. A training program in universal precautions for second-year medical students. *Acad. Med.* 1993 ;68(5) :3746.

[687] Ostrowsky BE, Trick WE, Sohn AH, et al. Control of vancomycinresistant enterococcus in health care facilities in a region. *N. Engl. J. Med.* 2001 ;344(19): 1427-33.

[688] Bonten MJ, Kollef MH, Hall JB. Risk factors for ventilator-associated pneumonia: from epidemiology to patient management. *Clin. Infect. Dis.* 2004;38(8):1 141-9.

[689] Lau JT, Fung KS, Wong TW, et al. SARS transmission among hospital workers in Hong Kong. *Emerg. Infect. Dis.* 2004;10(2):280-6.

[690] Talbot TR, Bradley SE, Cosgrove SE, Ruef C, Siegel JD, Weber DJ. Influenza vaccination of healthcare workers and vaccine allocation for healthcare workers during vaccine shortages. *Infect. Control Hosp. Epidemiol.* 2005;26(1 1):882-90.

[691] Harbarth S, Siegrist CA, Schira JC, Wunderli W, Pittet D. Influenza immunization: improving compliance of healthcare workers. *Infect. Control Hosp. Epidemiol.* 1998; 1 9(5):337-42.
[692] Bryant KA, Stover B, Cain L, Levine GL, Siegel J, Jarvis WR. Improving influenza immunization rates among healthcare workers caring for high- risk pediatric patients. *Infect. Control Hosp. Epidemiol.* 2004;25(1 1):912-7.
[693] Martinello RA, Jones L, Topal JE. Correlation between healthcare workers' knowledge of influenza vaccine and vaccine receipt. *Infect. Control Hosp. Epidemiol.* 2003 ;24(1 1):845-7.
[694] Goldrick B, Gruendemann B, Larson E. Learning styles and teaching/learning strategy preferences: implications for educating nurses in critical care, the operating room, and infection control. *Heart Lung.* 1 993;22(2): 176-82.
[695] Davis D, O'Brien MA, Freemantle N, Wolf FM, Mazmanian P, TaylorVaisey A. Impact of formal continuing medical education: do conferences, workshops, rounds, and other traditional continuing education activities change physician behavior or health care outcomes? *JAMA.* 1 999;282(9): 867-74.
[696] Carr H, and Hinson P. Education and Training. ed. APIC Text of Infection Control and Epidemiology. 2nd edition. Washington, DC: Association for Professionals in Infection Control and Epidemiology, Inc. (APIC); pp. 11-1; 2005.
[697] Caffarella RS. Planning Programs for Adult Learners: A Practical Guide for Educators, Trainers, and Staff Developers, Second Edition. In. San Francisco: Jossey-Bass; 2001.
[698] Sargeant J, Curran V, Jarvis-Selinger S, et al. Interactive on-line continuing medical education: physicians' perceptions and experiences. *J. Contin. Educ. Health Prof.* 2004;24(4) :227-36.
[699] Van Harrison R. Systems-based framework for continuing medical education and improvements in translating new knowledge into physicians' practices. *J. Contin. Educ. Health Prof.* 2004;24 Suppl 1:S50-62.
[700] Cole TB, Glass RM. Learning associated with participation in journal- based continuing medical education. *J. Contin. Educ. Health Prof.* 2004;24(4):205- 12.
[701] Diekema DJ, Albanese MA, Schuldt SS, Doebbeling BN. Blood and body fluid exposures during clinical training: relation to knowledge of universal precautions. *J. Gen. Intern. Med.* 1996;1 1(2):109-1 1.
[702] Diekema DJ, Schuldt SS, Albanese MA, Doebbeling BN. Universal precautions training of preclinical students: impact on knowledge, attitudes, and compliance. *Prev. Med.* 1995;24(6):580-5.

[703] Warren DK, Zack JE, Cox MJ, Cohen MM, Fraser VJ. An educational intervention to prevent catheter-associated bloodstream infections in a nonteaching, community medical center. *Crit. Care Med.* 2003;31(7):195963.
[704] Dubbert PM, Dolce J, Richter W, Miller M, Chapman SW. Increasing ICU staff handwashing: effects of education and group feedback. *Infect. Control Hosp. Epidemiol.* 1990;11(4):191-3.
[705] Avila-Aguero ML, Umana MA, Jimenez AL, Faingezicht I, Paris MM. Handwashing practices in a tertiary-care, pediatric hospital and the effect on an educational program. *Clin. Perform. Qual. Health Care.* 1998;6(2):702.
[706] Lai KK, Fontecchio SA, Kelley AL, Melvin ZS. Knowledge of the transmission of tuberculosis and infection control measures for tuberculosis among healthcare workers. *Infect. Control. Hosp. Epidemiol.* 1996; 17(3): 168-70.
[707] Koenig S, Chu J. Senior medical students' knowledge of universal precautions. *Acad. Med.* 1993;68(5):372-4.
[708] Babcock HM, Zack JE, Garrison T, et al. An educational intervention to reduce ventilator-associated pneumonia in an integrated health system: a comparison of effects. *Chest.* 2004; 125(6) :2224-31.
[709] McGuckin M, Taylor A, Martin V, Porten L, Salcido R. Evaluation of a patient education model for increasing hand hygiene compliance in an inpatient rehabilitation unit. *Am. J. Infect. Control.* 2004;32(4):235-8.
[710] Cirone N. Patient-education handbook. *Nursing.* 1997;27(8):44-5.
[711] Chase TM. Learning styles and teaching strategies: enhancing the patient education experience. *SCI Nurse.* 2001; 18:138-41.
[712] Jarvis WR. Handwashing--the Semmelweis lesson forgotten? *Lancet.* 1994;344(8933):131 1-2.
[713] Daniels IR, Rees BI. Handwashing: simple, but effective. *Ann. R. Coll. Surg. Engl.* 1999;81:117-8.
[714] Webster J, Faoagali JL, Cartwright D. Elimination of methicillin-resistant *Staphylococcus aureus* from a neonatal intensive care unit after hand washing with triclosan. *J. Paediatr. Child Health.* 1994;30(1):59-64.
[715] Zafar AB, Butler RC, Reese DJ, Gaydos LA, Mennonna PA. Use of 0.3% triclosan (Bacti-Stat) to eradicate an outbreak of methicillin-resistant *Staphylococcus aureus* in a neonatal nursery. *Am. J. Infect. Control.* 1995;23(3):200-8.
[716] Malik RK, Montecalvo MA, Reale MR, et al. Epidemiology and control of vancomycin-resistant enterococci in a regional neonatal intensive care unit. *Pediatr. Infect. Dis. J.* 1999;18(4):352-6.

[717] Pittet D, Boyce JM. Hand hygiene and patient care: pursuing the Semmelweis legacy. *Lancet Infect. Dis.* 2001:9-20.

[718] Lin CM, Wu FM, Kim HK, Doyle MP, Michael BS, Williams LK. A comparison of hand washing techniques to remove Escherichia coli and caliciviruses under natural or artificial fingernails. *J. Food Prot.* 2003;66(12):2296-301.

[719] Edel E, Houston S, Kennedy V, LaRocco M. Impact of a 5-minute scrub on the microbial flora found on artificial, polished, or natural fingernails of operating room personnel. *Nurs. Res.* 1998;47(1):54-9.

[720] Pottinger J, Burns S, Manske C. Bacterial carriage by artificial versus natural nails. *Am. J. Infect. Control.* 1989;17(6):340-4.

[721] Hedderwick SA, McNeil SA, Lyons MJ, Kauffman CA. Pathogenic organisms associated with artificial fingernails worn by healthcare workers. *Infect. Control Hosp. Epidemiol.* 2000;21(8):505-9.

[722] Passaro DJ, Waring L, Armstrong R, et al. Postoperative Serratia marcescens wound infections traced to an out-of- hospital source. *J. Infect. Dis.* 1997;175(4):992-5.

[723] Moolenaar RL, Crutcher JM, San Joaquin VH, et al. A prolonged outbreak of Pseudomonas aeruginosa in a neonatal intensive care unit: did staff fingernails play a role in disease transmission? *Infect. Control Hosp. Epidemiol.* 2000;2 1(2): 80-5.

[724] Parry MF, Grant B, Yukna M, et al. Candida osteomyelitis and diskitis after spinal surgery: an outbreak that implicates artificial nail use. *Clin. Infect. Dis.* 2001;32(3):352-7.

[725] Boszczowski I, Nicoletti C, Puccini DM, et al. Outbreak of extended spectrum beta-lactamase-producing Klebsiella pneumoniae infection in a neonatal intensive care unit related to onychomycosis in a health care worker. *Pediatr. Infect. Dis. J.* 2005;24(7):648-50.

[726] Trick WE, Vernon MO, Hayes RA, et al. Impact of ring wearing on hand contamination and comparison of hand hygiene agents in a hospital. *Clin. Infect. Dis.* 2003;36(1 1):1383-90.

[727] Pittet D, Dharan S, Touveneau S, Sauvan V, Perneger TV. Bacterial contamination of the hands of hospital staff during routine patient care. *Arch. Intern. Med.* 1999;159(8):821-6.

[728] Tenorio AR, Badri SM, Sahgal NB, et al. Effectiveness of gloves in the prevention of hand carriage of vancomycin-resistant enterococcus species by health care workers after patient care. *Clin. Infect. Dis.* 2001;32(5):8269.(s).

[729] Mast ST, Woolwine JD, Gerberding JL. Efficacy of gloves in reducing blood volumes transferred during simulated needlestick injury. *J. Infect. Dis.* 1993; 168(6): 1589-92.
[730] Medical Glove Guidance Manual. www.fda.gov/cdrh/dsma/gloveman/gloveman99.pdf
[731] Korniewicz DM, El-Masri M, Broyles JM, Martin CD, O'Connell K P. Performance of latex and nonlatex medical examination gloves during simulated use. *Am. J. Infect. Control.* 2002;30(2):133-8.
[732] Korniewicz DM, McLeskey SW. Latex allergy and gloving standards. *Semin. Perioper. Nurs.* 1 998;7(4):2 16-21.
[733] Ranta PM, Ownby DR. A review of natural-rubber latex allergy in health care workers. *Clin. Infect. Dis.* 2004;38(2):252-6.
[734] Korniewicz DM, Kirwin M, Cresci K, et al. Barrier protection with examination gloves: double versus single. *Am. J. Infect. Control.* 1994;22(1):12-5.
[735] Korniewicz DM, Kirwin M, Cresci K, Larson E. Leakage of latex and vinyl exam gloves in high and low risk clinical settings. *Am. Ind. Hyg. Assoc. J.* 1993;54(1):22-6.
[736] Rego A, Roley L. In-use barrier integrity of gloves: latex and nitrile superior to vinyl. *Am. J. Infect. Control.* 1999;27(5):405-10.
[737] Kotilainen HR, Brinker JP, Avato JL, Gantz NM. Latex and vinyl examination gloves. Quality control procedures and implications for health care workers. *Arch. Intern. Med.* 1989;149(12):2749-53.
[738] Korniewicz DM, Laughon BE, Butz A, Larson E. Integrity of vinyl and latex procedure gloves. *Nurs. Res.* 1989;38(3):144-6.
[739] OSHA. OSHA. Department of Labor: Occupational Safety and Health Administration. Occupational exposure to bloodborne pathogens: Final rule. 29 CFR Part 1910:1030 Federal Register 1991;56:64003-64182 Revised 2001 CFR 66 2001 :5317-25.
[740] CDC. Recommendations for preventing the spread of vancomycin resistance. Recommendations of the Hospital Infection Control Practices Advisory Committee (HICPAC). *MMWR. Recomm. Rep.* 1995;44 (RR- 12): 1-13.
[741] Olsen RJ, Lynch P, Coyle MB, Cummings J, Bokete T, Stamm WE. Examination gloves as barriers to hand contamination in clinical practice. *JAMA.* 1993;270(3):350-3.
[742] Doebbeling BN, Pfaller MA, Houston AK, Wenzel RP. Removal of nosocomial pathogens from the contaminated glove. Implications for glove reuse and handwashing. *Ann. Intern. Med.* 1988;109(5):394-8.

[743] Maki DG, McCormick RD, Zilz MA, et al. A MRSA outbreak in an SICU during universal precautions: new epidemiology for nosocomial MRSA. Abstract # 473 Presented at the 30th Annual Meeting of the Interscience Conference on Antimicrobial Agents and Chemotherapy (ICAAC), Chicago, Illinois October 2 1-24, 1990.

[744] Boyce JM, Jackson MM, Pugliese G, et al. Methicillin-resistant Staphylococcus aureus (MRSA): a briefing for acute care hospitals and nursing facilities. The AHA Technical Panel on Infections Within Hospitals. *Infect. Control Hosp. Epidemiol.* 1994;15(2):105-15.

[745] Boyce JM, Mermel LA, Zervos MJ, et al. Controlling vancomycinresistant enterococci. *Infect. Control Hosp. Epidemiol.* 1995; 16(11): 634-7.

[746] Gerding DN, Johnson S, Peterson LR, Mulligan ME, Silva J, Jr. Clostridium difficile-associated diarrhea and colitis. *Infect. Control Hosp. Epidemiol.* 1995;16(8):459-77.

[747] Cloney DL, Donowitz LG. Overgrown use for infection control in nurseries and neonatal intensive care units. *Am. J. Dis. Child.* 1986; 140(7):680-3.

[748] Pelke S, Ching D, Easa D, Melish ME. Gowning does not affect colonization or infection rates in a neonatal intensive care unit. *Arch. Pediatr. Adolesc. Med.* 1994; 148(10): 1016-20.

[749] Slaughter S, Hayden MK, Nathan C, et al. A comparison of the effect of universal use of gloves and gowns with that of glove use alone on acquisition of vancomycin-resistant enterococci in a medical intensive care unit. *Ann. Intern. Med.* 1996;125(6):448-56.

[750] Duquette-Petersen L, Francis ME, Dohnalek L, Skinner R, Dudas P. The role of protective clothing in infection prevention in patients undergoing autologous bone marrow transplantation. Oncol Nurs Forum. 1 999;26(8): 1319-24. http://www.ons.org.

[751] Sartori M, La Terra G, Aglietta M, Manzin A, Navino C, Verzetti G. Transmission of hepatitis C via blood splash into conjunctiva. *Scand. J. Infect. Dis.* 1993;25(2):270-1.

[752] Hosoglu S, Celen MK, Akalin S, Geyik MF, Soyoral Y, Kara IH. Transmission of hepatitis C by blood splash into conjunctiva in a nurse. *Am. J. Infect. Control.* 2003;31(8):502-4.

[753] CDC. Update: human immunodeficiency virus infections in health-care workers exposed to blood of infected patients. *MMWR Morb. Mortal. Wkly. Rep.* 1987;36(19):285-9.

[754] Keijman J, Tjhie J, Olde Damink S, Alink M. Unusual nosocomial transmission of Mycobacterium tuberculosis. *Eur. J. Clin. Microbiol. Infect. Dis.* 2001;20(1 1):808-9.

[755] Weaver GH. Value of the face mask and other measures. *JAMA*. 1918;70:76.
[756] Weaver GH. Droplet infection and its prevention by the face mask. *J. Infect. Dis.* 1919;24:218-30.
[757] Davidson IR, Crisp AJ, Hinwood DC, Whitaker SC, Gregson RH. Eye splashes during invasive vascular procedures. *Br. J. Radiol.* 1 995;68(805):39-41.
[758] Guidance for Industry and FDA Staff - Surgical Masks - Premarket Notification [5 10(k)] Submissions; Guidance for Industry and FDA. http://www.fda.gov/cdrh/ode/guidance/094.html
[759] National Institute for Occupational Health and Safety - Eye Protection for Infection Control. http://www.cdc.gov/niosh/topics/eye/eye-infectious.html
[760] Gala CL, Hall CB, Schnabel KC, et al. The use of eye-nose goggles to control nosocomial respiratory syncytial virus infection. *Jama*. 1986;256(1 9):2706-8.
[761] Agah R, Cherry JD, Garakian AJ, Chapin M. Respiratory syncytial virus (RSV) infection rate in personnel caring for children with RSV infections. Routine isolation procedure vs routine procedure supplemented by use of masks and goggles. *Am. J. Dis. Child.* 1987;141(6):695-7.
[762] Thorburn K, Kerr S, Taylor N, van Saene HK. RSV outbreak in a paediatric intensive care unit. *J. Hosp. Infect.* 2004;57(3):194-201.
[763] http://a257.g.akamaitech.net/7/257/2422/06jun20041800/edocket.access. g po.gov/2004/04-25183.htm
[764] Occupational Safety & Health Administration - Respiratory Protection. www.osha.gov/dcsp/ote/trng-materials/respirators/respirators.html
[765] Campbell DL, Coffey CC, Lenhart SW. Respiratory protection as a function of respirator fitting characteristics and fit-test accuracy. *Aihaj.* 2001 ;62(1):36-44.
[766] Lee K, Slavcev A, Nicas M. Respiratory protection against Mycobacterium tuberculosis: quantitative fit test outcomes for five type N95 filtering-facepiece respirators. *J. Occup. Environ. Hyg.* 2004; 1(1) :22-8.
[767] Coffey CC, Campbell DL, Zhuang Z. Simulated workplace performance of N95 respirators. *Am. Ind. Hyg. Assoc. J.* 1999;60(5):618-24.
[768] Coffey CC, Lawrence RB, Zhuang Z, Campbell DL, Jensen PA, Myers WR. Comparison of five methods for fit-testing N95 filtering-facepiece respirators. *Appl. Occup. Environ. Hyg.* 2002;17(10):723-30.
[769] National Personal Protective Technology Laboratory. www.cdc.gov/niosh/npptl/.
[770] McGowan JE, Jr. Nosocomial tuberculosis: new progress in control and prevention. *Clin. Infect. Dis.* 1995;21(3):489-505.

[771] Jarvis WR. Nosocomial transmission of multidrug-resistant Mycobacterium tuberculosis. *Am. J. Infect. Control.* 1995;23(2):146-51.

[772] CDC. Emergency Preparedness & Response. wwwbtcdcgov 2003.

[773] Anderson JD, Bonner M, Scheifele DW, Schneider BC. Lack of nosocomial spread of Varicella in a pediatric hospital with negative pressure ventilated patient rooms. *Infect. Control.* 1985;6(3):120-1.

[774] Brunell PA, Wood D. Varicella serological status of healthcare workers as a guide to whom to test or immunize. *Infect. Control Hosp. Epidemiol.* 1999;20(5):355-7.

[775] Saiman L, LaRussa P, Steinberg SP, et al. Persistence of immunity to varicella-zoster virus after vaccination of healthcare workers. *Infect. Control Hosp. Epidemiol.* 2001;22(5):279-83.

[776] Willy ME, Koziol DE, Fleisher T, et al. Measles immunity in a population of healthcare workers. *Infect. Control Hosp. Epidemiol.* 1994;15(1):12-7.

[777] Wright LJ, Carlquist JF. Measles immunity in employees of a multihospital healthcare provider. *Infect. Control Hosp. Epidemiol.* 1994;15(1):8-11.

[778] CDC. Updated U.S. Public Health Service Guidelines for the Management of Occupational Exposures to HBV, HCV, and HIV. *MMWR Recomm. Rep.* 2001;50 (RR-11):1-52.

[779] Do AN, Ciesielski CA, Metler RP, Hammett TA, Li J, Fleming PL. Occupationally acquired human immunodeficiency virus (HIV) infection: national case surveillance data during 20 years of the HIV epidemic in the United States. *Infect.Control Hosp. Epidemiol.* 2003;24(2):86-96.

[780] CDC. Update: universal precautions for prevention of transmission of human immunodeficiency virus, hepatitis B virus, and other bloodborne pathogens in health-care settings. *MMWR Morb. Mortal Wkly Rep.* 1988;37(24):377-82, 87-8.

[781] Davis MS. Occupational hazards of operating: opportunities for improvement. *Infect. Control Hosp. Epidemiol.* 1996;17(10):691-3.

[782] Gerberding JL. Procedure-specific infection control for preventing intraoperative blood exposures. *Am. J. Infect. Control.* 1993;21(6):364-7.

[783] Fry DE, Telford GL, Fecteau DL, Sperling RS, Meyer AA. Prevention of blood exposure. Body and facial protection. *Surg. Clin. North Am.* 1995;75(6):1141-57.

[784] Hansen ME. Bloodborne pathogens and procedure safety in interventional radiology. *Semin. Ultrasound CT MR.* 1998;19(2):209-14.

[785] Holodnick CL, Barkauskas V. Reducing percutaneous injuries in the OR by educational methods. *Aorn. J.* 2000;72(3):461-4, 8-72, 75-6.

[786] www.osha.gov/SLTC/bloodbornepathogens/index.html

[787] www.cdc.gov/niosh/2000-108.html
[788] National Insititute for Occupational Health and Safety - Safer Medical Device Implementation in Health Care Facilities. http://www.cdc.gov/niosh/topics/bbp/safer/
[789] www.cdc.gov/sharpssafety/resources.html.
[790] Catanzaro A. Nosocomial tuberculosis. *Am. Rev. Respir. Dis.* 1982; 125(5):559-62.
[791] Cepeda JA, Whitehouse T, Cooper B, et al. Isolation of patients in single rooms or cohorts to reduce spread of MRSA in intensive-care units: prospective two-centre study. *Lancet.* 2005 ;3 65(9456) :295-304.
[792] Mulin B, Rouget C, Clement C, et al. Association of private isolation rooms with ventilator-associated Acinetobacter baumanii pneumonia in a surgical intensive-care unit. *Infect. Control Hosp. Epidemiol.* 1997; 1 8(7):499-503.
[793] www.aia.org/aah_gd_hospcons.
[794] Raad I, Abbas J, Whimbey E. Infection control of nosocomial respiratory viral disease in the immunocompromised host. *Am. J. Med.* 1997;102(3A):48-52; discussion 3-4.
[795] Isaacs D, Dickson H, O'Callaghan C, Sheaves R, Winter A, Moxon ER. Handwashing and cohorting in prevention of hospital acquired infections with respiratory syncytial virus. *Arch.Dis. Child.* 1991;66(2):227-31.
[796] Chang VT, Nelson K. The role of physical proximity in nosocomial diarrhea. *Clin. Infect. Dis.* 2000;31(3):717-22.
[797] Byers KE, Anglim AM, Anneski CJ, et al. A hospital epidemic of vancomycin-resistant Enterococcus: risk factors and control. *Infect. Control Hosp. Epidemiol.* 2001 ;22(3): 140-7.
[798] Dassut B. The implementation of a commode cleaning and identification system. *Nurs Times.* 2004;100(8):47.
[799] Mayer RA, Geha RC, Helfand MS, Hoyen CK, Salata RA, Donskey CJ. Role of fecal incontinence in contamination of the environment with vancomycin-resistant enterococci. *Am. J. Infect. Control.* 2003 ;3 1 (4):22 1-5.
[800] Samore MH, Venkataraman L, DeGirolami PC, Arbeit RD, Karchmer AW. Clinical and molecular epidemiology of sporadic and clustered cases of nosocomial Clostridium difficile diarrhea. *Am. J. Med.* 1996;100(1):3240.
[801] Clabots CR, Johnson S, Olson MM, Peterson LR, Gerding DN. Acquisition of Clostridium difficile by hospitalized patients: evidence for colonized new admissions as a source of infection. *J. Infect. Dis.* 1992; 1 66(3):561 -7.

[802] Samore MH. Epidemiology of nosocomial clostridium difficile diarrhoea. *J. Hosp. Infect.* 1999;43 Suppl:S183-90.
[803] Tokars JI, Satake S, Rimland D, et al. The prevalence of colonization with vancomycin-resistant Enterococcus at a Veterans' Affairs institution. *Infect. Control Hosp. Epidemiol.* 1 999;20(3):171-5.
[804] Cone R, Mohan K, Thouless M, Corey L. Nosocomial transmission of rotavirus infection. *Pediatr. Infect. Dis. J.* 1988;7(2):103-9.
[805] Bruce BB, Blass MA, Blumberg HM, Lennox JL, del Rio C, Horsburgh CR, Jr. Risk of Cryptosporidium parvum transmission between hospital roommates. *Clin. Infect. Dis.* 2000;3 1(4): 947-50.
[806] Ford-Jones EL, Mindorff CM, Gold R, Petric M. The incidence of viral-associated diarrhea after admission to a pediatric hospital. *Am. J. Epidemiol.* 1990;131(4):711-8.
[807] Murray-Leisure KA, Geib S, Graceley D, et al. Control of epidemic methicillin-resistant Staphylococcus aureus. *Infect. Control Hosp. Epidemiol.* 1990;1 1(7):343-50.
[808] Jochimsen EM, Fish L, Manning K, et al. Control of vancomycin-resistant enterococci at a community hospital: efficacy of patient and staff cohorting. *Infect. Control Hosp. Epidemiol.* 1999;20(2):106-9.
[809] Sample ML, Gravel D, Oxley C, Toye B, Garber G, Ramotar K. An outbreak of vancomycin-resistant enterococci in a hematology-oncology unit: control by patient cohorting and terminal cleaning of the environment. *Infect. Control Hosp. Epidemiol.* 2002;23 (8):468-70.
[810] Podnos YD, Cinat ME, Wilson SE, Cooke J, Gornick W, Thrupp LD. Eradication of multi-drug resistant *Acinetobacter* from an Intensive Care Unit. *Surgical Infections.* 2001 ;2(2):297-301.
[811] Graham PL, 3rd, Morel AS, Zhou J, et al. Epidemiology of methicillin-susceptible Staphylococcus aureus in the neonatal intensive care unit. Infect Control Hosp. Epidemiol. 2002;23(1 1):677-82.
[812] Doherty JA, Brookfield DS, Gray J, McEwan RA. Cohorting of infants with respiratory syncytial virus. *J. Hosp. Infect.* 1998;38(3):203-6.
[813] Hall CB, Geiman JM, Douglas RG, Jr., Meagher MP. Control of nosocomial respiratory syncytial viral infections. *Pediatrics.* 1 978;62(5):728-32.
[814] Buffington J, Chapman LE, Stobierski MG, et al. Epidemic keratoconjunctivitis in a chronic care facility: risk factors and measures for control. *J. Am. Geriatr. Soc.* 1993;41(11):1177-81.

[815] Grehn M, Kunz J, Sigg P, Slongo R, Zbinden R. Nosocomial rotavirus infections in neonates: means of prevention and control. *J. Perinat. Med.* 1990;18(5):369-74.

[816] Tan YM, Chow PK, Tan BH, et al. Management of inpatients exposed to an outbreak of severe acute respiratory syndrome (SARS). *J. Hosp. Infect.* 2004;58(3):210-5.

[817] Talon D, Vichard P, Muller A, Bertin M, Jeunet L, Bertrand X. Modelling the usefulness of a dedicated cohort facility to prevent the dissemination of MRSA. *J. Hosp. Infect.* 2003;54(1):57-62.

[818] Hotchkiss JR, Strike DG, Simonson DA, Broccard AF, Crooke PS. An agent-based and spatially explicit model of pathogen dissemination in the intensive care unit. *Crit. Care Med.* 2005;33(1):168-76; discussion 253-4.

[819] Austin DJ, Bonten MJ, Weinstein RA, Slaughter S, Anderson RM. Vancomycin-resistant enterococci in intensive-care hospital settings: transmission dynamics, persistence, and the impact of infection control programs. *Proc. Natl. Acad. Sci. U. S. A.* 1999;96(12):6908-13.

[820] Kovner CT, Harrington C. Counting nurses. Data show many nursing homes to be short staffed. *Am. J. Nurs.* 2000;100(9):53-4.

[821] Mueller C. Staffing problems in long-term care. Let's do something about it! *J. Gerontol. Nurs.* 2003;29(3):3-4.

[822] Stats & facts. Nursing staff shortages in long-term care facilities. *Manag. Care Interface.* 2000;13(11):46-7.

[823] Mejias A, Chavez-Bueno S, Ramilo O. Human metapneumovirus: a not so new virus. *Pediatr. Infect. Dis. J.* 2004;23(1):1-7; quiz 8-10.

[824] Iwane MK, Edwards KM, Szilagyi PG, et al. Population-based surveillance for hospitalizations associated with respiratory syncytial virus, influenza virus, and parainfluenza viruses among young children. *Pediatrics.* 2004;113(6):1758-64.

[825] Ong GM, Wyatt DE, O'Neill HJ, McCaughey C, Coyle PV. A comparison of nested polymerase chain reaction and immunofluorescence for the diagnosis of respiratory infections in children with bronchiolitis, and the implications for a cohorting strategy. *J. Hosp. Infect.* 2001;49(2):122-8.

[826] von Linstow ML, Larsen HH, Eugen-Olsen J, et al. Human metapneumovirus and respiratory syncytial virus in hospitalized danish children with acute respiratory tract infection. *Scan. J. Infect. Dise.* 2004;36:578-84.

[827] Gehanno JF, Pestel-Caron M, Nouvellon M, Caillard JF. Nosocomial pertussis in healthcare workers from a pediatric emergency unit in France. *Infect. Control. Hosp. Epidemiol.* 1999;20(8):549-52.

[828] www.cdc.gov/flu/professionals/infectioncontrol/resphygiene.htm.
[829] Edlin BR, Tokars JI, Grieco MH, et al. An outbreak of multidrug-resistant tuberculosis among hospitalized patients with the acquired immunodeficiency syndrome. *N. Engl. J. Med.* 1992;326(23):1514-21.
[830] CDC. Update: Severe Acute Respiratory Syndrome --- Toronto, Canada, 2003. *MMWR.* 2003;52(23):547-50.
[831] Starke JR. Transmission of *Mycobacterium tuberculosis* to and from children and adolescents. *Seminars Pedi. Infect. Dis.* 2001; 12:115-23.
[832] Saiman L, Macdonald N, Burns JL, Hoiby N, Speert DP, Weber D. Infection control in cystic fibrosis: practical recommendations for the hospital, clinic, and social settings. *Am. J. Infect. Control.* 2000;28(5):3815. (s).
[833] COID. 2003 Report of the Committee on Infectious Diseases. In: Redbook. Elk Grove Village, IL: American Academy of Pediatrics; 2003.
[834] Lau JT, Lau M, Kim JH, Tsui HY, Tsang T, Wong TW. Probable secondary infections in households of SARS patients in Hong Kong. *Emerg. Infect. Dis.* 2004; 10(2):235-43.
[835] Hota B. Contamination, disinfection, and cross-colonization: are hospital surfaces reservoirs for nosocomial infection? *Clin. Infect. Dis.* 2004;39(8): 1182-9.
[836] Rutala WA, Weber DJ. Disinfection and sterilization in health care facilities: what clinicians need to know. *Clin. Infect. Dis.* 2004;39(5):702-9.
[837] Boyce JM, Opal SM, Chow JW, et al. Outbreak of multidrug-resistant *Enterococcus faecium* with transferable vanB class vancomycin resistance. J. *Clin. Microbiol.* 1 994;32(5): 1148-53.
[838] Engelhart S, Krizek L, Glasmacher A, Fischnaller E, Marklein G, Exner M. Pseudomonas aeruginosa outbreak in a haematology-oncology unit associated with contaminated surface cleaning equipment. *J. Hosp. Infect.* 2002;52(2):93-8.
[839] Denton M, Wilcox MH, Parnell P, et al. Role of environmental cleaning in controlling an outbreak of Acinetobacter baumannii on a neurosurgical intensive care unit. *J. Hosp. Infect.* 2004;56(2):106-10.
[840] Hollyoak V, Allison D, Summers J. Pseudomonas aeruginosa wound infection associated with a nursing home's whirlpool bath. *Commun. Dis. Rep. CDR. Rev.* 1995;5(7):R100-2.
[841] Malik RE, Cooper RA, Griffith CJ. Use of audit tools to evaluate the efficacy of cleaning systems in hospitals. *Am. J. Infect. Control.* 2003;3 1(3): 181-7.

[842] Ansari SA, Springthorpe VS, Sattar SA. Survival and vehicular spread of human rotaviruses: possible relation to seasonality of outbreaks. *Rev. Infect. Dis.* 1991;13(3):448-61.

[843] Kaatz GW, Gitlin SD, Schaberg DR, et al. Acquisition of Clostridium difficile from the hospital environment. *Am. J. Epidemiol.* 1988; 127(6): 1289-94.

[844] Mayfield JL, Leet T, Miller J, Mundy LM. Environmental control to reduce transmission of Clostridium difficile. Clin. Infect. Dis. 2000;3 1(4):995-1000.

[845] Dennehy PH. Transmission of rotavirus and other enteric pathogens in the home. *Pediatr. Infect. Dis. J.* 2000;19(10 Suppl):S103-5.

[846] Dennehy P. Rotavirus infections in infection control reference service. In: Abrutyn E, Goldmann D, Scheckler W, eds. Philadelphia: WE Saunders; 2001:821-3.

[847] Wilcox MH, Fawley WN, Wigglesworth N, Parnell P, Verity P, Freeman J. Comparison of the effect of detergent versus hypochlorite cleaning on environmental contamination and incidence of Clostridium difficile infection. *J. Hosp. Infect.* 2003;54(2):109-14.

[848] Rutala WA, Weber DJ, Committee HICPA. Guideline for Disinfection and Sterilization in Health-Care Facilities 2007 (in press).

[849] Bernards AT, Harinck HI, Dijkshoorn L, van der Reijden TJ, van den Broek PJ. Persistent Acinetobacter baumannii? Look inside your medical equipment. *Infect. Control. Hosp. Epidemiol.* 2004;25(1 1):1002-4.

[850] Neely AN, Weber JM, Daviau P, et al. Computer equipment used in patient care within a multihospital system: recommendations for cleaning and disinfection. *Am. J. Infect. Control.* 2005;33(4):233-7.

[851] Neely AN, Maley MP, Warden GD. Computer keyboards as reservoirs for Acinetobacter baumannii in a burn hospital. *Clin. Infect. Dis.* 1 999;29(5): 1358-60.

[852] Bures S, Fishbain JT, Uyehara CF, Parker JM, Berg BW. Computer keyboards and faucet handles as reservoirs of nosocomial pathogens in the intensive care unit. *Am. J. Infect. Control.* 2000;28(6):465-71.

[853] Brooks S, Khan A, Stoica D, et al. Reduction in vancomycin-resistant *Enterococcus* and *Clostridium difficile* infections following change to tympanic thermometers. *Infect. Control Hosp. Epidemiol.* 1998; 1 9(5):333-6.

[854] Jernigan JA, Siegman-Igra Y, Guerrant RC, Farr BM. A randomized crossover study of disposable thermometers for prevention of Clostridium difficile and other nosocomial infections. *Infect. Control Hosp. Epidemiol.* 1998; 1 9(7):494-9.

[855] Weinstein SA, Gantz NM, Pelletier C, Hibert D. Bacterial surface contamination of patients' linen: isolation precautions versus standard care. *Am. J. Infect. Control.* 1989;17(5):264-7.

[856] Pugliese G. Isolating and double-bagging laundry: is it really necessary? *Health Facil Manage.* 1989;2(2):16, 8-21.

[857]. (Accessed 2007, at

[858] Kiehl E, Wallace R, Warren C. Tracking perinatal infection: is it safe to launder your scrubs at home? *MCN Am. J. Matern. Child Nurs.* 1 997;22(4): 195-7.

[859] Jurkovich P. Home- versus hospital-laundered scrubs: a pilot study. *MCN Am. J. Matern. Child Nurs.* 2004;29(2):106-10.

[860] United States Environmental Protection Agency - Medical Waste. www.epa.gov/epaoswer/other/medical/

[861] www.cdc.gov/ncidod/dhqp/gl environinfection.html

[862] Maki DG, Alvarado C, Hassemer C. Double-bagging of items from isolation rooms is unnecessary as an infection control measure: a comparative study of surface contamination with single- and double- bagging. *Infect. Control.* 1986;7(1 1):535-7.

[863] CDC. Recommended antimicrobial agents for the treatment and postexposure prophylaxis of pertussis: 2005 CDC Guidelines. *MMWR Recomm. Rep.* 2005;54(RR-14):1-16.

[864] CDC. Prevention and control of meningococcal disease. Recommendations of the Advisory Committee on Immunization Practices (ACIP). *MMWR Recomm. Rep.* 2000;49(RR-7):1-10.

[865] CDC. Notice to Readers: Additional options for preventive treatment for persons exposed to inhalational anthrax. *MMWR Morb. Mortal Wkly. Rep.* 2001;50 (50):1142-51.

[866] CDC. Updated U.S. Public Health Service guidelines for the management of occupational *exposures to HIV and recommendations for postexposure prophylaxis. MMWR Recomm. Rep.* 2005;54(RR-9):1-17.

[867] Boyce JM. MRSA patients: proven methods to treat colonization and infection. *J. Hosp. Infect.* 2001;48 Suppl A:S9-14.

[868] Barrett FF, Mason EO, Jr., Fleming D. Brief clinical and laboratory observations. *J. Pediatr.* 1 979;94(5) :796-800.

[869] American Academy of Pediatrics. Guidelines for Perinatal Care. American Academy of Obstetricians and Gynecologists, 2002. Elk Grove Village, Il; 2002.

[870] Management of Multidrug-Resistant Organisms In Healthcare Settings, 2006. CDC, 2006. (Accessed 2007, at

[871] Kallen AJ, Wilson CT, Larson RJ. Perioperative intranasal mupirocin for the prevention of surgical-site infections: systematic review of the literature and meta-analysis. *Infect. Control Hosp. Epidemiol.* 2005;26(12):91 6-22.
[872] Carrier M, Marchand R, Auger P, et al. Methicillin-resistant Staphylococcus aureus infection in a cardiac surgical unit. *J. Thorac. Cardiovasc. Surg.* 2002;123(1):40-4.
[873] Tacconelli E, Carmeli Y, Aizer A, Ferreira G, Foreman MG, D'Agata EM. Mupirocin prophylaxis to prevent Staphylococcus aureus infection in patients undergoing dialysis: a meta-analysis. *Clin. Infect. Dis.* 2003;37(12): 1629-38.
[874] CDC. Immunization of health-care workers: recommendations of the Advisory Committee on Immunization Practices (ACIP) and the Hospital Infection Control Practices Advisory Committee (HICPAC). *MMWR Recomm. Rep.* 1997;46(RR18):1-42.
[875] Mahoney FJ, Stewart K, Hu H, Coleman P, Alter MJ. Progress toward the elimination of hepatitis B virus transmission among health care workers in the United States. *Arch. Intern. Med.* 1997;157(22):2601-5.
[876] Gladstone JL, Millian SJ. Rubella exposure in an obstetric clinic. *Obstet. Gynecol.* 1981 ;57(2): 182-6.
[877] Wilde JA, McMillan JA, Serwint J, Butta J, O'Riordan MA, Steinhoff MC. Effectiveness of influenza vaccine in health care professionals: a randomized trial. *JAMA.* 1999;281(10):908-13.
[878] Potter J, Stott DJ, Roberts MA, et al. Influenza vaccination of health care workers in long-term-care hospitals reduces the mortality of elderly patients. *J. Infect. Dis.* 1997;175(1): 1-6.
[879] Pearson ML, Bridges CB, Harper SA. Influenza vaccination of health-care personnel: recommendations of the Healthcare Infection Control Practices Advisory Committee (HICPAC) and the Advisory Committee on Immunization Practices (ACIP). *MMWR Recomm. Rep.* 2006;55(RR-2):116.
[880] Wright SW, Decker MD, Edwards KM. Incidence of pertussis infection in healthcare workers. *Infect. Control. Hosp. Epidemiol.* 1 999;20(2):120-3.
[881] Calugar A, Ortega-Sanchez IR, Tiwari T, Oakes L, Jahre JA, Murphy TV. Nosocomial pertussis: costs of an outbreak and benefits of vaccinating health care workers. *Clin. Infect. Dis.* 2006;42(7):981-8.
[882] www.fda.gov
[883] Campins-Marti M, Cheng HK, Forsyth K, et al. Recommendations are needed for adolescent and adult pertussis immunisation: rationale and strategies for consideration. *Vaccine.* 2001;20(5-6):641-6.
[884] www.cdc.gov/nip/recs/provisional_recs/default.htm

[885] CDC. Recommended childhood and adolescent immunization schedule -- United States, 2006. *MMWR Morb. Mortal Wkly. Rep.* 2006;54(Nos. 51 & 52):Q1-Q4.

[886] Recommended childhood and adolescent immunization schedule-- United States, 2006. *Pediatrics.* 2006;117(1):239-40.

[887] CDC. Recommended adult immunization schedule -- United States, October 2005-September 2006. *MMWR Morb. Mortal Wkly. Rep.* 2005;54(40):Q1-Q4; October 14.

[888] CDC. Prevention of Varicella Updated Recommendations of the Advisory Committee on Immunization Practices (ACIP). *MMWR Morb. Mortal Wkly. Rep.* 1999;48 (RR-6):1-5.

[889] McKenney D, Pouliot KL, Wang Y, et al. Broadly protective vaccine for Staphylococcus aureus based on an in vivo-expressed antigen. *Science.* 1999;284(5419): 1523-7.

[890] Shinefield H, Black S, Fattom A, et al. Use of a Staphylococcus aureus conjugate vaccine in patients receiving hemodialysis. *N. Engl. J. Med.* 2002;346(7):491-6.

[891] Abadesso C, Almeida HI, Virella D, Carreiro MH, Machado MC. Use of palivizumab to control an outbreak of syncytial respiratory virus in a neonatal intensive care unit. *J. Hosp. Infect.* 2004;58(1):38-41.

[892] George RH, Gully PR, Gill ON, Innes JA, Bakhshi SS, Connolly M. An outbreak of tuberculosis in a children's hospital. *J. Hosp. Infect.* 1986;8(2): 129-42.

[893] Simor AE, Lee M, Vearncombe M, et al. An outbreak due to multiresistant Acinetobacter baumannii in a burn unit: risk factors for acquisition and management. *Infect. Control Hosp. Epidemiol.* 2002;23(5):261-7.

[894] Puzniak LA, Leet T, Mayfield J, Kollef M, Mundy LM. To gown or not to gown: the effect on acquisition of vancomycin-resistant enterococci. *Clin. Infect. Dis.* 2002;35(1):18-25.

[895] Hanna H, Umphrey J, Tarrand J, Mendoza M, Raad I. Management of an outbreak of vancomycin-resistant enterococci in the medical intensive care unit of a cancer center. *Infect. Control Hosp. Epidem*iol. 2001;22(4):217-9.

[896] CDC. Recommendations for preventing transmission of infection with human T- lymphotropic virus type III/lymphadenopathy-associated virus in the workplace. *MMWR Morb. Mortal Wkly. Rep.* 1985;34(450:681-6, 91-5.

[897] CDC. Severe acute respiratory syndrome--Taiwan, 2003. *MMWR Morb. Mortal Wkly. Rep.* 2003;52(20):461-6.

[898] Capps JA. Measures for the prevention and control of respiratory infections in military camps. *JAMA* 1918;71:448-51.

[899] Thomas C. Efficiency of surgical masks in use in hospital wards. Report to the Control of Infection Subcommittee. *Guys Hosp. Rep.* 1961;110:157-67.

[900] Beck M, Antle BJ, Berlin D, et al. Wearing masks in a pediatric hospital: developing practical guidelines. *Can. J. Public Health.* 2004;95(4):256-7.

[901] Ryan MA, Christian RS, Wohlrabe J. Handwashing and respiratory illness among young adults in military training. *Am. J. Prev. Med.* 2001;21(2):79-83.

[902] Roberts L, Smith W, Jorm L, Patel M, Douglas RM, McGilchrist C. Effect of infection control measures on the frequency of upper respiratory infection in child care: a randomized, controlled trial. *Pediatrics.* 2000;105(4 Pt 1):738-42.js.

[903] White C, Kolble R, Carlson R, et al. The effect of hand hygiene on illness rate among students in university residence halls. *Am. J. Infect. Control.* 2003;31(6):364-70.

[904] Aiello AE, Larson EL. What is the evidence for a causal link between hygiene and infections? *Lancet. Infect. Dis.* 2002;2(2):103-10.

[905] www.aana.com/news.aspx?ucNavMenu_TSMenuTargetID=171&ucNavMenu_TSMenuTargetType=4&ucNavMenu_TSMenuID=6&id=1 613.

[906] Watanakunakorn C, Stahl C. Streptococcus salivarius meningitis following myelography. *Infect. Control Hosp. Epidemiol.* 1992; 13(8):454.

[907] Gelfand MS, Abolnik IZ. Streptococcal meningitis complicating diagnostic myelography: three cases and review. *Clin. Infect. Dis.* 1 995;20(3):582-7.

[908] Schlesinger JJ, Salit IE, McCormack G. Streptococcal meningitis after myelography. *Arch. Neurol.* 1 982;3 9(9): 576-7.

[909] Yaniv LG, Potasman I. Iatrogenic meningitis: an increasing role for resistant viridans streptococci? Case report and review of the last 20 years. *Scand. J. Infect. Dis.* 2000;32(6):693-6.

[910] Schlegel L, Merlet C, Laroche JM, Fremaux A, Geslin P. Iatrogenic meningitis due to Abiotrophia defectiva after myelography. *Clin. Infect. Dis.* 1999;28(1): 155-6.

[911] Schneeberger PM, Janssen M, Voss A. Alpha-hemolytic streptococci: a major pathogen of iatrogenic meningitis following lumbar puncture. Case reports and a review of the literature. *Infection.* 1 996;24(1):29-33.

[912] Veringa E, van Belkum A, Schellekens H. Iatrogenic meningitis by Streptococcus salivarius following lumbar puncture. *J. Hosp. Infect.* 1995;29(4):3 16-8.

[913] Couzigou C, Vuong TK, Botherel AH, Aggoune M, Astagneau P. Iatrogenic Streptococcus salivarius meningitis after spinal anaesthesia: need for strict application of standard precautions. *J. Hosp. Infect.* 2003;53(4):3 13-4.

[914] Torres E, Alba D, Frank A, Diez-Tejedor E. Iatrogenic meningitis due to Streptococcus salivarius following a spinal tap. *Clin. Infect. Dis.* 1993; 17(3):525-6.

[915] Trautmann M, Lepper PM, Schmitz FJ. Three cases of bacterial meningitis after spinal and epidural anesthesia. *Eur. J. Clin. Microbiol. Infect. Dis.* 2002;21(1):43-5.

[916] Baer ET. Iatrogenic meningitis: the case for face masks. *Clin. Infect. Dis.* 2000;31(2):519-21.

[917] Black SR, Weinstein RA. The case for face masks-zorro or zero? *Clin. Infect. Dis.* 2000;31(2):522-3.

[918] Philips BJ, Fergusson S, Armstrong P, Anderson FM, Wildsmith JA. Surgical face masks are effective in reducing bacterial contamination caused by dispersal from the upper airway. *Br. J. Anaesth.* 1992;69(4):4078.

[919] CDC. Guidelines for the Prevention of Intravascular Catheter-Related Infections. *MMWR.* 2002;5 1 (RR1 0)(1 0): 1-26.

[920] Catalano G, Houston SH, Catalano MC, et al. Anxiety and depression in hospitalized patients in resistant organism isolation. *South Med. J.* 2003;96(2): 141-5.

[921] Tarzi S, Kennedy P, Stone S, Evans M. Methicillin-resistant Staphylococcus aureus: psychological impact of hospitalization and isolation in an older adult population. *J. Hosp. Infect.* 2001 ;49(4):250-4.

[922] Kelly-Rossini L, Perlman DC, Mason DJ. The experience of respiratory isolation for HIV-infected persons with tuberculosis. *J. Assoc. Nurses AIDS Care.* 1996;Jan-Feb; 7(1):29-36.

[923] Knowles HE. The experience of infectious patients in isolation. *Nurs. Times.* 1993;89(30):53-6.

[924] Evans HL, Shaffer MM, Hughes MG, et al. Contact isolation in surgical patients: a barrier to care? *Surgery.* 2003; 134(2): 180-8.

[925] Kirkland KB, Weinstein JM. Adverse effects of contact isolation. *Lancet.* 1999;354(9185):1 177-8.

[926] Saint S, Higgins LA, Nallamothu BK, Chenoweth C. Do physicians examine patients in contact isolation less frequently? A brief report. *Am. J. Infect. Control.* 2003;31(6):354-6.

[927] Management of Multidrug-Resistant Organisms In Healthcare Settings, 2006. 2006. www.cdc.gov/ncidod/dhqp/pdf/ar/mdroGuideline2006.pdf

[928] Hall CB, Powell KR, MacDonald NE, et al. Respiratory syncytial viral infection in children with compromised immune function. *N. Engl. J. Med.* 1986;3 1 5(2):77-81.

[929] Lui SL, Luk WK, Cheung CY, Chan TM, Lai KN, Peiris JS. Nosocomial outbreak of parvovirus B19 infection in a renal transplant unit. *Transplantation.* 2001 ;71(1):59-64.

[930] Weinstock DM, Gubareva LV, Zuccotti G. Prolonged shedding of multidrug-resistant influenza A virus in an immunocompromised patient. *N. Engl. J. Med.* 2003;348(9):867-8.

[931] van Tol MJ, Claas EC, Heemskerk B, et al. Adenovirus infection in children after allogeneic stem cell transplantation: diagnosis, treatment and immunity. *Bone Marrow Transplant.* 2005;35 Suppl 1:S73-6.

[932] Wood DJ, David TJ, Chrystie IL, Totterdell B. Chronic enteric virus infection in two T-cell immunodeficient children. *J. Med. Virol.* 1988;24(4):435-44.

[933] 933. Mori I, Matsumoto K, Sugimoto K, et al. Prolonged shedding of rotavirus in a geriatric inpatient. *J. Med. Virol.* 2002;67(4):613-5.

[934] Cederna JE, Terpenning MS, Ensberg M, Bradley SF, Kauffman CA. Staphylococcus aureus nasal colonization in a nursing home: eradication with mupirocin. *Infect. Control Hosp. Epidemiol.* 1990;1 1(1):13-6.

[935] Kauffman CA, Terpenning MS, He X, et al. Attempts to eradicate methicillin-resistant Staphylococcus aureus from a long-term-care facility with the use of mupirocin ointment. *Am. J. Med.* 1993;94(4):371-8.

[936] Montecalvo MA, de Lencastre H, Carraher M, et al. Natural history of colonization with vancomycin-resistant Enterococcus faecium. *Infect. Control Hosp. Epidemiol.* 1995; 16(12): 680-5.

[937] D'Agata EM, et al. High rate of false-negative results of the rectal swab culture method in detection of gastrointestinal colonization with vancomycin-resistant enterococci. *Clin. Infect. Dis.* 2002;34(2): 167-72.

[938] Donskey CJ, Hoyen CK, Das SM, Helfand MS, Hecker MT. Recurrence of vancomycin-resistant Enterococcus stool colonization during antibiotic therapy. *Infect. Control Hosp. Epidemiol.* 2002;23 (8) :436-40.

[939] Scanvic A, Denic L, Gaillon S, Giry P, Andremont A, Lucet JC. Duration of colonization by methicillin-resistant Staphylococcus aureus after hospital discharge and risk factors for prolonged carriage. *Clin. Infect. Dis.* 2001 ;32(10): 1393-8.

[940] Noskin GA, Bednarz P, Suriano T, Reiner S, Peterson LR. Persistent contamination of fabric-covered furniture by vancomycin-resistant

enterococci: implications for upholstery selection in hospitals. *Am. J. Infect. Control.* 2000;28(4):31 1-3.

[941] Gerson SL, Parker P, Jacobs MR, Creger R, Lazarus HM. Aspergillosis due to carpet contamination. *Infect. Control Hosp. Epidemiol.* 1994;15(4 Pt 1):221-3.

[942] Taplin D, Mertz PM. Flower vases in hospitals as reservoirs of pathogens. *Lancet.* 1973;2(7841): 1279-81.

[943] Walsh TJ, Dixon DM. Nosocomial aspergillosis: environmental microbiology, hospital epidemiology, diagnosis and treatment. *Eur. J. Epidemiol.* 1989;5(2):131-42.

[944] Lass-Florl C, Rath P, Niederwieser D, et al. Aspergillus terreus infections in haematological malignancies: molecular epidemiology suggests association with in-hospital plants. *J. Hosp. Infect.* 2000;46(1):31-5.

[945] Raad I, Hanna H, Osting C, et al. Masking of neutropenic patients on transport from hospital rooms is associated with a decrease in nosocomial *aspergillosis during construction.* Infect. Control Hosp. Epidemiol. 2002;23(1):41-3.

[946] www.cms.hhs.gov/CLIA.

[947] Emori TG, Haley RW, Stanley RC. The infection control nurse in US hospitals, 1976-1977. Characteristics of the position and its occupant. *Am. J. Epidemiol.* 1980;1 1 1(5):592-607.

[948] Richet HM, Benbachir M, Brown DE, et al. Are there regional variations in the diagnosis, surveillance, and control of methicillin-resistant Staphylococcus aureus? *Infect. Control Hosp. Epidemiol.* 2003;24(5):33441.

[949] Anderson DJ, Kirkland KB, McDonald JR, et al. Results of a survey of work duties of 56 infection control professionals (ICPs): Are new guidelines needed for the staffing of infection control (IC) programs? Abstract #146. In: 16th Annual Society for Healthcare Epidemiology of America. Chicago, Ill; 2006.

[950] Harvey MA. Critical-care-unit bedside design and furnishing: impact on nosocomial infections. *Infect. Control Hosp. Epidemiol.* 1998;19(8):597601.

[951] Srinivasan A, Beck C, Buckley T, et al. The ability of hospital ventilation systems to filter Aspergillus and other fungi following a building implosion. *Infect. Control Hosp. Epidemiol.* 2002;23(9):520-4.

[952] Maragakis LL, Bradley KL, Song X, et al. Increased catheter-related bloodstream infection rates after the introduction of a new mechanical valve intravenous access port. *Infect. Control Hosp. Epidemiol.* 2006;27(1):67-70.

[953] Organizations JCoAoH. Comprehensive Accredication Manual for Hospitals: The Official Handbook. Oakbrook Terrace: JCAHO; 2007.

[954] Peterson LR, Noskin GA. New technology for detecting multidrugresistant pathogens in the clinical microbiology laboratory. *Emerg. Infect. Dis.* 2001;7(2):306-1 1.
[955] Diekema DJ, Doebbeling BN. Employee health and infection control. *Infect. Control Hosp. Epidemiol.* 1995; 16(5) :292-301.
[956] Rutala WA, Weber DJ, Healthcare Infection Control Practices Advisory Committee (HICPAC). Guideline for Disinfection and Sterilization in Health-Care Facilities. In preparation.
[957] Weems JJ, Jr. Nosocomial outbreak of Pseudomonas cepacia associated with contamination of reusable electronic ventilator temperature probes. *Infect. Control Hosp. Epidemiol.* 1993; 14(10): 583-6.
[958] Berthelot P, Grattard F, Mahul P, et al. Ventilator temperature sensors: an unusual source of Pseudomonas cepacia in nosocomial infection. *J. Hosp. Infect.* 1993;25(1):33-43.
[959] CDC. Bronchoscopy-related infections and pseudoinfections--New York, 1996 and 1998. *MMWR Morb. Mortal Wkly. Rep.* 1999;48(26):55760.
[960] Heeg P, Roth K, Reichl R, Cogdill CP, Bond WW. Decontaminated single-use devices: an oxymoron that may be placing patients at risk for cross-contamination. *Infect. Control Hosp. Epidemiol.* 2001 ;22(9): 542-9.
[961] www.fda.gov/cdrh/reprocessing/
[962] CDC. Prevention and Control of Influenza: Recommendations of the Advisory Committee on Immunization Practices (ACIP). *MMWR - Morbidity & Mortality Weekly Report.* 2003 ;52(RR08):1-36.
[963] Weinstock DM, Eagan J, Malak SA, et al. Control of influenza A on a bone marrow transplant unit. *Infect. Control Hosp. Epidemiol.* 2000;21(1 1):730-2.
[964] Cromer AL, Hutsell SO, Latham SC, et al. Impact of implementing a method of feedback and accountability related to contact precautions compliance. *Am. J. Infect. Control.* 2004;32(8):451-5.
[965] Eveillard M, Eb F, Tramier B, et al. Evaluation of the contribution of isolation precautions in prevention and control of multi-resistant bacteria in a teaching hospital. *J. Hosp. Infect.* 2001;47(2):1 16-24.
[966] Pfeiffer J, Gilmore G. The Text as an Orientation Tool. In: Pfeiffer J, ed. APIC Text of Infection Control and Epidemiology. Washingto, DC: Association for Professionals in Infection Control and Epidemiology, Inc. (APIC); 2000:7/1 - 7/8.
[967] Gaynes RP, Emori TG. Chapter 5: Surveillance for Nosocomial Infections. In: Abrutyn E, Goldmann DA, Scheckler WE, eds. Saunders Infection Control Reference Service. Philadelphia, PA: W.B. Saunders Company; 2001:40-4.

[968] CDC. Monitoring hospital-acquired infections to promote patient safety--United States, 1990-1999. *MMWR Morb. Mortal Wkly. Rep.* 2000;49(8): 149-53.

[969] Curran ET, Benneyan JC, Hood J. Controlling methicillin-resistant Staphylococcus aureus: a feedback approach using annotated statistical process control charts. *Infect. Control Hosp. Epidemiol.* 2002;23(1):13-8.

[970] Lanotte P, Cantagrel S, Mereghetti L, et al. Spread of Stenotrophomonas maltophilia colonization in a pediatric intensive care unit detected by monitoring tracheal bacterial carriage and molecular typing. *Clin. Microbiol. Infect.* 2003;9(11):1142-7.

[971] Coopersmith CM, Zack JE, Ward MR, et al. The impact of bedside behavior on catheter-related bacteremia in the intensive care unit. *Arch. Surg.* 2004;139(2):131-6.

[972] O'Brien KL, Beall B, Barrett NL, et al. Epidemiology of invasive group a streptococcus disease in the United States, 1995-1999. *Clin. Infect. Dis.* 2002;35(3):268-76.

[973] Nicolle LE, Dyck B, Thompson G, et al. Regional dissemination and control of epidemic methicillin-resistant Staphylococcus aureus. Manitoba Chapter of CHICA-Canada. *Infect. Control Hosp. Epidemiol.* 1999;20(3):202-5.

[974] Seybold U, Kourbatova EV, Johnson JG, et al. Emergence of community-associated methicillin-resistant Staphylococcus aureus USA300 genotype as a major cause of health care-associated blood stream infections. *Clin. Infect. Dis.* 2006;42(5):647-56.

[975] Bond WW, Favero MS, Petersen NJ, Gravelle CR, Ebert JW, Maynard JE. Survival of hepatitis B virus after drying and storage for one week. *Lancet.* 1981;1(8219):550-1.

[976] Ehrenkranz NJ, Alfonso BC. Failure of bland soap handwash to prevent hand transfer of patient bacteria to urethral catheters. *Infect. Control Hosp. Epidemiol.* 1991;12(11):654-62.

[977] Winnefeld M, Richard MA, Drancourt M, Grob JJ. Skin tolerance and effectiveness of two hand decontamination procedures in everyday hospital use. *Br. J. Dermatol.* 2000;143(3):546-50.

[978] Widmer AF. Replace hand washing with use of a waterless alcohol hand rub? *Clin. Infect. Dis.* 2000;31(1):136-43.

[979] Mortimer EA, Jr., Lipsitz PJ, Wolinsky E, Gonzaga AJ, Rammelkamp CH, Jr. Transmission of staphylococci between newborns. Importance of the hands to personnel. *Am. J. Dis. Child.* 1962;104:289-95.

[980] Casewell M, Phillips I. Hands as route of transmission for Klebsiella species. *Br. Med. J.* 1977;2(6098):1315-7.
[981] Ojajarvi J. Effectiveness of hand washing and disinfection methods in removing transient bacteria after patient nursing. *J. Hyg.* (Lond) 1 980;85(2): 193-203.
[982] Otter J, Havill N, Adams N, Joyce J. Extensive environmental contamination associated with patients with loose stools and MRSA colonization of the gastrointestinal tract. Abstract #159. In: the 16th annual scientific meeting of the Society for Healthcare Epidemiology of America. In. Chicago, Illinois; 2006.
[983] Weber DJ, Sickbert-Bennett E, Gergen MF, Rutala WA. Efficacy of selected hand hygiene agents used to remove Bacillus atrophaeus (a surrogate of Bacillus anthracis) from contaminated hands. *Jama.* 2003 ;289(10): 1274-7.
[984] Saiman L, Lerner A, Saal L, et al. Banning artificial nails from health care settings. *Am. J. Infect. Control.* 2002;30(4):252-4.
[985] Johnson S, Gerding DN, Olson MM, et al. Prospective, controlled study of vinyl glove use to interrupt Clostridium difficile nosocomial transmission. *Am. J. Med.* 1990;88(2):137-40.
[986] Neal JG, Jackson EM, Suber F, Edlich RF. Latex glove penetration by pathogens: a review of the literature. *J. Long Term Eff. Med. Implants.* 1 998;8(3-4):233-40.
[987] Broyles JM, O'Connell KP, Korniewicz DM. PCR-based method for detecting viral penetration of medical exam gloves. *J. Clin. Microbiol.* 2002;40(8):2725-8.
[988] Patterson JE, Vecchio J, Pantelick EL, et al. Association of contaminated gloves with transmission of Acinetobacter calcoaceticus var. anitratus in an intensive care unit. *Am. J. Med.* 1991;91(5):479-83.
[989] Goldmann DA. Epidemiology and prevention of pediatric viral respiratory infections in health-care institutions. *Emerg. Infect. Dis.* 2001;7(2):249-53.
[990] Gaggero A, Avendano LF, Fernandez J, Spencer E. Nosocomial transmission of rotavirus from patients admitted with diarrhea. *J. Clin. Microbiol.* 1992;30(12):3294-7.
[991] Merritt K, Hitchins VM, Brown SA. Safety and cleaning of medical materials and devices. *J. Biomed. Mater. Res.* 2000;53(2):131-6.
[992] Kampf G, Bloss R, Martiny H. Surface fixation of dried blood by glutaraldehyde and peracetic acid. *J. Hosp. Infect.* 2004;57(2):139-43.

[993] Weber DJ, Rutala WA. Role of environmental contamination in the transmission of vancomycin-resistant enterococci. *Infect. Control Hosp. Epidemiol.* 1997; 1 8(5):306-9.

[994] Byers KE, Durbin LJ, Simonton BM, Anglim AM, Adal KA, Farr BM. Disinfection of hospital rooms contaminated with vancomycin-resistant Enterococcus faecium. *Infect. Control Hosp. Epidemiol.* 1998;19(4):261-4.

[995] Martinez JA, Ruthazer R, Hansjosten K, Barefoot L, Snydman DR. Role of environmental contamination as a risk factor for acquisition of vancomycin-resistant enterococci in patients treated in a medical intensive care unit. *Arch. Intern. Med.* 2003;163(16):1905-12.

[996] EPA. Federal Insecticide, Fungicide, and Rodenticidal Act 7 U.S.C. 136 et seq. In: Agency EP, ed.

[997] Devine J, Cooke RP, Wright EP. Is methicillin-resistant Staphylococcus aureus (MRSA) contamination of ward-based computer terminals a surrogate marker for nosocomial MRSA transmission and handwashing compliance? *J. Hosp. Infect.* 2001;48(1):72-5.

[998] Sattar SA, Springthorpe S, Mani S, et al. Transfer of bacteria from fabrics to hands and other fabrics: development and application of a quantitative method using Staphylococcus aureus as a model. *J. Appl. Microbiol.* 2001;90(6):962-70.

[999] Shiomori T, Miyamoto H, Makishima K, et al. Evaluation of bedmakingrelated airborne and surface methicillin-resistant Staphylococcus aureus contamination. *J. Hosp. Infect.* 2002;50(1):30-5.

[1000] Whyte W, Baird G, Annand R. Bacterial contamination on the surface of hospital linen chutes. *J. Hyg.* (Lond) 1969;67(3):427-35.

[1001] Michaelsen GS. Designing Linen Chutes to Reduce Spread of Infectious Organisms. *Hospitals.* 1965;39:1 16-9.

[1002] Plott RT, Wagner RF, Jr., Tyring SK. Iatrogenic contamination of multidose vials in simulated use. A reassessment of current patient injection technique. *Arch. Dermatol.* 1990; 126(11): 1441-4.

[1003] Samandari T, Malakmadze N, Balter S, et al. A large outbreak of hepatitis B virus infections associated with frequent injections at a physician's office. *Infect. Control Hosp. Epidemiol.* 2005;26(9):745-50.

[1004] Comstock RD, Mallonee S, Fox JL, et al. A large nosocomial outbreak of hepatitis C and hepatitis B among patients receiving pain remediation treatments. *Infect. Control Hosp. Epidemiol.* 2004;25(7):576-83.

[1005] Germain JM, Carbonne A, Thiers V, et al. Patient-to-patient transmission of hepatitis C virus through the use of multidose vials during general anesthesia. *Infect. Control Hosp. Epidemiol.* 2005;26(9):789-92.

[1006] Macedo de Oliveira A, White KL, Leschinsky DP, et al. An outbreak of hepatitis C virus infections among outpatients at a hematology/oncology clinic. *Ann. Intern. Med.* 2005;142(11):898-902.

[1007] Hsu J, Jensen B, Arduino M, et al. Streptococcal Meningitis Following Myelogram Procedures. *Infect. Control Hosp. Epidemiol.* 2007;28(5):61417.

[1008] Srinivasan A, Song X, Ross T, Merz W, Brower R, Perl TM. A prospective study to determine whether cover gowns in addition to gloves decrease nosocomial transmission of vancomycin-resistant enterococci in an intensive care unit. *Infect. Control Hosp. Epidemiol.* 2002;23(8):424-8.

[1009] Nichols WG, Corey L, Gooley T, Davis C, Boeckh M. Parainfluenza virus infections after hematopoietic stem cell transplantation: risk factors, response to antiviral therapy, and effect on transplant outcome. *Blood.* 2001;98(3):573-8.

[1010] Elizaga J, Olavarria E, Apperley J, Goldman J, Ward K. Parainfluenza virus 3 infection after stem cell transplant: relevance to outcome of rapid diagnosis and ribavirin treatment. *Clin. Infect. Dis.* 2001;32(3):413-8.

[1011] Oishi I, Kimura T, Murakami T, et al. Serial observations of chronic rotavirus infection in an immunodeficient child. *Microbiology and Immunology.* 1991;35(11):953-61.

[1012] Fierobe L, Lucet JC, Decre D, et al. An outbreak of imipenem-resistant Acinetobacter baumannii in critically ill surgical patients. *Infect. Control Hosp. Epidemiol.* 2001;22(1):35-40.

[1013] Montesinos I, Salido E, Delgado T, Lecuona M, Sierra A. Epidemiology of methicillin-resistant Staphylococcus aureus at a university hospital in the Canary Islands. *Infect. Control Hosp. Epidemiol.* 2003;24(9):667-72.

[1014] Poutanen SM, Vearncombe M, McGeer AJ, Gardam M, Large G, Simor AE. Nosocomial acquisition of methicillin-resistant Staphylococcus aureus during an outbreak of severe acute respiratory syndrome. *Infect. Control Hosp. Epidemiol.* 2005;26(2):134-7.

[1015] Yap FH, Gomersall CD, Fung KS, et al. Increase in methicillin-resistant Staphylococcus aureus acquisition rate and change in pathogen pattern associated with an outbreak of severe acute respiratory syndrome. *Clin. Infect. Dis.* 2004;39(4):511-6.

[1016] Layton MC, Perez M, Heald P, Patterson JE. An outbreak of mupirocin-resistant Staphylococcus aureus on a dermatology ward associated with an environmental reservoir. *Infect. Control Hosp. Epidemiol.* 1993;14(7):36975.

[1017] Gilmore A, Stuart J, Andrews N. Risk of secondary meningococcal disease in health-care workers. *Lancet.* 2000;356(9242):1654-5.

[1018] www.cdc.gov/flu/avian/index.htm
[1019] www.hhs.gov/pandemicflu/plan/pdf/S04.pdf
[1020] Ehresmann KR, Hedberg CW, Grimm MB, Norton CA, MacDonald KL, Osterholm MT. An outbreak of measles at an international sporting event with airborne transmission in a domed stadium. *J. Infect. Dis.* 1995; 171(3):679-83.
[1021] Gustafson TL, Lavely GB, Brawner ER, Jr., Hutcheson RH, Jr., Wright PF, Schaffner W. An outbreak of airborne nosocomial varicella. *Pediatrics.* 1 982;70(4):550-6.
[1022] Hyams PJ, Stuewe MC, Heitzer V. Herpes zoster causing varicella (chickenpox) in hospital employees: cost of a casual attitude. *Am. J. Infect. Control.* 1984;12(1):2-5.
[1023] Pavelchak N, DePersis RP, London M, et al. Identification of factors that disrupt negative air pressurization of respiratory isolation rooms. *Infect. Control Hosp. Epidemiol.* 2000;2 1(3): 191-5.
[1024] Rice N, Streifel A, Vesley D. An evaluation of hospital special-ventilation-room pressures. *Infect. Control Hosp. Epidemiol.* 2001 ;22(1): 1923.
[1025] Hutton MD, Stead WW, Cauthen GM, Bloch AB, Ewing WM. Nosocomial transmission of tuberculosis associated with a draining abscess. *J. Infect. Dis.* 1990;161(2):286-95.
[1026] Frampton MW. An outbreak of tuberculosis among hospital personnel caring for a patient with a skin ulcer. *Ann. Intern. Med.* 1992;1 17(4):312-3.
[1027] Ammari LK, Bell LM, Hodinka RL. Secondary measles vaccine failure in healthcare workers exposed to infected patients. *Infect. Control. Hosp. Epidemiol.* 1993;14(2):81-6.
[1028] Behrman A, Schmid DS, Crivaro A, Watson B. A cluster of primary varicella cases among healthcare workers with false-positive varicella zoster virus titers. *Infect. Control Hosp. Epidemiol.* 2003 ;24(3):202-6.
[1029] Josephson A, Gombert ME. Airborne transmission of nosocomial varicella from localized zoster. *J. Infect. Dis.* 1988;158(1):238-41.
[1030] Brodkin RH. Zoster Causing Varicella. Current Dangers Of Contagion Without Isolation. *Arch. Dermatol.* 1963;88:322-4.
[1031] Suzuki K, Yoshikawa T, Tomitaka A, Matsunaga K, Asano Y. Detection of aerosolized varicella-zoster virus DNA in patients with localized herpes zoster. *J. Infect. Dis.* 2004;189(6):1009-12.
[1032] Ruuskanen O, Salmi TT, Halonen P. Measles vaccination after exposure to natural measles. *J. Pediatr.* 1978;93(1):43-6.

[1033] Berkovich S, Starr S. Use of live-measles-virus vaccine to abort an expected outbreak of measles within a closed population. *N. Engl. J. Med.* 1963;269:75-7.

[1034] CDC. Measles, mumps, and rubella--vaccine use and strategies for elimination of measles, rubella, and congenital rubella syndrome and control of mumps: recommendations of the Advisory Committee on Immunization Practices (ACIP). *MMWR Recomm. Rep.* 1998;47(RR-8):157.

[1035] CDC. General recommendations on immunization: recommendations of the Advisory Committee on Immunization Practices (ACIP). *MMWR Morb. Mortal. Wkly. Rep.* 2006;55(RR-15):1-48.

[1036] Watson B, Seward J, Yang A, et al. Postexposure effectiveness of varicella vaccine. *Pediatrics.* 2000;105(1 Pt 1):84-8.

[1037] Salzman MB, Garcia C. Postexposure varicella vaccination in siblings of children with active varicella. *Pediatr. Infect. Dis.* J 1998; 1 7(3):256-7.

[1038] CDC. Vaccinia (smallpox) vaccine: recommendations of the Advisory Committee on Immunization Practices (ACIP), 2001. *MMWR. Recomm. Rep.* 2001;50(RR-10):1-25; quiz CE1-7.

[1039] Fulginiti VA, Papier A, Lane JM, Neff JM, Henderson DA. Smallpox vaccination: a review, part I. Background, vaccination technique, normal vaccination and revaccination, and expected normal reactions. *Clin. Infect. Dis.* 2003;37(2):241-50.

[1040] Dixon CW. Smallpox in Tripolitania, 1946: an epidemiological and clinical study of 500 cases, including trials of penicillin treatment. *J. Hyg.* (Lond) 1948;46:351-77.

[1041] Murray WA, Streifel AJ, O'Dea TJ, Rhame FS. Ventilation for protection of immune compromised patients. *ASHRAE Transactions.* 1 988;94: 1185.

[1042] Rutala WA, Jones SM, Worthington JM, Reist PC, Weber DJ. Efficacy of portable filtration units in reducing aerosolized particles in the size range of Mycobacterium tuberculosis. *Infect. Control Hosp. Epidemiol.* 1995;16(7):391-8.

[1043] Mandell GL, Bennett JE, Dolin R. Mandell, Douglas and Bennett's Principles and Practice of Infectious Diseases. GL Mandell, JE Bennett, R Dolin, Eds. 5th edition. Churchill Livingstone, Philadelphia, 2000. 2000.

[1044] Control of Communicable Diseases Manual. DL Heymann Ed. 18th edition, American Public Health Association, Washington, DC 2005. 2005.

[1045] Vreden SG, Visser LG, Verweij JJ, et al. Outbreak of amebiasis in a family in The Netherlands. *Clin. Infect. Dis.* 2000;31(4):1 101-4.

[1046] Thacker SB, Kimball AM, Wolfe M, Choi K, Gilmore L. Parasitic disease control in a residential facility for the mentally retarded: failure of selected isolation procedures. *Am. J. Public Health.* 1981;71(3):303-5.

[1047] Sampathkumar P. West Nile virus: epidemiology, clinical presentation, diagnosis, and prevention. *Mayo Clin. Proc.* 2003 ;78(9): 1137-43; quiz 44.

[1048] Ruben B, Band JD, Wong P, Colville J. Person-to-person transmission of Brucella melitensis. *Lancet.* 1991 ;337(8732): 14-5.

[1049] Vandercam B, Zech F, de Cooman S, Bughin C, Gigi J, Wauters G. Isolation of Brucella melitensis from human sperm. *Eur. J. Clin. Microbiol. Infect. Dis.* 1990;9(4):303-4.

[1050] Robichaud S, Libman M, Behr M, Rubin E. Prevention of laboratory-acquired brucellosis. *Clin. Infect. Dis.* 2004;38(12):e1 19-22.

[1051] Troy CJ, Peeling RW, Ellis AG, et al. Chlamydia pneumoniae as a new source of infectious outbreaks in nursing homes. *Jama.* 1997;277(15): 12 14-8.

[1052] Ekman MR, Grayston JT, Visakorpi R, Kleemola M, Kuo CC, Saikku P. An epidemic of infections due to Chlamydia pneumoniae in military conscripts. *Clin. Infect. Dis.* 1993; 17(3) :420-5.

[1053] Eickhoff TC. An outbreak of surgical wound infections due to Clostridium perfringens. *Surg. Gynecol. Obstet.* 1962;1 14:102-8.

[1054] Kohn GJ, Linne SR, Smith CM, Hoeprich PD. Acquisition of coccidioidomycosis at necropsy by inhalation of coccidioidal endospores. *Diagn. Microbiol. Infect. Dis.* 1992;15(6):527-30.

[1055] Wright PW, Pappagianis D, Wilson M, et al. Donor-related coccidioidomycosis in organ transplant recipients. *Clin. Infect. Dis.* 2003;37(9): 1265-9.

[1056] Maitreyi RS, Dar L, Muthukumar A, et al. Acute hemorrhagic conjunctivitis due to enterovirus 70 in India. *Emerg. Infect. Dis.* 1999;5(2):267-9.

[1057] CDC. Acute hemorrhagic conjunctivitis outbreak caused by Coxsackievirus A24--Puerto Rico, 2003. *MMWR Morb. Mortal Wkly. Rep.* 2004;53(28):632-4.

[1058] Faden H, Wynn RJ, Campagna L, Ryan RM. Outbreak of adenovirus type 30 in a neonatal intensive care unit. *J. Pediatr.* 2005;146(4):523-7.

[1059] Chaberny IE, Schnitzler P, Geiss HK, Wendt C. An outbreak of epidemic keratoconjunctivtis in a pediatric unit due to adenovirus type 8. *Infect. Control Hosp. Epidemiol.* 2003 ;24(7):514-9.

[1060] Warren D, Nelson KE, Farrar JA, et al. A large outbreak of epidemic keratoconjunctivitis: problems in controlling nosocomial spread. *J. Infect. Dis.* 1989;160(6):938-43.
[1061] www.cdc.gov/ncidod/dvrd/cjd/qa_cjd_infection_control.htm
[1062] Wang CY, Wu HD, Hsueh PR. Nosocomial transmission of cryptococcosis. *N. Engl. J. Med.* 2005;352(12):1271-2.
[1063] Beyt BE, Jr., Waltman SR. Cryptococcal endophthalmitis after corneal transplantation. *N. Engl. J. Med.* 1978;298(15):825-6.
[1064] Widdowson MA, Glass R, Monroe S, et al. Probable transmission of norovirus on an airplane. *Jama.* 2005;293(15):1859-60.
[1065] CDC. Prevention of Hepatitis A Through Active or Passive Immunization: Recommendations of the Advisory Committee on Immunization Practices (ACIP). *MMWR Recomm. Rep.* 1999;48(RR-12):1-37.
[1066] Rosenblum LS, Villarino ME, Nainan OV, et al. Hepatitis A outbreak in a neonatal intensive care unit: risk factors for transmission and evidence of prolonged viral excretion among preterm infants. *J. Infect. Dis.* 1991; 1 64(3):476-82.
[1067] Carl M, Kantor RJ, Webster HM, Fields HA, Maynard JE. Excretion of hepatitis A virus in the stools of hospitalized hepatitis patients. *J. Med. Virol.* 1982;9(2):125-9.
[1068] Robson SC, Adams S, Brink N, Woodruff B, Bradley D. Hospital outbreak of hepatitis E. *Lancet.* 1 992;3 39(8806): 1424-5.
[1069] Arvin A, Whitley R. Herpes Simplex virus infections in Infectious Diseases of the Fetus and Newborn Infant, ed. Remington JS and Klein JO. Fifth Edition. WB Saunders Co., Philadelphia, PA. 2001.
[1070] Enright AM, Prober CG. Neonatal herpes infection: diagnosis, treatment and prevention. *Semin. Neonatol.* 2002;7(4):283-91.
[1071] Esper F, Boucher D, Weibel C, Martinello RA, Kahn JS. Human metapneumovirus infection in the United States: clinical manifestations associated with a newly emerging respiratory infection in children. *Pediatrics.* 2003;111(6 Pt 1):1407-10.
[1072] Colodner R, Sakran W, Miron D, Teitler N, Khavalevsky E, Kopelowitz J. Listeria moncytogenes cross-contamination in a nursery. *Am. J. Infect. Control.* 2003;3 1(5):322-4.
[1073] Farber JM, Peterkin PI, Carter AO, Varughese PV, Ashton FE, Ewan EP. Neonatal listeriosis due to cross-infection confirmed by isoenzyme typing and DNA fingerprinting. *J. Infect. Dis.* 1991;163(4):927-8.

[1074] Schuchat A, Lizano C, Broome CV, Swaminathan B, Kim C, Winn K. Outbreak of neonatal listeriosis associated with mineral oil. *Pediatr. Infect. Dis. J.* 1991;10(3):183-9.

[1075] Pejaver RK, Watson AH, Mucklow ES. Neonatal cross-infection with Listeria monocytogenes. *J. Infect.* 1993 ;26(3):301-3.

[1076] Jain SK, Persaud D, Perl TM, et al. Nosocomial malaria and saline flush. *Emerg. Infect. Dis.* 2005;1 1(7):1097-9.

[1077] Abulrahi HA, Bohlega EA, Fontaine RE, al-Seghayer SM, al-Ruwais AA. Plasmodium falciparum malaria transmitted in hospital through heparin locks. *Lancet.* 1997;349(9044):23-5.

[1078] Al-Saigul AM, Fontaine RE, Haddad Q. Nosocomial malaria from contamination of a multidose heparin container with blood. *Infect. Control Hosp. Epidemiol.* 2000;21(5):329-30.

[1079] Piro S, Sammud M, Badi S, Al Ssabi L. Hospital-acquired malariatransmitted by contaminated gloves. *J. Hosp. Infect.* 2001 ;47(2): 156-8.

[1080] Book LS, Overall JC, Jr., Herbst JJ, Britt MR, Epstein B, Jung AL. Clustering of necrotizing enterocolitis. Interruption by infection-control measures. *N. Engl. J. Med.* 1977;297(18):984-6.

[1081] Rotbart HA, Levin MJ. How contagious is necrotizing enterocolitis? *Pediatr. Infect. Dis.* 1983;2(5):406-13.

[1082] Rotbart HA, Levin MJ, Yolken RH, Manchester DK, Jantzen J. An outbreak of rotavirus-associated neonatal necrotizing enterocolitis. *J. Pediatr.* 1983;103(3):454-9.

[1083] Gerber AR, Hopkins RS, Lauer BA, Curry-Kane AG, Rotbart HA. Increased risk of illness among nursery staff caring for neonates with necrotizing enterocolitis. *Pediatr. Infect. Dis.* 1 985;4(3):246-9.

[1084] Sanchez MP, Erdman DD, Torok TJ, Freeman CJ, Matyas BT. Outbreak of adenovirus 35 pneumonia among adult residents and staff of a chronic care psychiatric facility. *J. Infect. Dis.* 1997;176(3):760-3.(s).

[1085] Singh-Naz N, Brown M, Ganeshananthan M. Nosocomial adenovirus infection: molecular epidemiology of an outbreak. *Pediatr. Infect. Dis. J.* 1993;12(1 1):922-5.

[1086] Uemura T, Kawashitam T, Ostuka Y, Tanaka Y, Kusubae R, Yoshinaga M. A recent outbreak of adenovirus type 7 infection in a chronic inpatient facility for the severely handicapped. *Infect. Control Hosp. Epidemiol.* 2000;21(9):559-60.

[1087] Nuorti JP, Butler JC, Crutcher JM, et al. An outbreak of multidrug-resistant pneumococcal pneumonia and bacteremia among unvaccinated nursing home residents. *N. Engl. J. Med.* 1998;338(26):1861-8.

[1088] Houff SA, Burton RC, Wilson RW, et al. Human-to-human transmission of rabies virus by corneal transplant. *N. Engl. J. Med.* 1979;300(11):603-4.

[1089] CDC. Human Rabies Prevention - United States, 1999 Recommendations of the Advisory Committee on Immunization Practices (ACIP). *MMWR.* 1999;48 (RR-1):1-21.

[1090] Hayden FG. Rhinovirus and the lower respiratory tract. *Rev. Med. Virol.* 2004; 14(1): 17-31.

[1091] Valenti WM, Clarke TA, Hall CB, Menegus MA, Shapiro DL. Concurrent outbreaks of rhinovirus and respiratory syncytial virus in an intensive care nursery: epidemiology and associated risk factors. *J. Pediatr.* 1982; 100(5):722-6.

[1092] Chidekel AS, Rosen CL, Bazzy AR. Rhinovirus infection associated with serious lower respiratory illness in patients with bronchopulmonary dysplasia. *Pediatr. Infect. Dis. J.* 1997;16(1):43-7.

[1093] Drusin LM, Ross BG, Rhodes KH, Krauss AN, Scott RA. Nosocomial ringworm in a neonatal intensive care unit: a nurse and her cat. *Infect. Control Hosp. Epidemiol.* 2000;21(9):605-7.

[1094] Lewis SM, Lewis BG. Nosocomial transmission of Trichophyton tonsurans *tinea corporis in a rehabilitation hospital. Infect. Control Hosp.* Epidemiol. 1997; 18(5):322-5.

[1095] Saiman L, Jakob K, Holmes KW, et al. Molecular epidemiology of staphylococcal scalded skin syndrome in premature infants. *Pediatr. Infect. Dis. J.* 1998;17(4):329-34.

[1096] Ramage L, Green K, Pyskir D, Simor AE. An outbreak of fatal nosocomial infections due to group A streptococcus on a medical ward. *Infect. Control. Hosp. Epidemiol.* 1996; 17(7) :429-31.

[1097] Kakis A, Gibbs L, Eguia J, et al. An outbreak of group A Streptococcal infection among health care workers. *Clin. Infect. Dis.* 2002;35(11): 1353-9.

[1098] Schwartz B, Elliott JA, Butler JC, et al. Clusters of invasive group A streptococcal infections in family, hospital, and nursing home settings. *Clin. Infect. Dis.* 1992;15(2):277-84.

[1099] National Communicable Disease Center. Isolation Techniques for Use in Hospitals. 1st ed. Washington, DC: US Government Printing Office;. PHS publication no 2054 1970.

[1100] CDC. Isolation Techniques for Use in Hospitals. 2nd ed. Washington, DC: US Government Printing Office;1975. HHS publication no. (CDC) 80-8314. 1975.

[1101] Garner JS, Simmons BP. CDC Guideline for Isolation Precautions in Hospitals. Atlanta, GA: US Department of Health and Human Services, Public Health Service, Centers for Disease Control; 1983. HHS publication no. (CDC) 83-83 14. *Infect. Control.* 1983;4:245-325.

[1102] Lynch P, Jackson MM, Cummings MJ, Stamm WE. Rethinking the role of isolation practices in the prevention of nosocomial infections. *Ann. Intern. Med.* 1987;107(2):243-6.

In: Hospital-Acquired Infections
Editor: Julia B. Wilcox, pp. 237-294

ISBN: 978-1-60692-728-1
© 2009 Nova Science Publishers, Inc.

Chapter 2

HEALTH-CARE-ASSOCIATED INFECTIONS IN HOSPITALS: LEADERSHIP NEEDED FROM HHS TO PRIORITIZE PREVENTION PRACTICES AND IMPROVE DATA ON THESE INFECTIONS[*]

United States Government Accountability Office

WHAT GAO FOUND

CDC has 13 guidelines for hospitals on infection control and prevention, which cover a variety of topics, and in these guidelines CDC recommends almost 1,200 practices for implementation to prevent HAIs and related adverse events. Most of the practices are sorted into five categories—from strongly recommended for implementation to not recommended—primarily on the basis of the strength of the scientific evidence for each practice. Over 500 practices are strongly recommended. CDC and AHRQ have conducted some activities to promote implementation of recommended practices, but these activities are not based on a clear prioritization of the practices. Prioritization may consider not only the strength of the evidence, but also other factors that can affect implementation, such as cost and organizational obstacles. In addition to CDC, AHRQ has reviewed scientific evidence for certain HAI-related practices, but the efforts of the two agencies have not been coordinated.

---

[*] This is an edited, excerpted and augmented edition of a United States Government Accountability Office publication, Report GAO-08-283, dated March 2008.

The infection control standards required by CMS and hospital-accrediting organizations—the Joint Commission and the Healthcare Facilities Accreditation Program of the American Osteopathic Association (AOA)— describe the fundamental components of a hospital's infection control program. These components include the active prevention, control, and investigation of infections. The standards are far fewer in number than the recommended practices in CDC's guidelines and generally do not require that hospitals implement all recommended practices in CDC's infection control and prevention guidelines. CMS, the Joint Commission, and AOA assess compliance with their infection control standards through direct observation of hospital activities and review hospital policy documents during on-site surveys.

Multiple HHS programs collect data on HAIs, but limitations in the scope of information they collect and a lack of integration across the databases maintained by these separate programs constrain the utility of the data. Three agencies within HHS currently collect HAI-related data for a variety of purposes in databases maintained by four separate programs: CDC's National Healthcare Safety Network program, CMS's Medicare Patient Safety Monitoring System, CMS's Annual Payment Update program, and AHRQ's Healthcare Cost and Utilization Project. Each of the four databases presents only a partial view of the extent of the HAI problem because each focuses its data collection on selected types of HAIs and collects data from a different subset of hospital patients across the country. GAO did not find that the agencies were taking steps to integrate data across the four databases by creating linkages across the databases, such as creating common patient identifiers. Creating linkages across the HAI-related databases could enhance the availability of information to better understand where and how HAIs occur. Although CDC officials have produced national estimates of HAIs, those estimates derive from assumptions and extrapolations that raise questions about the reliability of those estimates.

WHY GAO DID THIS STUDY

According to the Centers for Disease Control and Prevention (CDC), health-care-associated infections (HAI) are estimated to be 1 of the top 10 causes of death in the United States. HAIs are infections that patients acquire while receiving treatment for other conditions. GAO was asked to examine (1) CDC's guidelines for hospitals to reduce or prevent HAIs and what the Department of Health and Human Services (HHS) does to promote their implementation, (2) Centers for Medicare & Medicaid Services' (CMS) and hospital accrediting organizations' required standards for hospitals to reduce or prevent HAIs and how compliance is assessed, and (3) HHS programs that collect data related to HAIs and integration of the data across HHS. GAO reviewed documents and interviewed officials from CDC, CMS, the Agency for Healthcare Research and Quality (AHRQ), and accrediting organizations.

WHAT GAO RECOMMENDS

GAO recommends that the Secretary of HHS identify priorities among the recommended practices in CDC's guidelines and establish greater consistency and compatibility of the data collected across HHS on HAIs. HHS generally agreed with GAO's recommendations. In response to comments from the Joint Commission, GAO clarified its discussion of Joint Commission activities; in addition, it incorporated technical comments from the Joint Commission and AOA.

ABBREVIATIONS

ABCs	Active Bacterial Core Surveillance
AHRQ	Agency for Healthcare Research and Quality
AOA	Healthcare Facilities Accreditation Program of the American Osteopathic Association
APIC	Association for Professionals in Infection Control and Epidemiology
APU	Annual Payment Update
BSI	bloodstream infection
CDC	Centers for Disease Control and Prevention
CMS	Centers for Medicare & Medicaid Services
COP	condition of participation
DRA	Deficit Reduction Act of 2005
DRG	diagnosis-related group
FDA	Food and Drug Administration
HAI	health-care-associated infection
HCUP	Healthcare Cost and Utilization Project
HHS	Department of Health and Human Services
HICPAC	Healthcare Infection Control Practices Advisory Committee
ICD-9	International Classification of Diseases, Ninth Revision

MDRO	multidrug-resistant organism
MPSMS	Medicare Patient Safety Monitoring System
MRSA	methicillin-resistant *Staphylococcus aureus*
NHSN	National Healthcare Safety Network
NNIS	National Nosocomial Infections Surveillance
PSI	Patient Safety Indicator
PSO	Patient Safety Organization
SCIP	Surgical Care Improvement Project
SHEA	Society for Healthcare Epidemiology of America
SSI	surgical site infection
UTI	urinary tract infection
VAP	ventilator-associated pneumonia
VRE	vancomycin-resistant enterococci
WHO	World Health Organization

March 31, 2008

The Honorable Henry Waxman
Chairman
Committee on Oversight and Government Reform
House of Representatives

Dear Mr. Chairman:

According to the Centers for Disease Control and Prevention (CDC), healthcare-associated infections (HAI) are estimated to be 1 of the top 10 causes of death in the United States. HAIs, as defined by CDC, are infections that patients acquire while receiving treatment for other conditions.[1] For example, a patient may acquire an infection from bacteria on a device used to treat them, such as a needle or tube to deliver medicine, fluids, or blood. According to CDC, the most common HAIs are urinary tract infection (UTI), surgical site infection (SSI), pneumonia, and bloodstream infection (BSI). Some HAIs can be caused by bacteria that have become resistant to multiple antimicrobial drugs.[2] One example of such a bacterium is methicillin-resistant *Staphylococcus aureus*, or MRSA, which causes infections that are resistant to treatment with usual antibiotics, including methicillin, and can be serious and potentially life-threatening. MRSA can cause a wide variety of infections, including skin infections, BSIs, SSIs, and pneumonia.

HAIs can be expensive. In 2005 the average payment for a hospitalization in Pennsylvania was over six times higher for patients who contracted a hospital-acquired infection than for patients who did not acquire infections, according to a report by the Pennsylvania Health Care Cost Containment Council.[3] A 2007 study of 1.69 million patients who were discharged from 77 hospitals found that the additional cost of treating a patient with an HAI averaged $8,832.[4] The costs of HAIs are borne not only by the patients who suffer infections, but also by those who pay for care, such as the Centers for Medicare & Medicaid Services (CMS). According to the American Hospital Association, Medicare paid for over one-third of all hospital costs in 2005.[5] Hospitals may also incur some of the cost because they are not fully reimbursed for the cost of the extra care attributable to HAIs.

Although not all HAIs are preventable, public and private organizations have established standards and other activities aimed at controlling and preventing them. CMS has established health and safety standards— known as conditions of participation (COP)—with which hospitals must comply in order to be eligible for payment by Medicare and Medicaid and which include the COP for infection control.[6] Hospitals may choose one of two ways to show that they have met these or equivalent standards: they may be certified by a state agency under agreement with CMS to survey the hospital's compliance with the COPs or they may be accredited by one of two private organizations—the Joint Commission or the Healthcare Facilities Accreditation Program of the American Osteopathic Association (AOA).[7] Most hospitals are accredited by the Joint Commission.[8] Other activities within the Department of Health and Human Services (HHS) aimed at addressing the problem of HAIs in hospitals include the development of guidelines by CDC, which contain recommended practices that hospitals may adopt, and several databases in different parts of HHS that contain information about HAIs in hospitals. According to the Institute of Medicine, prevention of HAIs through implementation of evidence-based guidelines can lead to improvements in quality of care.[9] Furthermore, the collection of national data on these infections can provide a benchmark for individual hospitals to gauge their performance and design targeted interventions.

Federal and state lawmakers are also concerned about HAIs and have taken action to reduce them. With the passage of the Deficit Reduction Act of 2005 (DRA),[10] the Congress took steps to revise the way Medicare pays hospitals so that beginning on October 1, 2008, they would not receive higher payments for patients that acquire certain preventable conditions (including any of three HAIs) during their hospital stay.[11] The HAI-related preventable conditions that CMS identified in the final regulation implementing subsection 500 1(c) of the DRA were UTIs caused by catheters, infections caused by vascular catheters, and mediastinitis following coronary artery bypass graft surgery.[12] According to Consumers Union—a nonprofit organization that has a campaign to stop HAIs—23 state legislatures have enacted laws that require public reporting of hospital HAI rates or HAI-related information.[13]

In light of congressional activity in this area and concerns you raised about how to prevent or reduce HAIs in hospitals, we examined (1) CDC's guidelines for hospitals to reduce or prevent HAIs, and what HHS does to promote their implementation, (2) CMS's and the accrediting organizations' required standards for hospitals to reduce or prevent HAIs, and how compliance is assessed, and (3) HHS programs that collect data related to HAIs in hospitals, and the extent the data are integrated across HHS.

In general, to conduct our work, we reviewed documents and interviewed HHS agency officials, including officials from CDC, CMS, the Agency for Healthcare Research and Quality (AHRQ), and the Food and Drug Administration (FDA).

To identify CDC's guidelines for hospitals related to HAIs as well as assess their content, we reviewed CDC's infection control and prevention guidelines issued between 1981 and 2007. To determine the extent to which HHS promotes CDC's guidelines, we asked CDC officials about the activities they undertake to promote their guidelines, and we interviewed officials from AHRQ. We reviewed minutes of the Healthcare Infection Control Practices Advisory Committee (HICPAC), a federal advisory body appointed by the Secretary of HHS that provides recommendations to the Secretary and CDC and includes members from government agencies and private organizations.[14] In addition, we interviewed officials from CDC, CMS, FDA, and AHRQ. We interviewed selected experts in the field of infection control, including individuals from private organizations that represent health professionals in infection control and develop materials to support their work, such as the Society for Healthcare Epidemiology of America (SHEA) and the Association for Professionals in Infection Control and Epidemiology (APIC). We also reviewed the World Health Organization's (WHO) guideline on hand hygiene.[15]

To determine CMS's and the accrediting organizations' required standards for hospitals to reduce or prevent HAIs and how compliance is assessed, we reviewed CMS's COPs for hospitals and the Joint Commission's and AOA's standards for hospitals and interviewed officials from CMS, the Joint Commission, and AOA. We reviewed CMS's interpretive guidelines, which describe the COPs and provide survey procedures used to determine compliance with them and can be found primarily in CMS's *State Operations Manual*.[16] In addition, we reviewed CMS's revised interpretive guidelines for the infection control COP, which were published in November 2007, during the course of our work.[17] We also reviewed the Joint Commission's and AOA's hospital standards manuals. For the purpose of this chapter, we refer to the guidance that CMS provides about its COPs in the interpretive guidelines, and that the Joint Commission and AOA provide about their standards in their respective manuals, as "standards interpretations." Our review focused on CMS's infection control COP and the standards the Joint Commission and AOA have in the infection control chapters of their respective manuals. We obtained the following information from each organization: the number of hospitals surveyed by each organization during the first quarter of 2007, and the number of hospitals surveyed by each organization during the first quarter of 2007 that were cited as noncompliant with one of the standards on infection control. Using the data we obtained from these officials, we calculated the percentage of hospitals surveyed by each organization that were noncompliant with at least one infection control standard for the first quarter of 2007. Based on information obtained from and discussions with each organization, we determined that the data CMS, the Joint Commission, and AOA provided to us were sufficiently reliable for the purposes of this chapter.

To identify HHS programs that routinely collect and maintain in designated databases information that relates specifically to HAIs, we interviewed officials at CDC, CMS, AHRQ, and FDA, and reviewed relevant documents. To describe and assess the programs HHS has that collect data related to HAIs and determine the extent to which the data are integrated, we reviewed agency manuals and other relevant documents that explain the programs that collect the data, examined related publications and data analyses conducted by the agencies based on the data collected, and reviewed HICPAC meeting minutes from March 2004 to June 2007. We also interviewed officials of CDC, CMS, FDA, and AHRQ responsible for each agency's HAI data collection efforts. We obtained data reported from these HAI-related databases, and based on relevant documents and discussion with agency officials we determined that the data were sufficiently reliable for the purposes of this chapter.

We examined only guidelines, standards, and databases that apply to HAIs in acute care hospitals other than critical access hospitals and did not examine guidelines, standards, or databases that might apply to community-acquired infections or health care workers. We did not independently assess the clinical evidence that supports CDC's infection control and prevention guidelines. We describe CMS's, the Joint Commission's, and AOA's infection control standards, the standards interpretations, and the survey process, but we did not observe the survey process. We conducted this performance audit from January 2007 to March 2008, in accordance with generally accepted government auditing standards. Those standards require that we plan and perform the audit to obtain sufficient, appropriate evidence to provide a reasonable basis for our findings and conclusions based on our audit objectives. We believe that the evidence obtained provides a reasonable basis for our findings and conclusions based on our audit objectives.

RESULTS IN BRIEF

CDC has 13 guidelines for hospitals on infection control and prevention, and in these guidelines CDC recommends almost 1,200 practices for implementation to prevent HAIs and related adverse events. The guidelines cover such topics as prevention of catheter-associated UTIs, prevention of SSIs, and hand hygiene. An example of a recommended practice in the hand hygiene guideline is the recommendation that health care workers decontaminate their hands before having direct contact with patients. Most of the practices are sorted into five categories—from strongly recommended for implementation to not recommended— primarily on the basis of the strength of the scientific evidence for each practice. Over 500 practices are strongly recommended. CDC and AHRQ have conducted some activities to promote implementation of recommended practices, such as disseminating the guidelines and providing research funds. However, these steps have not been guided by a prioritization of recommended practices. One factor to consider in prioritization is strength of evidence, as CDC has done. In addition to strength of evidence, an AHRQ study identified other factors to consider in prioritizing recommended practices, such as costs or organizational obstacles. Furthermore, the efforts of the two agencies have not been coordinated. For example, we found that CDC and AHRQ both conducted reviews of evidence for HAI-related practices, such as hand hygiene. Although this could have been an opportunity for coordination, an official from the HHS Office of the Secretary told us that no one within the office is responsible for coordinating infection control activities across HHS.

While CDC's infection control guidelines describe specific clinical practices recommended to reduce HAIs, the infection control standards that CMS and the accrediting organizations require as part of the hospital certification and accreditation processes describe the fundamental components of a hospital's infection control program. These components include the active prevention, control, and investigation of infections. Examples of standards and corresponding standards interpretations that hospitals must follow include educating hospital personnel about infection control and having infection control policies in place. The standards are far fewer in number than the recommended practices in CDC's guidelines—for example, CMS's infection control COP contains two standards. Furthermore, CMS and the accrediting organizations generally do not require that hospitals implement all recommended practices in CDC's infection control and prevention guidelines. Only the Joint Commission and AOA have standards that require the implementation of certain practices recommended in CDC's infection control guidelines. For example, the Joint Commission and AOA require hospitals to annually offer influenza vaccinations to health care workers, whereas CMS's interpretive guidelines, or standards interpretations, are more general, stating that hospitals should adopt policies and procedures based as much as possible on national guidelines that address hospital-staff-related issues, such as evaluating hospital staff immunization status for designated infectious diseases. CMS, the Joint Commission, and AOA assess compliance with their infection control standards through direct observation of hospital activities and review of hospital policy documents during on-site surveys.

Multiple HHS programs collect data on HAIs, but limitations in the scope of information they collect and the lack of integration across the databases maintained by these separate programs constrain the utility of the data. Three agencies within HHS—CDC, CMS, and AHRQ—currently collect HAI-related data for a variety of purposes in databases maintained by four separate programs: CDC's National Healthcare Safety Network (NHSN) program, CMS's Medicare Patient Safety Monitoring System (MPSMS), CMS's Annual Payment Update (APU) program, and AHRQ's Healthcare Cost and Utilization Project (HCUP). Each of these databases presents only a partial view of the extent of the HAI problem because each focuses its data collection on selected types of HAIs and collects data from a different subset of hospital patients across the country. Although officials from the various HHS agencies discuss HAI data collection with each other, we did not find that the agencies were taking steps to integrate any of the existing data by creating linkages across the databases, such as creating common patient identifiers. Creating linkages across the HAIrelated databases could enhance the availability of information to better understand where and how HAIs occur. Although none of the databases collect data on the incidence of HAIs for a nationally representative sample of hospital patients, CDC officials have produced national estimates of HAIs. However, those estimates derive from assumptions and extrapolations that raise questions about the reliability of those estimates.

In order to help reduce HAIs in hospitals, we are calling for stronger leadership from HHS by recommending that the Secretary of HHS take action to prioritize prevention practices and improve data about HAIs. In commenting on a draft of this chapter, HHS generally agreed with our recommendations. In terms of our first recommendation, HHS's comments indicated that CMS welcomed the opportunity to work with CDC to review and prioritize recommendations for infection control and would consider whether to incorporate some of the recommendations into CMS's hospital COPs. HHS's comments also noted that the COPs currently lack the specificity of guidance and recommendations issued by HHS agencies, including CDC's recommendations for infection control. In terms of our second recommendation, HHS's comments acknowledged the need for greater consistency and compatibility of the data collected on HAIs and identified some steps CMS would take to implement this recommendation. HHS also provided technical comments, which we incorporated as appropriate. In response to comments from the Joint Commission, we clarified the discussion of Joint Commission activities; in addition, we incorporated technical comments from the Joint Commission and AOA.

BACKGROUND

CDC has developed several guidelines for hospitals that describe and recommend practices to prevent or control HAIs, such as hand washing or the use of alcohol-based hand rubs, isolation of infected patients, proper sterilization of equipment, provision of antibiotics to patients before surgery, and annual vaccination of health care workers for influenza. Standards from CMS and hospital accrediting organizations provide a means for assessing hospital compliance with infection control standards that are also aimed at preventing or controlling HAIs.

CDC's Infection Control and Prevention Guidelines

CDC issues both guidelines and guidance relevant to infection control and prevention in hospitals. Guidelines are based on scientific evidence, whereas guidance is usually provisional and limited in its supporting evidence. CDC's infection control and prevention guidelines set forth recommended practices, summarize the applicable scientific evidence and research, and contain contextual information and citations for relevant studies and literature.

Most of CDC's infection control and prevention guidelines are developed in conjunction with HICPAC, an advisory body created in 1992 by the Secretary of HHS. According to its charter, HICPAC provides CDC and the Secretary with (1) advice and guidance on the practice of infection control and strategies for surveillance,[18] prevention, and control of HAIs and related events in health care facilities; and (2) advice on the periodic updating of existing HAI guidelines, the development of new guidelines and evaluations, and other HAI policy statements.[19] HICPAC currently consists of 14 voting members from various infection control disciplines throughout the United States, a designated staff person from CDC, and 15 nonvoting liaison members from government agencies and private organizations.

When CDC and HICPAC select a topic for an infection control and prevention guideline, they begin with internal discussions. After selecting a topic, HICPAC members and CDC conduct research on the topic, which includes identifying and evaluating clinical studies relevant to the topic and developing recommended practices, as appropriate. The draft guidelines are written and reviewed by HICPAC members; circulated to outside experts to validate the content; and sent to other federal agencies for review and approval.[20] Afterward, HICPAC members resolve issues raised during review in face-to-face meetings or conference calls with HICPAC members who wrote the guideline. The approved document is published in the *Federal Register* for a 45- to 60-day public comment period, after which comments are reviewed by HICPAC members. CDC publishes the final guideline in its *Morbidity and Mortality Weekly Report*, on its Web site, or through a professional journal.

CMS's and the Accrediting Organizations' Standards for Hospitals

Hospital compliance with CMS's or the accrediting organizations' standards, including those related to infection control, is assessed on a regular basis. Unannounced on-site surveys, conducted by surveyors from CMS or the accrediting organizations, are a major component in the process by which hospitals' compliance with health and safety standards is assessed. Standards interpretations are given by CMS primarily in its *State Operations Manual*,[21] which is arranged by COP; by the Joint Commission in its *Comprehensive Accreditation Manual for Hospitals: The Official Handbook*, which identifies rationales and performance expectations that are used to measure each standard and is organized into 11 chapters of safety and quality standards such as "Medication Management" and "Leadership;" and by AOA's standards manual, *Accreditation Requirements for Healthcare Facilities*, which provides explanations for surveyors and the scoring procedures along with its standards and is organized into 32 chapters. Based on the information documented during the survey, surveyors from each organization assess a hospital's compliance with the standards.[22] Hospitals are required to correct instances of noncompliance found during the survey. CMS's policy is to survey hospitals every 3 years; however, this policy is contingent on CMS's budget. In fiscal year 2007, CMS set a goal to survey hospitals on average once every 4.5 years, with no more than 6 years elapsing between surveys for any one hospital. Both the Joint Commission and AOA survey hospitals at least once every 3 years.

The Joint Commission has additional components in its standards and survey process. First, it issues National Patient Safety Goals, which are requirements intended to promote specific improvements in patient safety. Officials at the Joint Commission told us that the goals are updated annually and derive primarily from informal recommendations made in the Joint Commission's safety newsletter, *Sentinel Event Alert*, recommendations from the Sentinel Event Advisory Group, sentinel events reported to the Joint Commission, and a review of the patient safety literature. The goals target problem areas in health care, such as reducing the risk of patient injury resulting from a fall or encouraging patients' active involvement in their own care. Each goal is reviewed during the on- site survey to determine compliance with it. Second, the Joint Commission conducts several "tracers" as part of its hospital surveys, during which the care provided to selected patients is followed or "traced" through the hospital in the same sequence in which the patient received it. Other requirements that a hospital must meet to be accredited by the Joint Commission include conducting an annual self-assessment of the hospital's compliance with the Joint Commission standards and submitting data for selected measures of clinical performance, some of which are related to HAIs.

CDC HAS 13 INFECTION CONTROL AND PREVENTION GUIDELINES CONTAINING ALMOST 1,200 RECOMMENDED PRACTICES, BUT ACTIVITIES ACROSS HHS TO PROMOTE IMPLEMENTATION ARE NOT GUIDED BY PRIORITIZATION OF PRACTICES

CDC has 13 guidelines for hospitals on infection control and prevention, and in these guidelines CDC recommends almost 1,200 specific clinical practices for implementation to prevent HAIs and related adverse events. The practices generally are sorted into five categories—from strongly recommended for implementation to not recommended—primarily on the basis of the strength of the scientific evidence for each practice. Over 500 practices are strongly recommended. Within HHS, CDC and AHRQ conduct some activities to promote the implementation of recommended practices, but the activities are not based on clear prioritization of the practices, which may consider not only the strength of the evidence, but also other factors that can affect implementation, such as cost or organizational obstacles.

CDC Has 13 Infection Control and Prevention Guidelines, Which Contain Almost 1,200 Recommended Practices, and over 500 of Them Are Strongly Recommended

CDC has 13 infection control and prevention guidelines, which contain 1,198 specific clinical practices that CDC recommends for preventing HAIs.[23] (See table 1.) The hand hygiene guideline, for example, strongly recommends that health care workers decontaminate their hands before having direct contact with patients. The number of recommended practices for each guideline varies. For example, the

2003 guideline outlining environmental infection control practices contains 329 recommended practices, whereas the 2006 guideline for influenza vaccination of health care personnel has 6 recommended practices. The earliest of the guidelines, which was on catheter-associated UTIs, was published in February 1981, and as of December 2007, the most recent, a revision of the guideline for isolation precautions, was published in June 2007.

Table 1. CDC's Infection Control and Prevention Guidelines, with Number of Recommended Practices, Issued between 1981 and 2007

	Guideline (issue date)	Total number of recommended practices
1	Guideline for Prevention of Catheter-associated Urinary Tract Infections (1981)	24
2	Guideline for Infection Control in Health Care Personnel (1998)	183
3	Guideline for Prevention of Surgical Site Infection (1999)	63
4	Guidelines for Preventing Opportunistic Infections among Hematopoietic Stem Cell Transplant	a
5	Guidelines for the Prevention of Intravascular Catheter-Related Infections (2002)	111
6	Guideline for Hand Hygiene in Health-Care Settings (2002)	42
7	Recommendations for Using Smallpox Vaccine in a Pre-Event Vaccination Program (2003)	b
8	Guidelines for Environmental Infection Control in Health-Care Facilities (2003)	329
9	Guidelines for Preventing Health-Care-Associated Pneumonia (2003)	208
10	Guidelines for Preventing the Transmission of Mycobacterium Tuberculosis in Health-Care	b
11	Influenza Vaccination of Health-Care Personnel (2006)	6
12	Management of Multidrug-Resistant Organisms in Healthcare Settings (2006)	80
13	Guideline for Isolation Precautions: Preventing Transmission of Infectious Agents in Healthcare	152
	Total	1,198

Source: GAO analysis of CDC guidelines.

[a] For the purpose of this table, we do not include a count of the recommended practices in this guideline because the guideline is targeted to a specific patient population that not all hospitals treat. However, for the hospitals that do treat such patients, this guideline provides at least another 164 recommended practices.

[b] The practices in these guidelines are not organized in a way that supports counting the total number of practices.

The practices in these 13 guidelines are categorized primarily based on the strength of the scientific evidence, and these categories have changed over time. Basing the categories on the strength of the evidence means that the more highly recommended practices have more and better scientific support indicating their effectiveness than those practices that are not as highly recommended. Seven of the guidelines published between 2002 and 2007 used five categories: (1) strongly recommended for implementation and strongly supported by well-designed experimental, clinical, or epidemiological studies; (2) strongly recommended for implementation and supported by some experimental, clinical, or epidemiologic studies and a strong theoretical rationale; (3) suggested for implementation by suggestive clinical or epidemiologic studies; (4) additional practices, including federal, state, and other requirements; and (5) not recommended due to insufficient evidence or lack of consensus regarding efficacy.[24] Over 500 practices in these 7 guidelines fall into one of the two strongly recommended categories. Six of the 7 guidelines identify 82 practices that are not recommended, due to a lack of evidence supporting a recommendation. (See table 2.) For example, the 2003 guideline for preventing health-care-associated pneumonia identifies 45 practices that are not recommended. The four guidelines issued between 1981 and 2000 ranked recommended practices into between three and five categories.[25] The 2003 guideline on smallpox vaccine and the 2005 guideline on mycobacterium tuberculosis contain recommended practices, but they are not categorized.[26]

In general, CDC took an average of about 3 years to develop each guideline—ranging from less than 1 year to 6 years. CDC officials agreed that the amount of time it took to prepare a guideline has been long. CDC reported that it has been developing one guideline that is still in draft form—the Guideline for Disinfection and Sterilization in Healthcare Facilities—for over 7 years.[27] This guideline has taken a long time to develop, in part, according to CDC officials, because the agency had to coordinate with other agencies involved in the oversight of disinfection and sterilization products. CDC officials said they were working to reduce the time it takes to develop guidelines by issuing shorter and more focused guidelines.

Table 2. Number of Practices in the Seven CDC Infection Control and Prevention Guidelines That Used the Five Categories, by Category Recommended practices

Guideline	Strongly recommended and strongly supported (Category 1)	Strongly recommended and supported (Category 2)	Suggested for implementation (Category 3)	Total number of recommended practices	Additional practices including federal, state, and other requirements[a] (Category 4)	Not recommended practices Category 5
Guidelines for the Prevention of Intravascular Catheter-Related infections (2002)	39	39	33	111	3	8
Guideline for Hand Hygiene in Health-Care Settings (2002)	9	20	13	42	2	2
Guidelines for Environmental Infection Control in Health-Care Facilities (2003)	10	134	185	329	94	16
Guidelines for Preventing Health-Care-Associated Pneumonia (2003)	28	97	83	208	1	45
Influenza Vaccination of Health-Care Personnel (2006)	1	3	2	6	0	0

Table 2. (Continued).

Guideline	Strongly recommended and strongly supported (Category 1)	Strongly recommended and supported (Category 2)	Suggested for implementation (Category 3)	Total number of recommended practices	Additional practices including federal, state, and other requirements[a] (Category 4)	Not recommended practices (Category 5)
Management of Multidrug-Resistant Organisms in Healthcare Settings (2006)	2	60	18	80	1	4
Guideline for Isolation Precautions: Preventing Transmission of Infectious Agents in Healthcare Settings (2007)	21	83	48	152	3	7
Total by category	110	436	382	928	104	82

Source: GAO analysis of CDC guidelines.

Notes: CDC has 13 infection control guidelines, of which about half are categorized using the five categories displayed in this table. More than 84 percent of the practices in Category 4 are, for example, Occupational Safety and Health Administration workplace standards, building and engineering standards, or administrative plans or procedures.

[a] For the purpose of this table, Category 4 excludes a count of practices that CDC also classified as recommended.

CDC and AHRQ Have Taken Steps to Promote Implementation of Practices to Reduce HAIs but Lack Prioritization of These Practices to Guide Their Actions

CDC officials identified some activities that the agency has undertaken to promote the implementation of the recommended practices in its guidelines.[28] CDC disseminates its infection control guidelines by publishing them in the *Morbidity and Mortality Weekly Report*, posting them on CDC's Web site, and distributing training videos. CDC has also provided some funding support to groups that are developing ways to implement selected recommendations in CDC infection control guidelines. For example, through its Prevention Epicenter Program,[29] CDC provided financial support and technical assistance to a study that was assessing the effect of an intervention to prevent catheter-associated BSIs. The researchers reviewed participating hospitals' policies and procedures on a commonly used catheter, updated them to reflect CDC's *Guidelines for the Prevention of Intravascular Catheter-Related Infections*, and implemented an intervention designed to educate staff about the importance of implementing a group of selected recommendations in that guideline.[30] In a similar effort, CDC provided technical support and funding to the Pittsburgh Regional Healthcare Initiative, which reportedly has demonstrated a 68 percent decline in BSIs over a 4-year period among intensive care unit patients.[31]

AHRQ officials also reported undertaking some initiatives to promote implementation of practices aimed at reducing HAIs. In 2007, AHRQ issued a report that evaluated several strategies, such as clinician and patient education, for possible use in hospitals to increase implementation of specified infection prevention practices related to catheterization, surgical antibiotic prophylaxis, central lines, and ventilator-associated pneumonia (YAP) interventions.[32] Although researchers were unable to reach any firm conclusions regarding actionable strategies to prevent HAIs, they identified four strategies worth additional study.[33] In addition, through its Accelerating Change and Transformation in Organizations and Networks program, in September 2007, AHRQ funded several studies to improve the implementation of practices that are known to minimize HAIs and to identify the challenges to implementing those practices.[34] The program will implement clinician training at 72 hospitals that is designed to facilitate change in clinician behaviors and habits, care processes, and the safety culture of the participating hospitals. In a document summarizing this initiative, AHRQ acknowledges that the problem is not the lack of knowledge of infection control techniques, but rather the inability to translate the knowledge into social and behavioral changes that can be sustained in health care organizations.

While CDC and AHRQ have taken steps to promote the implementation of practices to reduce HAIs, these steps have not been guided by a prioritization of recommended practices. As WHO has indicated in its hand hygiene guideline, when there is a large number of practices it is important to prioritize them. One factor to consider in prioritization is strength of evidence, which CDC has primarily relied on to categorize its recommended practices. However, a 2001 AHRQ study suggested other factors to consider in prioritizing recommended practices. This study rated 79 patient safety practices—including 22 practices that were related to HAIs—on their potential to improve patient safety. The study examined not only strength of the evidence, but also such factors as

- the potential magnitude of impact of the practice on mitigating patient death or disability,
- the financial cost of implementing the practice,
- the complexity of implementing the practice,
- the organizational and technical obstacles, and
- the risk that other negative consequences could occur if the practice were put into place.

In addition to CDC, AHRQ has reviewed scientific evidence for certain practices related to HAIs, but the efforts of the two agencies have not been coordinated. For example, both agencies independently examined various aspects of the evidence related to improving hand hygiene compliance, such as the selection of hand hygiene products and health care worker education. Although this could have been an opportunity for coordination, an official from the HHS Office of the Secretary told us that no one within the office is responsible for coordinating infection control activities across HHS.[35]

CMS'S AND ACCREDITING ORGANIZATIONS' REQUIRED HOSPITAL STANDARDS DESCRIBE COMPONENTS OF INFECTION CONTROL PROGRAMS, AND COMPLIANCE WITH THESE STANDARDS IS ASSESSED THROUGH ON-SITE SURVEYS

The infection control standards that CMS, the Joint Commission, and AOA require as part of the hospital certification and accreditation processes vary in number and content among the organizations, and generally describe the fundamental components of a hospital infection control program, that is, the active prevention, control, and investigation of infections. Examples of standards and corresponding standards interpretations that hospitals must follow include educating hospital personnel about infection control and having infection control policies in place. CMS, the Joint Commission, and AOA standards generally do not require that hospitals implement all recommended practices in CDC's infection control and prevention guidelines. Only the Joint Commission and AOA have standards that require the implementation of certain practices recommended in CDC's infection control guidelines. For example, the Joint Commission and AOA require hospitals to annually offer influenza vaccinations to health care workers, which is recommended in CDC's *Influenza Vaccination of Health Care Personnel* guideline. CMS, the Joint Commission, and AOA assess compliance with their infection control standards through direct observation of hospital activities and review of hospital policy documents during on-site surveys.

Standards for Hospitals on Infection Control Required by CMS and Accrediting Organizations Describe Components of Infection Control Programs

CMS, Joint Commission, and AOA standards for hospital certification and accreditation include standards on infection control. In contrast to CDC's infection control guidelines, which describe clinical practices recommended to reduce HAIs, the CMS, Joint Commission, and AOA standards and their interpretations—which include the performance expectations and explain the standards—describe the fundamental components of a hospital's infection control program, the overall goal of which is the prevention, control, and investigation of infections.

CMS's infection control COP, the Joint Commission's chapter on infection control, and AOA's chapter on infection control have varying numbers of standards, some of which have been updated more recently than others. (See app. II for CMS's, Joint Commission's, and AOA's infection control standards for hospitals.)

- CMS's infection control COP contains two standard-level requirements and has not substantially changed since 1986.[36] CMS's *State Operations Manual: Appendix A* provides guidance to surveyors in assessing compliance with the COP and explains its intent. CMS issued revised guidance to surveyors for assessing the infection control COP on November 21, 2007, with an immediate effective date.
- The Joint Commission has 10 infection control standards in the infection control chapter of its manual, the *Comprehensive Accreditation Manual*

for Hospitals: The Official Handbook.[37] The Joint Commission describes its standards as broad, overarching compliance principles. The Joint Commission manual provides hospitals with information about the accreditation process, including how to comply with the 10 standards in the infection control chapter, and presents a rationale for each standard and "elements of performance," which describe the specific requirements for a hospital to be in compliance with a standard. There are a total of 48 elements of performance associated with the standards in the infection control chapter, ranging from 2 to 8 per standard. In 2006 the Joint Commission began revising its hospital standards, including the infection control standards. These revisions, which the Joint Commission officials described as clarifications to existing standards, will take effect on January 1, 2009.[38] The Joint Commission manual also describes other requirements hospitals must meet to be accredited by the Joint Commission, such as the eight National Patient Safety Goals for 2008, one of which relates to HAIs and requires hospitals to (1) comply with the current WHO hand hygiene guideline or CDC hand hygiene guideline[39] and (2) manage as a "sentinel event" all identified cases of unanticipated death or major permanent loss of function associated with an HAI.[40]

- AOA has 51 standards in the "Infection Control" chapter of its *Accreditation Requirements for Healthcare Facilities* manual, which also provides guidance to surveyors in applying AOA's standards, and these were last updated in 2005.[41] AOA officials also told us they anticipated updating this chapter to reflect CMS's revised infection control COP guidance.

As a whole, the CMS, Joint Commission, and AOA standards and their interpretations describe similar required elements of hospital infection control programs. Similarities include the following:

- The infection control program is hospitalwide.
- The hospital designates a person or persons as responsible for the infection control program.
- The hospital develops policies to control and reduce infections.
- The hospital educates health care personnel, patients, and family members about infection control.
- The hospital conducts surveillance activities, which include infection-related data collection and analysis.

- The hospital evaluates the effectiveness of infection control activities and modifies or updates the infection control program as needed.

However, there are also differences between the CMS, Joint Commission, and AOA infection control standards and their interpretations. One example is that the CMS and AOA standards specify that the hospital should maintain a log of infections and communicable diseases detected at the hospital, whereas the Joint Commission has several standards whose elements of performance state that hospitals should collect infection control surveillance data. Another difference is the extent to which the standards and their interpretations require implementation of practices recommended in CDC's infection control guidelines. The CMS, Joint Commission, and AOA standards generally do not require that hospitals implement all required practices in CDC's infection control and prevention guidelines. While CMS's and the accrediting organizations' standards interpretations make general references to incorporating guidelines into the hospital's infection control activities, only the Joint Commission and AOA have standards that require the implementation of certain practices recommended in CDC's infection control guidelines. The CMS standards interpretations have a more general statement that a hospital with a comprehensive hospitalwide infection control program should adopt policies and procedures based as much as possible on national guidelines. For example:

- As noted previously, a Joint Commission National Patient Safety Goal requires hospitals to implement selected practices in either CDC's or WHO's hand hygiene guideline.[42] AOA has a standard on hand washing that requires hospitals to have policies and procedures on practices related to hand decontamination and the prevention of HAIs, some of which are also recommended in CDC's guidelines, such as the elimination of artificial nails for staff working in intensive care units. The CMS standards interpretations are more general, stating that hospitals should adopt policies and procedures based on national guidelines that, among other things, address the mitigation of risks that contribute to HAIs by, for example, promoting hand washing hygiene among staff and employees, including use of alcohol-based hand sanitizers.
- Two AOA standards require hospitals to comply with certain practices recommended in CDC's guidelines that reduce surgical site infections and prevent central venous catheter–related infections. The CMS and Joint Commission standards and their interpretations are not as specific. The CMS standards interpretations state that a hospital with a comprehensive infection control program should adopt policies and procedures that address the mitigation of risk

associated with HAIs, including surgery-related infections and device-associated infections. The Joint Commission standards interpretations state that hospitals set goals that include minimizing the risk of transmitting infections associated with the use of procedures, medical equipment, and medical devices and implement methods such as appropriate sterilization techniques to reduce those risks.

- Both the Joint Commission and AOA standards incorporate recommendations from CDC's guideline *Influenza Vaccination of Health-Care Personnel* by requiring hospitals to annually offer influenza vaccinations to health care workers. In contrast, the CMS standards interpretations are more general, stating that hospitals should adopt policies and procedures that address hospital-staff-related issues, such as evaluating hospital staff immunization status for designated infectious diseases, as recommended by CDC and its Advisory Committee on Immunization Practices.

Compliance with Required Infection Control Standards Is Assessed through Observation and Document Review during on-Site Surveys of Hospitals

During on-site surveys, CMS, Joint Commission, or AOA surveyors assess compliance with their respective infection control standards by directly observing patient care, interviewing hospital staff, and reviewing key infection control documents, such as the hospital's infection control plan. In addition, the Joint Commission's surveyors assess compliance with the infection control standards by conducting an infection control system tracer, which is designed to address a hospital's overall system for detecting and preventing infections. Joint Commission officials noted that they foster compliance with the practices for reducing HAIs by using a "systems-based" approach.[43] Throughout each on-site survey, CMS, the Joint Commission, and AOA surveyors document noncompliance with the standards that they observe. For example, CMS, Joint Commission, and AOA officials told us that surveyors document observations of poor hand hygiene (e.g., a health care worker not washing his or her hands).

Based on the results of the surveys, CMS and the accrediting organizations assess a hospital's compliance with the infection control standards. CMS, Joint Commission, and AOA surveyors are required to cite all instances of noncompliance. At the end of each survey, CMS surveyors review the observations of noncompliance for each standard and determine whether to cite the hospital at the condition level or the standard level based on the nature (i.e., severity) and extent (i.e., prevalence) of the noncompliance. A CMS-surveyed hospital is required to develop a corrective action plan within 10 days of receiving a report documenting the noncompliance found during a survey.[44] The Joint Commission assesses each of the elements of performance that constitute the infection control standards as satisfactory, partially compliant, or insufficient. The entire standard is assessed as not compliant if the hospital has insufficient compliance with any of the corresponding elements of performance or if the hospital is partially compliant with 35 percent or more of the elements of performance. Joint Commission–surveyed hospitals have 45 days from receipt of the survey results to submit a report to the Joint Commission that describes the steps the hospitals took to become compliant with any standards that were assessed as not compliant.[45] The AOA standards are assessed on a scale from 1 to 4, which varies by standard, where 1 indicates full compliance and 4 indicates noncompliance. AOA-surveyed hospitals have 30 days to report to AOA on the steps they took to become compliant with standards assessed as noncompliant that indicate immediate jeopardy or are at the CMS condition level and 60 days to address other standards assessed as noncompliant. Among the surveys conducted in the first quarter of 2007, 12.6 percent of state-agencysurveyed hospitals, 17.6 percent of Joint Commission–surveyed hospitals, and 22.2 percent of AOA-surveyed hospitals were cited as noncompliant with one of the respective organizations' standards on infection control.[46]

Between regular surveys, limited information about compliance with the infection control standards may be identified through validation and complaint surveys of hospitals conducted by state survey agencies. State survey agencies conduct validation surveys for CMS on a small number of Joint Commission–accredited hospitals within 60 days of their last Joint Commission survey and compare the results of the two surveys.[47] For example, in fiscal year 2006, state agencies conducted validation surveys at 67 hospitals. State survey agencies conduct complaint surveys in response to complaints made by patients, family members, or health care providers.[48] In the first quarter of calendar year 2007, state survey agencies conducted 1,119 complaint surveys in 828 hospitals, and infection control deficiencies were found at 3.5 percent of the hospitals.

Information about hospital compliance with infection control standards is generally not publicly reported on Web sites, although the Joint Commission reports compliance with its National Patient Safety Goals on its Web site. It reported that in calendar year 2006, 91.2 percent of the hospitals surveyed that year were compliant with the goal related to implementing CDC's hand hygiene guideline, and 100 percent were compliant with the goal related to managing all identified cases of unanticipated death or major permanent loss of function associated with an HAI as a sentinel event. The rate reported by the Joint Commission in 2006 for adherence to hand hygiene practices was much higher than some studies had reported. For example, in the 2002 *Guideline for Hand Hygiene in Health-Care Settings*, CDC cited several observational studies of health care workers and reported the average adherence across the studies to be 40 percent.[49] The Joint Commission's surveyors assess this requirement by interviewing and observing hospital employees and would assess a hospital as noncompliant with the requirement if the surveyors observed noncompliance three or more times. Joint Commission officials acknowledged that their assessment mechanism might not sufficiently measure compliance because hospital staff could be on their best behavior when surveyors were present. Joint Commission officials told us they anticipated publishing in 2008 examples of different ways to measure adherence to hand hygiene as well as tools and training materials that hospitals could use to improve their hand hygiene compliance.

MULTIPLE HHS PROGRAMS COLLECT DATA ON HAIS, BUT LACK OF INTEGRATION OF AVAILABLE DATA AND OTHER PROBLEMS LIMIT UTILITY OF THE DATA

Three agencies within HHS—CDC, CMS, and AHRQ—currently collect HAI-related data for a variety of purposes in four separate databases, but each of these databases presents only a partial view of the extent of the HAI problem. Each database focuses its data collection on selected types of HAIs and collects data from a different subset of hospital patients across the country. Although officials from the various HHS agencies discuss HAI data collection with each other, we did not find that the agencies were taking steps to integrate any of the existing data by creating linkages across the databases such as standardizing patient identifiers or other data items. Creating linkages across the HAI-related databases could enhance the availability of information to better understand where and how HAIs occur. Although none of the databases collect data on the incidence of HAIs for a nationally representative sample of hospital patients, CDC officials have produced national estimates of HAIs. However, those estimates derive from assumptions and extrapolations that raise questions about the reliability of those estimates.

MULTIPLE HHS AGENCIES COLLECT DIFFERENT DATA ON HAIs, BUT THESE DATA PRESENT ONLY A PARTIAL VIEW OF THE EXTENT OF THE PROBLEM

Three agencies within HHS currently collect HAI-related data in four separate databases, which were created for a variety of purposes. These are the databases associated with CDC's National Healthcare Safety Network (NHSN), CMS's Medicare Patient Safety Monitoring System (MPSMS), CMS's Annual Payment Update (APU) program, and AHRQ's Healthcare Cost and Utilization Project (HCUP).

The most detailed source of information on HAIs within HHS is the NHSN database.[50] CDC established the NHSN database in 2005 to combine the data it had previously collected on HAIs through the National Nosocomial Infections Surveillance (NNIS) system with data from two other related databases.[51] CDC instituted NNIS as a voluntary program in the 1970s to assist hospitals that wanted to monitor their HAI rates. CDC analyzed the data submitted by those hospitals—which tended to be disproportionately large hospitals, many of them academic medical centers—in order to provide the hospitals with a benchmark HAI rate against which to compare their own rates. In addition, CDC drew on these data to publicly report aggregate trends in selected HAIs, and it continues to do that with the data being submitted to the NHSN database.[52] Many of the hospitals that voluntarily participated in the NNIS database have continued to submit HAI data voluntarily to the NHSN database. CDC is working with a number of states implementing mandatory programs for hospitals to submit HAI-related data, using NHSN as the designated mechanism by which hospitals must submit their data.[53] As a result, by the end of December 2007, approximately 1,000 hospitals were enrolled in the NHSN database, some of which continued to participate by choice while others enrolled in the NHSN program because of state mandates.[54]

The NHSN program provides hospitals with substantial flexibility to determine the scope of their HAI data collection efforts. Participating hospitals can choose which types of HAIs they will submit data on from among those for which the NHSN program has developed detailed definitions and protocols, including such device-associated infections as central-line-associated BSIs, catheter-associated UTIs, and VAP, as well as procedure-related HAIs such as SSIs and postprocedure pneumonia. Hospitals also choose the specific hospital units (typically different kinds of intensive care units) to monitor for device-associated HAIs and the specific surgical procedures to monitor for SSIs and postprocedure pneumonia. Hospital staff are supposed to follow the detailed definitions and protocols that the NHSN program specifies to identify which patients currently under treatment have developed one of the targeted infections. Hospitals also have to provide at least some HAI data for 6 months of the year to maintain their enrollment in the NHSN program.[55]

The MPSMS database provides CMS with information on national trends in the incidence of selected adverse events among hospitalized Medicare beneficiaries, including a number of different types of HAIs. Beginning with hospital discharges from 2002, CMS has collected these data from the medical records selected for annual random samples of approximately 25,000 Medicare inpatients,[56] though the list of specific adverse events monitored has varied over time. A CMS contractor receives copies of these medical records after the patients' discharge from the hospital, and the contractor's abstractors[57] follow CMS's detailed protocols to extract and record specific information on each patient in the sample. These data elements are then entered into algorithms that determine which patients meet CMS's case selection criteria for experiencing the adverse event and for being at risk for the adverse event. For example, the abstractors would determine which of the sampled patients had a central line catheter inserted during that hospital stay and which of those patients had laboratory reports indicating a BSI not present at admission, which together would allow the calculation of the rate of central-line-associated BSIs.[58] Since 2004, HHS has publicly reported some of the rates of adverse events from the MPSMS database in the *National Healthcare Quality Report* and *National Healthcare Disparity Report*, both of which are issued annually by AHRQ.

The APU program implemented a financial incentive for hospitals to submit to CMS data that are used to calculate hospital performance on measures of the quality of care they provide. The APU program receives quality-related data from hospitals on a quarterly basis for a range of medical conditions and, in 2007, began to require submission of information on three specific surgical infection prevention measures.[59] Hospitals paid under Medicare's inpatient prospective payment system receive a higher rate of payment if they submit these quality data that address their performance on recommended care practices. During fiscal year 2008, 3,270 hospitals will receive this higher level of payment, which represents 93 percent of hospitals eligible to participate in the APU program.[60] For patients who underwent specified surgical procedures, hospital staff review their medical records after discharge and, following detailed protocols from CMS, extract and record items of information that relate to three infection prevention practices that are associated with reduced risks of acquiring an SSI: (1) providing antibiotics within 1 hour of the surgery, (2) selecting appropriate antibiotics to prevent surgical infections, and (3) stopping the administration of the antibiotics within 24 hours of the end of the surgery. This information in turn is entered into algorithms that determine what proportion of patients who met CMS's criteria for designation as eligible for these infection prevention measures actually received them.

CMS publicly reports these results for each hospital individually on its Web site, Hospital Compare, along with state and national averages for comparison.[61]

AHRQ sponsored the development of the HCUP databases to create a national information resource of patient-level health care data. One of the HCUP databases assembles a sample of patient hospital discharge data from 37 states and converts them to a uniform format that enables the application of AHRQ's 20 Patient Safety Indicators (PSI)—including two that relate to HAIs—to an approximate national sample of all hospital patients.[62] The two PSIs related to HAIs involve (1) "selected infections due to medical care," which focuses on infections caused by intravenous lines and catheters, and (2) postoperative sepsis among patients undergoing elective surgery.[63] The PSIs are designed to identify patient safety issues by using the kinds of data that are available in hospital discharge data sets—specifically International Classification of Diseases, Ninth Revision (ICD-9), diagnostic and procedure codes, as well as patient demographics and admission and discharge status—and can be used with the HCUP database without collecting any additional information from patient medical records. However, these indicators are intended to be used as quality improvement tools to highlight aggregate patterns, and so they do not identify specific instances of adverse events with a high degree of precision.[64] AHRQ has posted national estimates for these two indicators—along with the other PSIs—on its Web site, showing the trend from 1994 to 2004.[65]

Two HHS agencies collect, or plan to collect, some limited additional information about HAIs in other HHS databases. FDA obtains data on deaths or serious injuries related to the use of medical devices and stores them in the Manufacturer and User Facility Device Experience Database.

A small portion of these adverse events may involve HAIs.[66] FDA uses these data to identify devices whose safety warrants closer scrutiny, such as might be warranted for heart valves that were not properly sterilized by the manufacturer. AHRQ is developing a database on adverse events, including HAIs, that will assemble data voluntarily submitted by hospitals to multiple Patient Safety Organizations (PSO).[67] AHRQ officials told us that they planned to disseminate aggregate results derived from the PSOs in an annual report.[68]

Table 3. Selected Characteristics of HHS Databases that Contain HAI-Related Information

Responsible agency and database	HAI-related data collected	Population for which data are collected	Hospital role in collecting data	Type of HAI information published by HHS
CDC's National Healthcare Safety Network (NHSN)	Infection types • central-line-associated BSI • catheter-associated UTI • VAP • postprocedure pneumonia • SSI • MDRO[a] • other[b]	Most hospitals report on patients in selected critical care units and those undergoing selected procedures such as coronary bypass surgery and colon surgery.	Hospital staff conduct medical review of signs, symptoms, and laboratory and radiological test results while patient is an inpatient. Hospital staff enter electronic information into database over the Internet.	CDC publishes rate of infection by type of infection and type of hospital unit or procedure for hospitals, in aggregate.
CMS's Medicare Patient Safety Monitoring System (MPSMS)	Infection types[c] • central-line-associated BSI • catheter-associated UTI • postoperative pneumonia • antibiotic-associated *C. difficile* • MRSA • VRE	National sample of hospitalized Medicare patients.	Hospital staff send a copy of sampled medical records to CMS, which are reviewed by contract abstractors.	AHRQ publishes nationallevel data on percentage of Medicare patients who experience selected infection types in two annual reports.[d]

Table 3. (Continued).

Responsible agency and database	HAI-related data collected	Population for which data are collected	Hospital role in collecting data	Type of HAI information published by HHS
CMS's Annual Payment Update (APU) database	Practices to prevent or reduce SSIs • providing antibiotics within 1 hour of surgery • selecting appropriate antibiotics to prevent surgical infections • stopping the administration of the antibiotics within 24 hours of end of surgery	National inpatient population for selected surgical procedures.[a]	Medical record review by hospital staff after patient's discharge. The hospital sends data to a CMS contractor.	CMS posts on a public Web site the proportion of patients receiving recommended practice, by hospital, as well as the state and national average.
AHRQ's Healthcare Cost and Utilization Project (HCUP) database, Nationwide Inpatient Sample	Infection types • postoperative sepsisf • "infection due to medical care" (focused on intravenous and catheter infections)	A sample of inpatients in hospitals in 37 states.	HCUP obtains hospital discharge data with ICD-9 diagnostic and procedure codes from statewide data systems.	AHRQ posts on its Web site national-level data on the proportion of patients with ICD-9 codes indicative of the two infection types.

Sources: GAO analysis of CDC, CMS, and AHRQ information.

Notes: BSI is bloodstream infection; *C. difficile* is *Clostridium difficile*; ICD-9 is International Classification of Diseases, Ninth Revision; MDRO is multidrug-resistant organism; MRSA is methicillin-resistant *Staphylococcus aureus*; SSI is surgical site infection; UTI is urinary tract infection; VAP is ventilator-associated pneumonia; and VRE is vancomycin-resistant enterococci.

[a] For patients whose infections are laboratory-confirmed, NHSN collects data on the pathogens identified, and for specified pathogens (including those responsible for MRSA and VRE), the result of any testing of their resistance to specific antibiotics. Participating hospitals have the option to report separately the number of times in a given month that they tested specimens of any of eight specified organisms for resistance to selected antibiotics, as well as the results of those tests. From these data, NHSN produces rates of antimicrobial resistance relative to the number of nonduplicative specimens tested (i.e., excluding

multiple tests for the same organism in the same patient). This part of NHSN does not distinguish between MDRO infections acquired in the hospital and community-acquired infections present at admission.

[b] Hospitals can choose to submit to NHSN data on other types of HAIs, such as skin and soft tissue infections, cardiovascular system infections, and gastrointestinal system infections. CDC does not provide data collection protocols for these types of infections, but they can be entered into NHSN as "custom events" using definitions provided separately by CDC.

[c] In 2007, CMS added catheter-associated UTIs, VAP, MRSA, and VRE to MPSMS and dropped insertion-site infections associated with central vascular catheters, BSIs, and postoperative-associated UTIs.

[d] The two annual reports are *The National Healthcare Quality Report* and *The National Healthcare Disparities Report*.

[e] The three practice measures are assessed for certain categories of surgeries: coronary artery bypass graft; other cardiac surgery; colon surgery; hip arthroplasty; knee arthroplasty; abdominal hysterectomy; vaginal hysterectomy; and vascular surgery.

[f] The rate of postoperative sepsis is computed only for patients undergoing elective surgeries.

Each of the four main HHS databases that currently collect information about HAIs presents only a partial view of the extent of the problem. None of them can provide information on the full range of HAIs, because each focuses its data collection on selected types of HAIs (see table 3).[69] In addition, none of the databases can address the frequency of even these selected HAIs for the nation as a whole, because each collects data from different subsets of the nationwide population of hospital patients. Although two databases—NHSN and MPSMS—address many of the same types of HAIs, the former provides information only from selected units of hospitals that participate in the NHSN program (which do not represent hospitals nationwide) while the latter provides information only on a representative sample of Medicare inpatients (i.e., MPSMS does not provide information on non-Medicare patients). The APU program does not collect information on patients with HAIs, but instead tracks the implementation of practices intended to prevent SSIs. The other three databases attempt to identify patients who developed infections as a result of their hospital stay using different data sources and varying approaches. The methods employed by the NHSN, MPSMS, and HCUP databases range from concurrent review of patient care as patients are treated in the hospital, to retrospective review of patient medical records after patients are discharged, to analyses of diagnostic codes recorded electronically in patient billing data.

The four databases also apply different sets of procedures to ensure the validity of their data, and each set has its own limitations. For the NHSN program, CDC requires participating hospitals to agree to its detailed instructions for identifying patients with HAIs, but CDC currently has no process in place to check how thoroughly and consistently those instructions are followed.[70] For the MPSMS program, CMS relies on internal procedures performed by a contractor that collects the data to routinely monitor the interrater reliability of its abstractors. However, CMS has not assessed the completeness or accuracy of the information in patient medical records that the MPSMS database measures rely on and how that might affect the HAI rates reported by the MPSMS program. CMS requires hospitals that submit APU data to have a small sample of their cases checked each quarter by a CMS contractor.[71] The contractor assesses the accuracy with which the hospital abstracted its APU data from patient medical records. AHRQ's HCUP database relies on ICD-9 codes filed with patient bills.[72] Many hospitals have their ICD-9 coding periodically checked by outside auditors, but the reason is to determine accuracy for billing purposes, not whether patients experienced HAIs.

Among the four databases, NHSN collects the most clinically detailed information about HAIs, but those data nonetheless have important limitations. Among the strengths of the NHSN database is that it presents detailed information on HAI rates across different types of hospital units and multiple types of HAIs. Moreover, its procedures for identifying patients with HAIs draw on the wider range of clinical information available while patients are still in the hospital, as opposed to retrospective reviews of patient medical records after discharge. On the other hand, the NHSN database is much more limited than any of the other databases in terms of the patient population that it represents. Because the hospitals that submit data either do so by choice or, for a limited number of states, by mandate, this group of hospitals is not representative of hospitals nationwide, as a random sample would be. In addition, the data these hospitals supply do not reflect the experience of many of their patients. For example, the hospitals that participate in the NHSN program report device-related HAIs such as central-line-associated BSIs and VAP for selected hospital units such as different types of intensive care units (e.g., coronary, burn, surgical, medical). In addition, most of the hospitals that participate in the NHSN program report procedure-based HAIs such as SSIs and postprocedure pneumonia for a relatively small number of specific procedures. For example, during March 2007, 225 hospitals reported SSIs for colon surgery and 133 did so for coronary bypass surgery, but only 11 hospitals reported SSIs for appendix surgery and 10 for gallbladder surgery.

Available Data Are Not Integrated across Programs to Use Them to Their Full Potential

Although officials from the various HHS agencies discuss HAI data collection with each other, we did not find that the agencies were taking steps to integrate any of the existing data from the four databases that collect HAI-related data. This integration could involve creating linkages between existing data by, for example, creating common patient identifiers in the different databases so that data on the same individuals found in multiple databases could be pulled together, or creating "crosswalks" that could specify in detail how related data fields in the various databases are similar or different. We found that the most extensive exchange of information across the three HHS agencies that collect HAI data occurred through the participation of their representatives in HICPAC. HICPAC generally holds 2-day meetings three times per year, and at each meeting the members from the participating HHS agencies typically provide a summary of their HAI-related activities. Our review of HICPAC minutes from 2004 through 2007 identified numerous instances of officials describing what their own agency was doing to collect HAI data, but we did not find in the HICPAC meeting minutes any evidence that the agencies had taken action to create greater compatibility among the databases or to address gaps in information across the databases. Outside of HICPAC meetings, HHS officials provided other examples of communication and outreach among HHS agencies taking place in relation to various databases. For example, the MPSMS program has a technical expert panel that includes representatives from CDC and AHRQ. Similarly, CMS, CDC, and AHRQ are represented on the steering committee for the public-private Surgical Care Improvement Project (SCIP), which developed the HAI-related measures used in the APU program.[73] These group discussions allow agency officials to discuss and explain their different approaches for collecting HAI data, but the focus of these meetings is still on the individual database, rather than on creating linkages from one database to another.

Creating mechanisms for linking data across the HAI-related databases could enhance the availability of information to better understand where and how HAIs occur. A case in point concerns information collected by two of the databases on surgical-related HAIs. Approximately 500 hospitals already submit data to APU on surgical processes of care and to NHSN on surgical infection rates for some of the same patients, but these data are not currently linked. As a consequence, the potential benefit of using the existing data to monitor the extent to which compliance with the recommended surgical care processes leads to actual improvements in surgical infection rates has not been realized. Officials at CDC reported that they approached CMS about developing mechanisms for linking NHSN data with APU data. To do this, CDC officials suggested that CDC and CMS agree to collect uniform patient identifiers. Officials at CMS reported that although they recognized the potential benefits of linking the APU data with the data in related HHS databases, CMS is currently focused on managing the expansion of the APU program.

Data Limitations Preclude Development of Reliable National Estimates

HHS cannot use its HAI-related databases to produce reliable national estimates of HAI rates, even for the selected types of HAIs monitored, because none of the databases collect data on the incidence of HAIs for a nationally representative sample of hospital patients. Two of the databases—APU and HCUP—come close to covering a national population for selected HAIs, but the APU database collects data on practices intended to prevent HAIs among surgery patients, not on the number of HAIs that occur. In addition, although the information in HCUP relates to the incidence of some HAIs, its reliance on diagnostic codes recorded in claims data substantially reduces the reliability of that information.[74] The other two databases—NHSN and MPSMS—collect clinical data on the incidence of selected HAIs, but their data do not derive from a representative sample of the national hospital patient population because NHSN is limited to selected units of participating hospitals that do not represent hospitals nationwide and MPSMS is limited to Medicare patients. (See table 3.)

Recent concerns about the magnitude of HAIs caused by the drug-resistant pathogen MRSA have further highlighted limitations in HHS's databases for estimating HAI rates. In June 2007, APIC, the professional association for infection control professionals, released the results of a survey it conducted that showed that 46 of every 1,000 patients in those hospitals had tested positive for MRSA.[75] This was a much higher rate than had previously been estimated by clinicians. The NHSN database has some information about the frequency of MRSA infections, as well as other MDROs, but this information is limited to the subset of patients for whom each hospital submits data, based on the particular hospital units, infection types, and procedures that it has chosen to report to NHSN. Thus, the NHSN database does not provide information on the overall proportion of patients in a given hospital who were found to have a MRSA infection.[76] The MPSMS program has begun to collect, but has not yet reported, data on the incidence of hospital-acquired MRSA infections within the Medicare inpatient population.[77] However, a CMS official responsible for the program acknowledged that the ability of the MPSMS program to detect patients with MRSA infections is limited by its reliance on retrospective review of patients' medical records.

The varying content and methods used to collect and report data on HAIs for HHS's four databases also preclude HHS from combining data from the databases to produce reliable estimates on either selected HAIs or an overall HAI rate. Even the databases that collect data on the same types of HAIs calculate and report rates in different ways that cannot be reconciled. For example, the MPSMS program reported that 1.7 percent of all the Medicare patients that had a central line inserted in 2004 experienced a central-line-associated BSI. In contrast, the NHSN program reported the mean number of central-line-associated BSIs detected during 2006 by different types of intensive care units, calculated as the number of infections per 1,000 days of central line use. This ranged from 1.5 per 1,000 days in inpatient medical/surgical wards to 6.8 per 1,000 days in burn intensive care units. HHS might be able to develop approaches for linking data across its different databases, such as by developing common data collection methods and specifications or creating crosswalks between the specifications for different databases. However, until that is done, the information on HAI rates from each of the three databases collecting that information stands alone.

CDC officials have produced national estimates of HAIs, but those estimates derive from assumptions and extrapolations that raise questions about the reliability of those estimates. Most recently, in 2007, CDC officials published estimates of the aggregate incidence of HAIs and deaths attributable to HAIs in 2002—which included an estimate of 99,000 HAIrelated deaths per year.[78] These estimates rested on two key assumptions. The first assumption was that data from 283 hospitals reporting to the NNIS program (the predecessor program to NHSN) were indicative of hospital rates nationwide, even though the authors acknowledged that the NNIS hospitals were not randomly selected and their rates could differ from those of U.S. acute care hospitals as a whole. The second assumption was that 2002 NNIS data on SSIs could be used to estimate rates for all other types of HAIs, based on the relative frequency of SSIs compared to other types of HAIs observed in a portion of NNIS hospitals during the 1990s.[79] In 2004, CDC officials announced plans for conducting a national survey designed to collect more up-to-date data on hospitalwide incidence of all types of HAIs in a sample of hospital discharges, but they subsequently decided not to proceed with those plans. CDC officials told us they were developing plans to obtain similar data by adding questions on HAIs to the National Hospital Discharge Survey conducted by CDC's National Center for Health Statistics.[80] CDC officials said they planned to put questions about HAIs into the National Hospital Discharge Survey starting in 2010. However, CDC officials stated that they planned first to pilot test several different approaches for collecting HAI data through the National Hospital Discharge Survey, and it was too early to say what specific information they would collect through this process.

CONCLUSIONS

HAIs in hospitals can cause needless suffering and death. Federal authorities and private organizations have undertaken a number of activities to address this serious problem; however, to date, these activities have not gained sufficient traction to be effective. Current activities at the federal level include guidelines with recommended practices issued by CDC, required standards for hospitals set by CMS, and HAI-related data collected through multiple HHS databases. Private-sector organizations, such as the Joint Commission and AOA, have also set infection control standards for hospitals. With the passage of the DRA by the Congress, hospitals will be encouraged to reduce certain HAIs, because beginning in October 2008 CMS will stop paying hospitals higher payments for patients that acquire them.

We identified two possible reasons for the lack of effective actions to control HAIs to date. First, although CDC's guidelines are an important source for its recommended practices on how to reduce HAIs, the large number of recommended practices and lack of department-level prioritization have hindered efforts to promote their implementation. The guidelines we reviewed contain almost 1,200 recommended practices for hospitals, including over 500 that are strongly recommended—a large number for a hospital trying to implement them. A few of these are required by CMS's or accrediting organizations' standards or their standards interpretations, but it is not reasonable to expect CMS or accrediting organizations to require additional practices without a prioritization. Although CDC has categorized the practices on the basis of the strength of the scientific evidence, there are other factors to consider in developing priorities. For example, work by AHRQ suggests factors such as costs or organizational obstacles that could be considered. The lack of coordinated prioritization may have resulted in duplication of effort by CDC and AHRQ in their reviews of scientific evidence on HAIrelated practices.

Second, HHS has not effectively used the HAI-related data it has collected through multiple databases across the department to provide a complete picture about the extent of the problem. Limitations in the databases, such as nonrepresentative samples, hinder HHS's ability to produce reliable national estimates on the frequency of different types of HAIs. In addition, currently collected data on HAIs are not being combined to maximize their utility. For example, data on surgical infection rates and data on surgical processes of care are collected for some of the same patients in two different databases that are not linked. HHS has made efforts to use the currently collected data to understand the extent of the problem of HAIs, but the lack of linkages across the various databases results in a lost opportunity to gain a better grasp of the problem of HAIs.

HHS has multiple methods to influence hospitals to take more aggressive action to control or prevent HAIs, including issuing guidelines with recommended practices, requiring hospitals to comply with certain standards, releasing data to expand information about the nature of the problem, and soon, using hospital payment methods to encourage the reduction of HAIs. Prioritization of CDC's many recommended practices can help guide their implementation, and better use of currently collected data on HAIs could help HHS—and hospitals themselves—monitor efforts to reduce HAIs. Unfortunately, leadership from the Secretary of HHS is currently lacking to do this. Without such leadership, the department is unlikely to be able to effectively leverage its various methods to have a significant effect on the suffering and death caused by HAIs.

RECOMMENDATIONS FOR EXECUTIVE ACTION

In order to help reduce HAIs in hospitals, the Secretary of HHS should take the following two actions:

1. Identify priorities among CDC's recommended practices and determine how to promote implementation of the prioritized practices, including whether to incorporate selected practices into CMS's conditions of participation (COP) for hospitals.

2   Establish greater consistency and compatibility of the data collected across HHS on HAIs to increase information available about HAIs, including reliable national estimates of the major types of HAIs.

COMMENTS FROM HHS AND ACCREDITING ORGANIZATIONS AND OUR EVALUATION

We obtained written comments on our draft chapter from HHS, which appear in appendix III. HHS generally agreed with our recommendations and noted its appreciation for our efforts in developing this chapter. The comments addressed both of our recommendations.

In terms of our first recommendation, HHS's comments indicated that CMS welcomed the opportunity to work with CDC to review and prioritize recommendations for infection control and would consider whether to incorporate some of the recommendations into CMS's hospital COPs. HHS stated that COPs represent minimum health and safety requirements and the two standards in the infection control COP have a broad reach for assessing a hospital's infection control program. HHS's comments also noted that the COPs currently lack the specificity of guidance and recommendations issued by HHS agencies, including CDC's recommendations for infection control.

In terms of our second recommendation, HHS's comments acknowledged the need for greater consistency and compatibility of data collected on HAIs and identified three actions CMS would take. First, CMS will work with other HHS agencies to evaluate opportunities for consolidating and coordinating national data collection programs. Second, CMS will implement consensus-based measures whenever possible. Third, CMS will require the collection of data that facilitate linkages between databases, including Medicare beneficiary and hospital patient identifiers in the APU program. HHS's comments also noted that CDC has recently begun moving toward greater alignment with CMS.

HHS's comments also noted other activities under way that the department believes would improve the collection of HAI-related data. For example, as part of implementing section 5001(c) of the DRA, hospitals are required to begin reporting "present on admission" data—diagnoses that are present in patients at the time of admission—in order to determine whether the selected preventable conditions were acquired prior to the hospitalization. We noted this activity in the chapter, and we believe that it is too early to know the extent of information that will be generated on HAIs or how it will be used by HHS agencies. HHS's comments also indicated that CMS is evaluating an update to the diagnostic and procedure coding system, which could offer clearer and more detailed information than the current system, and also noted the benefits of employing industry data standards for electronic health care data exchanges to facilitate reporting of HAI-related data to both CDC and CMS. In our chapter, we did not assess the effect of these activities because they have not been implemented.

We also obtained comments on a draft of this chapter from representatives of the Joint Commission and AOA. The Joint Commission concurred with our findings that it would be beneficial to have more accurate estimates of HAIs and that prioritization of practices to guide actions in preventing HAIs is a valuable and necessary undertaking. However, it noted that other actions, such as cultural changes in health care organizations, clear strategies for implementation, and a concerted, multifaceted effort by many stakeholders, are needed to reduce HAIs. We agree that such actions are important in reducing HAIs, and that better prioritization of the many recommended practices would facilitate the process the Joint Commission describes. The Joint Commission also provided two comments related to the section of the chapter that discusses hospital infection control standards. First, it commented that our chapter places too great a focus on the number of standards, and pointed out the benefit of the Joint Commission's systems-based approach. It expressed a concern that a reader could perceive that the Joint Commission has fewer expectations for hospitals than CMS or AOA. That was not our intention, and we have modified the chapter to note the Joint Commission's systems-based approach to foster compliance with practices to reduce HAIs. Second, the Joint Commission said that the chapter indicates that their standards are less specific in that they have not adopted certain CDC recommendations, but they noted that many of the CDC guidelines cannot be implemented without additional research or translation into concrete, actionable steps. In the draft, we described some activities being undertaken by CDC and AHRQ to promote implementation of recommended practices to reduce HAIs, including studies funded by AHRQ, and we added a clarification to the text to note the importance of translating knowledge into social and behavioral changes that can be sustained. Furthermore, we believe that clearer prioritization can help efforts to promote the implementation of practices to reduce HAIs.

HHS, the Joint Commission, and AOA provided technical comments, which we incorporated as appropriate.

Sincerely yours,

Cynthia A. Bascetta
Director, Health Care

APPENDIX I: OTHER CDC ACTIVITIES DESIGNED TO REDUCE OR PREVENT HEALTH-CARE-ASSOCIATED INFECTIONS

In addition to developing infection control and prevention guidelines and recommendations, the Centers for Disease Control and Prevention (CDC) provides leadership in outbreak investigations, surveillance, and laboratory research and prevention of health-care-associated infections (HAI). According to officials, CDC's work in the area of outbreak investigations has led to new knowledge on ways to prevent HAIs. For example, in 2006, CDC investigated an outbreak of eye inflammation that was occurring in patients who recently had cataract surgery at a hospital in Maine. The outcome of this investigation led to the development of recommended practices for cleaning and sterilizing intraocular surgical instruments developed by the American Society of Cataract and Refractive Surgery and the American Society of Ophthalmic Registered Nurses.

CDC's surveillance, research, and demonstration projects measure the effect of HAIs, adverse drug events, and other complications of health care. CDC has funded many activities through its Prevention Epicenter Program, which began in 1997 and is devoted to improving the detection, reporting, and prevention of HAIs, antimicrobial resistance, and other adverse events in health care. For example, CDC funded a multicenter trial research project and found that daily bathing with chlorhexidine, an antiseptic, reduces the incidence of methicillin-resistant *Staphylococcus aureus* (MRSA), vancomycin-resistant enterococci (VRE),[81]and bloodstream infection (BSI). In addition, CDC has collaborated with three public hospitals in Chicago to develop a clinical data warehouse using the hospitals' information systems, which enabled the hospitals to develop a series of quality improvement strategies to decrease antimicrobial resistance and improve antibiotic prescribing and infection control practices.

Finally, CDC provides direct support and assistance to external groups involved in many HAI prevention activities. CDC has funded and collaborated with the Pittsburgh Veterans Affairs Medical Center to reduce MRSA infections by more than 60 percent in its health care units. The success of this project has led CDC and the Department of Veterans Affairs to initiate similar efforts across all VA hospitals. In addition, CDC is represented on the Surgical Care Improvement Project (SCIP) steering committee. SCIP is a national public-private partnership to reduce surgical complications that is sponsored by the Centers for Medicare & Medicaid Services. CDC told us that they have worked with SCIP to develop quality measures and market the project. Finally, CDC has provided technical assistance to the Institute for Healthcare Improvement, a not-for-profit organization working to improve global health care, in the development of the institute's hand hygiene "bundle" and MRSA infection prevention "bundle" guides.

APPENDIX II: CENTERS FOR MEDICARE & MEDICAID SERVICES' (CMS) CONDITION OF PARTICIPATION: INFECTION CONTROL

The conditions of participation (COP) for hospitals, including the infection control COP as well as the survey protocols and interpretive guidelines that accompany the COPs, are contained in Appendix A of CMS's *State Operations Manual*.[82] CMS issued revised interpretive guidelines for the infection control COP on November 21, 2007.[83]

The COP on infection control (42 C.F.R. § 482.42) (2007) states that

The hospital must provide a sanitary environment to avoid sources and transmission of infections and communicable diseases. There must be an active program for the prevention, control, and investigation of infections and communicable diseases.

(a) Standard: Organization and policies. A person or persons must be designated as infection control officer or officers to develop and implement policies governing control of infections and communicable diseases.

(1) The infection control officer or officers must develop a system for identifying, reporting, investigating, and controlling infections and communicable diseases of patients and personnel.

(2) The infection control officer or officers must maintain a log of incidents related to infections and communicable diseases.

(b) Standard: Responsibilities of chief executive officer, medical staff, and director of nursing services. The chief executive officer, the medical staff, and the director of nursing services must—

(1) Ensure that the hospital-wide quality assurance program and training programs address problems identified by the infection control officer or officers; and

(2) Be responsible for the implementation of successful corrective action plans in affected problem areas.

In addition, CMS officials said that the quality assessment and performance improvement COP, which can be found at 42 C.F.R. § 482.21 (2007), can also affect infection control.[84]

APPENDIX III: COMMENTS FROM THE DEPARTMENT OF HEALTH AND HUMAN SERVICES

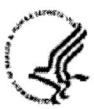

DEPARTMENT OF HEALTH & HUMAN SERVICES

Office of the Assistant Secretary
for Legislation

Washington, D.C. 20201

FEB 19 2008

Ms. Cynthia A. Bascetta
Director, Health Care
U.S. Government Accountability Office
Washington, DC 20548

Dear Ms. Bascetta:

Enclosed are comments on the Government Accountability Office (GAO) Draft Report, "Health-Care-Associated Infections in Hospitals: Leadership Needed From HHS to Prioritize Prevention Practices and Improve Data on These Infections" (GAO-08-283).

The Department appreciates the opportunity to review and comment on this report before its publication.

Sincerely,

Vincent Ventimiglia
Assistant Secretary for Legislation

GENERAL COMMENTS OF THE DEPARTMENT OF HEALTH AND HUMAN SERVICES (HHS) ON THE U.S. GOVERNMENT ACCOUNTABILITY OFFICE'S (GAO) DRAFT REPORT ENTITLED: "HEALTH-CARE-ASSOCIATED INFECTINS IN HOSPITALS: LEADERSHIP NEEDED FROM HHS TO PRIORITIZE PREVENTION PRACTICES AND IMPROVE DATA ON THESE INFECTIONS" (GAO-08-283).

The Department appreciates GAO's efforts to ensure that the Centers for Medicare & Medicaid Services (CMS) collaborates with other Health and Human Services (HHS) agencies to--(1) identify and potentially codify infection control practices to prevent health-care-associated infections (HAIs); and (2) develop linkages between the various HHS data collection systems to facilitate the collection and analysis of national HAI data.

As a condition of their participation in the Medicare and Medicaid programs, hospitals must comply with all of CMS's minimum regulatory health and safety requirements, called conditions of participation (CoPs), including the CoP for infection control.

The CoP for infection control requires hospitals to provide a sanitary environment to avoid sources and transmission of infections and communicable diseases and to have an active program for the prevention, control, and investigation of infections and communicable diseases. Hospitals must designate at least one infection control officer to develop and implement policies governing control of infections and communicable diseases. That officer must develop a system for identifying, reporting, investigating, and controlling infections and communicable diseases of patients and personnel; and maintain a log of incidents related to infections and communicable diseases. Further, each hospital's chief executive officer, medical staff, and director of nursing services is responsible for ensuring that the hospital-wide quality and training programs address problems identified by the infection control officer(s) and for implementation of successful corrective action plans in affected problem areas.

As the GAO report notes, CMS has developed interpretive guidelines for CoPs that describe the CoPs and provide survey procedures. Medicare/Medicaid providers utilize these guidelines to determine how to implement the requirements in the CoPs. The CMS guidelines for the hospital infection control CoP (CMS State Operations Manual, Appendix A: http://www.cms.hhs.gov/Manuals/IOM/itemdetail.asp?filterType=none&filterByDID=-99&sortByDID=1&sortOrder=ascending&itemID=CMS1201984&intNumPerPage=10) reference some of the CDC recommendations that hospitals can use to ensure they are in compliance with the requirements of the CoP. For example, the Guidelines cite the CDC "Guidelines for Prevention and Control of Nosocomial Infections" and "Guidelines for Preventing the Transmission of Tuberculosis in Health Care Facilities." The Guidelines state that hospitals should provide a safe environment, "consistent with nationally recognized infection control precautions, such as the current CDC recommendations for the identified infection and/or communicable disease...."

Although CMS does not have specific infection control requirements, such as hand hygiene or sterilization standards, we cite noted improper practices that do not follow nationally recognized standards (such as CDC strongly recommended practices) at our standard-level requirement for preventing and controlling infections. In a plan of correction, we would expect a hospital to demonstrate that it had implemented recognized practices to address the improper practices and that it had incorporated the corrective actions into its quality assessment and performance improvement program to ensure sustainability.

GENERAL COMMENTS OF THE DEPARTMENT OF HEALTH AND HUMAN SERVICES (HHS) ON THE U.S. GOVERNMENT ACCOUNTABILITY OFFICE'S (GAO) DRAFT REPORT ENTITLED: "HEALTH-CARE-ASSOCIATED INFECTINS IN HOSPITALS: LEADERSHIP NEEDED FROM HHS TO PRIORITIZE PREVENTION PRACTICES AND IMPROVE DATA ON THESE INFECTIONS" (GAO-08-283).

Thus, although our CoPs have only two standards, the standards have an extremely broad reach when it comes to assessing a hospital's infection control program, and we routinely cite observed infection control breaches, even when such breaches have not resulted in a known infection.

In regard to the collection of HAI data, it is important to note that these data collection programs are designed in some cases for very different purposes. For example, the Reporting Hospital Quality Data for Annual Payment Update (RHQDAPU) program is designed to produce hospital level estimates. Under the RHQDAPU Program, participating hospitals report several infection-related measures. These include SCIP-Inf-1 Prophylactic Antibiotic Received Within One Hour Prior to Surgical Incision, SCIP-Inf-2 Prophylactic Antibiotic Selection for Surgical Patients, and SCIP-Inf-3 Prophylactic Antibiotics Discontinued Within 24 Hours After Surgery End Time. These measures are currently publicly reported on CMS's Hospital Compare website. In addition, under Medicare's Quality Improvement Organization Program, selected hospitals receive technical assistance to improve their performance for these and additional measures. The rare nature of selected HAI measures and the current burden of data collection preclude the production of reliable hospital level estimates for these relatively rare events for sampled data. Nevertheless, CMS acknowledges the need for greater consistency and compatibility of the collected data on HAI's.

One advance in the collection of HAI data will occur when we move from the current coding system, ICD-9-CM to an updated system, ICD-10. CMS is currently evaluating this move. Identifying hospital-acquired conditions requires clear and detailed diagnosis codes. The current coding system, ICD-9-CM, is three decades old. It is outdated, and has numerous instances of broad and vague codes. Attempts to add this detail to ICD-9-CM are constrained by a lack of room to expand. This has a negative impact on CMS' attempts to identify cases with a hospital-acquired condition. ICD-10 codes are more precise and capture information using medical terminology used by current medical practitioners. Examples of problems with ICD-9-CM that impact our current effort with hospital-acquired conditions that have been rectified with ICD-10 include the following examples.

- Pressure ulcers – We selected pressure ulcers as one of our hospital-acquired conditions. This condition is both high cost and high frequency. There are prevention guidelines for pressure ulcers. Unfortunately, ICD-9-CM does not provide enough detail to clearly identify the exact location, size, or depth of the pressure ulcer. Using trend data, one cannot tell if the pressure ulcer is getting better or worse (increasing in size or depth). ICD-9-CM has nine codes that identify the generic part of the body with the pressure ulcer. It provides no information of the size, depth, or exact location of the pressure ulcer. ICD-10-CM has 60 codes that identify the size, depth, and location of the pressure ulcer.
- Hospital-acquired Infections – ICD-9-CM does not have unique codes that identify specific types of bacterial infections which are resistant to antibiotics, such as MRSA infections. MRSA infections are captured through a combination of at least three separate codes under ICD-9-CM. This includes a vague code that captures all types of infections that are resistant to antibiotics.

GENERAL COMMENTS OF THE DEPARTMENT OF HEALTH AND HUMAN SERVICES (HHS) ON THE U.S. GOVERNMENT ACCOUNTABILITY OFFICE'S (GAO) DRAFT REPORT ENTITLED: "HEALTH-CARE-ASSOCIATED INFECTINS IN HOSPITALS: LEADERSHIP NEEDED FROM HHS TO PRIORITIZE PREVENTION PRACTICES AND IMPROVE DATA ON THESE INFECTIONS" (GAO-08-283).

ICD-10 has more detail in each code as to the type and location of the infection. The next draft of ICD-10 will have detailed codes that would indicate whether the patient had a MRSA infection or was colonized with MRSA, but suffering no current infection. The ability to expand ICD-10 to capture detailed information on additional conditions is also one of the strengths of ICD-10.

- Septicemia – CMS is evaluating the selection of septicemia as one of the hospital-acquired condition. ICD-9-CM codes are quite problematic in capturing septicemia cases. Multiple, overlapping codes are required to identify these cases. This makes coding, reporting, and data analysis of septicemia difficult. ICD-10 codes are much improved and clearly identify septicemia cases.
- Falls and trauma -ICD-9-CM codes are vague and do not describe whether an injury, such as a leg fracture, occurs on the right or left leg. ICD-9-CM also does not provide information on whether the encounter is for the initial treatment of the fracture or for subsequent care. ICD-10 has detailed codes that identify the nature of the injury, whether it was to the left or right extremity, and whether the treatment is toward a new or earlier fracture. ICD-10 also provides greater detail as to where the injury occurred (e.g., the patient room, corridor, operating room, bathroom). This detail is not present in ICD-9-CM.
- Foreign body left in after surgery (never event) – ICD-9-CM has one vague code that captures the fact that a complication developed as a result of a device being inadvertently left in a patient after surgery. ICD-10 codes provides much greater detail and describes the type of complication that results from this never event. The codes describe the type of complication such as an obstruction, perforation, infection, or adhesions. The codes also clearly describe the type of procedure performed that resulted in the device being inadvertently left in a patient, such as an endoscopic procedure or an open procedure. This more detailed information provides a more definitive picture of the nature of the complication resulting from the never event.

There are many other parts of ICD-10 that provide clear and concise codes to capture events and conditions important for health care delivery. ICD-10 has codes that describe under-dosing and over-dosing patients. This information would provide valuable information on patient outcomes. With more precise codes, CMS could add additional hospital-acquired provisions to our proposals.

Another advance in the collection of HAI data is the recent requirement for the collection of Present on Admission data as part of hospital submitted Medicare claims. The Deficit Reduction Act (DRA) required CMS to select certain conditions for which Medicare will no longer pay an additional amount when that condition is acquired during a hospitalization. The DRA further requires that the selected conditions be reasonably preventable through the application of evidence-based guidelines. CMS has closely collaborated with CDC on the selection of these conditions, with particular attention to identifying evidence-based guidelines that are consistent with CDC's recommended practices. Thus, this Medicare payment provision is closely tied to CDC's prioritized practices.

GENERAL COMMENTS OF THE DEPARTMENT OF HEALTH AND HUMAN SERVICES (HHS) ON THE U.S. GOVERNMENT ACCOUNTABILITY OFFICE'S (GAO) DRAFT REPORT ENTITLED: "HEALTH-CARE-ASSOCIATED INFECTINS IN HOSPITALS: LEADERSHIP NEEDED FROM HHS TO PRIORITIZE PREVENTION PRACTICES AND IMPROVE DATA ON THESE INFECTIONS" (GAO-08-283).

As a prerequisite for implementing this Medicare payment provision, the DRA also requires hospitals to begin reporting present on admission (POA) indicator data to identify whether the selected conditions are acquired during a hospitalization. CMS' approach to POA indicator reporting is consistent with the standards set forth in the ICD-9-CM guidelines, which are maintained by CDC. CMS' collection of POA data will generate increased information about hospital-acquired conditions, including infections, which can be used by CDC and others to inform and disseminate reliable national estimates of these conditions.

Finally, CMS, under its Quality Improvement Organization 9th Statement of Work, will include as components of the Patient Safety Theme, measures relevant to health-care associated infections in hospitals. These measures will include a Surgical Care Improvement Project (SCIP) measure on the use of prophylactic antibiotics and a measure on the incidence of Methcillin-Resistant Staphylococcus aureus (MRSA). This work is being conducted in collaboration with CDC.

CMS is committed to ensuring that all patients in Medicare and Medicaid participating hospitals receive quality health care and appreciates the GAO's support in helping HHS achieve that goal.

GAO Recommendations:

In order to reduce HAIs in hospitals, the Secretary should--

1. Identify priorities among CDC's recommended practices and determine how to promote the prioritized practices, including whether to incorporate selected practices into CMS's conditions of participation for hospitals; and

2. Establish greater consistency and compatibility of the data collected across HHS on HAIs to increase information available about HAIs, including reliable national estimates of the major types of HAIs.

CMS Response:

Medicare/Medicaid CoPs are broadly written, minimum health and safety requirements that providers and suppliers must meet to participate in Medicare and Medicaid. As a result, CoPs lack the specificity of the guidance and recommendations issued by HHS agencies, including the CDC recommendations for infection control. CMS continuously evaluates the CoPs for all Medicare/Medicaid providers to determine whether they need to be updated, for example, to reflect more current standards of practice. We welcome the opportunity to work with the CDC to review and prioritize its recommendations. When the recommendations are prioritized, CMS will consider whether to incorporate some of the recommendations into the hospital CoPs.

CMS will take the following actions to establish consistency and compatibility of the data collected across HHS on HAIs:

GENERAL COMMENTS OF THE DEPARTMENT OF HEALTH AND HUMAN SERVICES (HHS) ON THE U.S. GOVERNMENT ACCOUNTABILITY OFFICE'S (GAO) DRAFT REPORT ENTITLED: "HEALTH-CARE-ASSOCIATED INFECTINS IN HOSPITALS: LEADERSHIP NEEDED FROM HHS TO PRIORITIZE PREVENTION PRACTICES AND IMPROVE DATA ON THESE INFECTIONS" (GAO-08-283).

(1) Work with other HHS agencies to evaluate opportunities for consolidating and coordinating national data collection programs.

(2) Implement consensus-based measures definitions, such as using National Quality Forum endorsed measures in the APU program, whenever possible.

(3) Require collection of data that facilitate linkage between databases, including Medicare beneficiary ID and Hospital patient ID in the APU program.

CMS will be mindful of the burden to hospitals and the need for collecting reliable national level HAI estimates in its national data collection programs. We appreciate the GAO's efforts in developing this report on prioritizing HAI prevention practices and improving HAI data collection.

Page 35, Paragraph 3, Line 1 The GAO draft report states "Although officials from the various HHS agencies discuss HAI data collection with each other, we did not find that the agencies were taking steps to integrate any of the existing data from the four databases that collect HAI-related data."

- Most recently, CDC has taken steps toward definitional alignment with CMS, and CDC has taken steps toward enabling CMS-SCIP data imports into NHSN. Also, the HHS Patient Safety Task Force made efforts toward integrating patient safety reporting to multiple agencies through a common portal.

- In recent years, the Health Level Seven (HL7) data standards organization has developed a XML file format for electronic exchanges of structured clinical documents. The HL7 standard, known as Clinical Document Architecture (CDA), is designed for use in exchange of clinical records, such as continuity of care records and patient history and physical examination findings. The versatility of the CDA standard has led to additional uses, including HIPAA-mandated electronic claims attachments that CMS has developed with HL7 for use in claims processing. All electronic claims attachment documents promulgated by CMS are CDA documents. CDC is using CDA as the file format for information system developers to use in enabling their systems to report healthcare associated infection (HAI) data from hospitals to CDC's National Healthcare Safety Network (NHSN). The clinical, financial, and public health uses of CDA are evidence of the importance this industry standard has already achieved as a specification for data exchanges between disparate systems.

GENERAL COMMENTS OF THE DEPARTMENT OF HEALTH AND HUMAN SERVICES (HHS) ON THE U.S. GOVERNMENT ACCOUNTABILITY OFFICE'S (GAO) DRAFT REPORT ENTITLED: "HEALTH-CARE-ASSOCIATED INFECTINS IN HOSPITALS: LEADERSHIP NEEDED FROM HHS TO PRIORITIZE PREVENTION PRACTICES AND IMPROVE DATA ON THESE INFECTIONS" (GAO-08-283).

- One important benefit of adopting an industry standard solution for electronic healthcare data exchanges is that it facilitates communication and reuse of data already collected for some other purpose. CDA calls for use of standard healthcare vocabulary in the documents that are exchanged. This requirement is an integral part of enabling interoperability between sending and receiving systems. Another important benefit is enabling technical features for importing files from one system to another and distributing data into the second system's database to be reused for a variety of files that conform to the standard format. For example, CDA documents can be imported and parsed into a database using the same technical features regardless of whether the document carries data about a clinical outcome, such as a healthcare associated infection, or a process of care, such as use of an antimicrobial agent to prevent a surgical site infection.

- This latter benefit points to why adoption of an industry standard file format, in particular CDA, would be advantageous for CDC in its monitoring of HAIs through NHSN and CMS in its monitoring of process of care, such as surgical care, through its CART tool and the Annual Payment Update database. A CDA import function, under development for the NHSN application, will enable CDC's system to be used to import HAI data reported via a CDA document. The same function will lend itself for use in importing a process of care measurement data if those data are conveyed using the CDA file format. The CART tool generates proprietary XML files, i.e., files that do not conform to specifications of a standards development organization such as HL7. At the relatively low cost of converting the proprietary format used in the CART tool to the industry-standard CDA file format, the process of care data collected for the Annual Payment Update database, including Surgical Care Improvement Program (SCIP) data, would be available for importation into NHSN and linkage with the outcome data. In other words, migration to CDA across CDC and CMS systems will enable hospitals participating in both systems to readily combine patient-level process and outcome data.

REFERENCES

[1] In general, HAIs are distinct from community-acquired infections, that is, infections that patients may have acquired before entering the hospital.
[2] Antimicrobial resistance is the result of microbes changing in ways that reduce or eliminate the effectiveness of drugs, chemicals, or other agents to cure or prevent infections.

[3] See Pennsylvania Health Care Cost Containment Council, *Hospital-Acquired Infections in Pennsylvania* (Harrisburg, Pa.: November 2006).
[4] See D. Murphy et al., *Dispelling the Myths: The True Cost of Healthcare-Associated Infections* (Washington, D.C., Association for Professionals in Infection Control and Epidemiology, February 2007).
[5] Medicare is a federal health insurance program that serves over 42 million elderly and certain disabled beneficiaries and pays for health care needs, such as inpatient hospital stays and physician visits.
[6] See 42 C.F.R. § 482.1 (2007).
[7] Section 1865(b)(1) of the Social Security Act also provides that any other national accreditation body that meets certain requirements as determined by HHS may accredit hospitals.
[8] In calendar year 2007, about 81 percent of hospitals were accredited by the Joint Commission, state survey agencies certified approximately 16 percent of hospitals, and less than 2 percent were accredited by AOA. Less than 1 percent of hospitals were accredited by both the Joint Commission and AOA. The Joint Commission was formerly known as the Joint Commission on Accreditation of Healthcare Organizations or "JCAHO."
[9] See K. Adams et al., *Priority Areas for National Action: Transforming Health Care Quality*, Institute of Medicine of the National Academies (Washington, D.C.: The National Academies Press, 2003).
[10] Pub. L. No. 109-171, § 5001(c), 120 Stat. 4, 30.
[11] Under Medicare, hospitals generally receive fixed payments for inpatient stays based on diagnosis-related groups (DRG), a system that classifies stays by patient diagnoses and procedures. Some DRGs take account of certain comorbidities or complications associated with a diagnosis or procedure and pay at a higher rate than would otherwise be paid for the diagnosis or procedure. In a final regulation implementing section 500 1(c) of the DRA, CMS identified certain preventable conditions it would not consider as a comorbidity or complication that would lead to the higher payment. See 72 Fed. Reg. 47130, 47200-2 17 (Aug. 22, 2007). The DRA also requires hospitals to indicate the diagnoses that were present in patients at the time of admission in order for CMS to determine if a preventable condition developed during a patient's hospital stay.
[12] Mediastinitis is inflammation of the area between the lungs (the heart, the large blood vessels, the trachea, the esophagus, the thymus gland, and connective tissues). Additional preventable conditions that will no longer result in higher payments to hospitals include hospital-acquired injuries, such as fractures, pressure ulcers, objects left in the body during surgery, air embolisms, and

blood incompatibility. CMS plans to propose additional conditions in the fiscal year 2009 Hospital Inpatient Prospective Payment Systems proposed rule. See 72 Fed. Reg. 47130 (Aug. 22, 2007).

[13] See Consumers Union, "State Hospital Infection Disclosure Laws," available at http://www.consumersunion.org/campaigns/stophospitalinfections/learn.html, accessed on March 10, 2008.

[14] Representatives from the following government agencies are nonvoting members of HICPAC: CDC, CMS, AHRQ, FDA, the National Institutes of Health, and the Health Resources and Services Administration.

[15] See World Health Organization, WHO Guidelines on Hand Hygiene in Healthcare (Advanced Draft): Global Patient Safety Challenge 2005-2006: Clean Care Is Safer Care (Geneva, Switzerland, 2006).

[16] HHS officials noted that the interpretive guidelines are used by Medicare and Medicaid providers, such as hospitals, critical access hospitals, hospices, nursing homes, and home health agencies, to determine how to implement the requirements in the COPs.

[17] Throughout this report, where we refer to the interpretive guidelines for infection control we are referring to the most recent revision.

[18] Public health surveillance is defined as the ongoing systematic collection, analysis, and interpretation of health data for purposes of improving health and safety.

[19] The creation of HICPAC is authorized under section 222 of the Public Health Service Act (codified at 42 U.S.C. §217a). The committee is governed by the provisions of the Federal Advisory Committee Act, Pub. L. No. 92-463, 86 Stat. 770 (1972), (codified at 5 U.S.C. App. 2), which sets forth standards for the formation and use of an advisory committee.

[20] In addition, CDC circulates the draft guideline to experts outside of CDC for comment as part of an Office of Management and Budget initiative to respond to concerns about whether diverse experts and members of the public are provided with sufficient opportunities to comment on influential scientific information or highly influential assessment documents. CDC's infection control and prevention guidelines are considered highly influential documents.

[21] Appendix A of the *State Operations Manual* contains the COPs for hospitals and is available at http://www.cms.hhs.gov/GuidanceforLawsAndRegulations/08_Hospitals.asp, downloaded on May 14, 2007.

[22] As we noted in a previous report, due to the Joint Commission's unique legal status, CMS has limited oversight authority over the Joint Commission's hospital accreditation program. See GAO, *Medicare: CMS Needs*

Additional Authority to Adequately Oversee Patient Safety in Hospitals, GAO-04-850 (Washington, D.C.: July 20, 2004).

[23] CDC has issued four infection control guidance documents for hospitals: (1) Infection Control Guidance for the Prevention and Control of Influenza in Acute-Care Facilities, (2) Interim Guidance for the Use of Masks to Control Influenza Transmission, (3) Respiratory Hygiene/Cough Etiquette, and (4) Guidelines on Public Reporting of Healthcare-Associated Infections. While the title of this fourth guidance document includes the word "guidelines," CDC officials consider this document to be guidance.

[24] CDC placed some of the practices in these seven guidelines in two categories.

[25] Recommended practices related to *Guideline for Prevention of Catheter-associated Urinary Tract Infections* issued in 1981 were categorized as (1) strongly recommended, (2) moderately recommended, and (3) weakly recommended for adoption. *Guideline for Infection Control in Health Care Personnel* issued in 1998 and *Guideline for Prevention of Surgical Site Infection* issued in 1999 used a slightly different four-tier ranking system of (1) strongly recommended and strongly supported by well-designed experimental or epidemiologic studies, (2) strongly recommended based on strong rationale and suggestive evidence, (3) suggested for implementation based on suggestive clinical or epidemiologic studies, and (4) no recommendation or unresolved issue. *Guidelines for Preventing Opportunistic Infections among Hematopoietic Stem Cell Transplant Recipients* issued in 2000 used an evidence-based rating system to determine strength of recommendations and another evidence-based system to determine quality of evidence. Using the first system, the recommendations were categorized as (1) strongly recommended, (2) generally recommended, (3) optional, (4) generally not recommended, and (5) never recommended.

[26] These two guidelines were created outside of HICPAC by another CDC advisory committee—the Advisory Committee on Immunization Practices—and CDC's Division of Tuberculosis Elimination.

[27] CDC has been drafting this guideline since 2000, and CDC officials told us they expected to publish the guideline in 2008.

[28] This section addresses efforts to facilitate or encourage implementation of recommended practices, as distinct from requiring hospitals to adopt these practices by incorporating them in the standards set by CMS, the Joint Commission, and AOA.

[29] CDC began the Prevention Epicenter Program in 1997 as a way to collaborate with academic institutions to investigate the epidemiology and prevention of HAIs. More information on CDC's Prevention Epicenter Program and other HAI-related activities can be found in app. I.

[30] Studies have demonstrated reductions in HAIs when selected recommended practices are implemented as a group or "bundle." The Institute for Healthcare Improvement and the Michigan Health and Hospital Association Keystone Intensive Care Unit Project have also employed the bundle approach with success. See P. Pronovost et al., "An Intervention to Decrease Catheter-Related Bloodstream Infections in the ICU," *The New England Journal of Medicine*, vol. 355, no. 26 (2006): 2725–2732.

[31] See C. Muto et al., "Reduction in Central Line-Associated Bloodstream Infections among Patients in Intensive Care Units—Pennsylvania, April 2001–March 2005," *Morbidity and Mortality Weekly Report*, vol. 54, no. 40 (2005): 1013–1016.

[32] See S. R. Ranji et al., Closing the Quality Gap: A Critical Analysis of Quality Improvement Strategies, Volume 6—Prevention of Healthcare-Associated Infections, AHRQ Publication No. 04(07)-0051-6 (Rockville, Md., January 2007).

[33] The four strategies were (1) use of printed or computer-based reminders with automatic stop orders to reduce unnecessary urethral catheterization; (2) printed or computer-based reminders to improve surgical antibiotic prophylaxis; (3) active educational interventions with use of checklists to improve adherence to central line insertion practices; and (4) active educational interventions such as tutorials to improve adherence to preventive interventions for ventilator-associated pneumonia.

[34] According to AHRQ, this program develops and diffuses scientific evidence about what works and does not work to improve health care delivery systems.

[35] Although HICPAC includes representation from multiple HHS agencies as well as from private organizations, it is not responsible for coordinating the activities of these groups and functions as an advisory body to the Secretary of HHS.

[36] The infection control COP is found in 42 C.F.R. § 482.42 (2007). CMS officials said that the quality assessment and performance improvement COP, which can be found at 42 C.F.R. § 482.21 (2007), can also affect infection control. The quality assessment and performance improvement COP states that the hospital must develop, implement, and maintain an effective, ongoing, hospitalwide, data-driven quality assessment and performance

[37] improvement program that reflects all of the hospital's departments and services.
Joint Commission officials said that standards in other chapters of their manual could also affect infection control, such as standards in the "Provision of Care" chapter, the "Treatment and Services" chapter, the "Medication Management" chapter, the "Improving Organization Performance" chapter, the "Leadership" chapter, and the "Management of the Environment of Care" chapter.

[38] Prior to the revisions that will take effect on January 1, 2009, the Joint Commission added a standard requiring hospitals to immunize staff and licensed independent practitioners against influenza. This standard took effect on January 1, 2007.

[39] Prior to 2008, the Joint Commission's National Patient Safety Goal included only the CDC hand hygiene guideline.

[40] The Joint Commission defines a sentinel event as an unexpected occurrence involving death or serious physical or psychological injury, or the risk thereof. To "manage as a sentinel event" for this goal is to determine why the patient acquired the infection and why the patient died or suffered serious injury as a result of the infection.

[41] AOA officials said that standards in other chapters of their manual could also affect infection control, including the chapters on "Medical Staff," "Physical Environment," "Quality Assessment and Performance Improvement," "Cardiovascular Services," and "Special Care Units." The "Medical Staff" chapter describes the activities of the infection control committee, which is required in the "Infection Control" chapter.

[42] The selected practices in CDC's and WHO's hand hygiene guidelines are those in the categories of (1) strongly recommended and strongly supported; (2) strongly recommended and supported; and (3) additional practices, including federal, state, and other requirements.

[43] The Joint Commission officials noted that a systems-based approach includes learning the root causes of infections and developing processes to mitigate their recurrence, and uses an epidemiologic approach that includes surveillance, control, and prevention.

[44] CMS told us that if the hospital is cited at the condition level, surveyors revisit the hospital to determine if the hospital is in compliance with the COPs, including whether the previously cited noncompliance has been corrected. Hospitals that are cited for condition- level noncompliance may lose their ability to participate in Medicare if the noncompliance is not corrected. If a hospital is noncompliant with a standard-level requirement, the state

surveyors review the hospital's corrective action plan to determine if the plan is likely to correct the noncompliance and prevent reoccurrence.

[45] Joint Commission officials told us that a hospital's failure to submit this report could eventually lead to the loss of accreditation.

[46] During the first quarter of 2007, state survey agencies surveyed 190 hospitals, the Joint Commission surveyed 329 hospitals, and AOA surveyed 9 hospitals.

[47] In a prior GAO report, we recommended that CMS increase the number of validation surveys it conducts to at least 5 percent of all Joint Commission–accredited hospitals. See GAO-04-850.

[48] To evaluate complaints, CMS decides which COP(s) to assess during an on-site survey; the state agency conducts the on-site survey of the identified COP(s); and based on the results of the survey, CMS decides whether a full hospital survey is needed.

[49] Adherence rates in the studies ranged from 5 to 81 percent. CDC notes that the methods used for defining and observing adherence varied by study. See J. M. Boyce et al., "Guideline for Hand Hygiene in Health-Care Settings: Recommendations of the Healthcare Infection Control Practices Advisory Committee and the HICPAC/SHEA/APIC/IDSA Hand Hygiene Task Force," *Morbidity and Mortality Weekly Report*, vol. 51, no. RR-16 (2002): 1–44.

[50] CDC operates other databases that may collect some HAI-related data, but they are not as comprehensive as NHSN. For example, the Active Bacterial Core Surveillance (ABCs) program collects data on six specific bacterial pathogens from 10 designated geographic locations. In 9 of these locations, CDC collects data on the incidence of both community- associated and health-care-associated (including hospital-onset) infections through laboratory results and medical record review. The 9 sites from which CDC collects MRSA data are the state of Connecticut; eight counties in the Atlanta metropolitan area; three counties in the San Francisco Bay area; one county in the Denver metropolitan area; three counties in the Portland, Oregon, metropolitan area; one county in the Rochester, New York, metropolitan area; Baltimore, Maryland; Davidson County (Nashville), Tennessee; and Ramsey County (St. Paul), Minnesota.

[51] The other two are the Dialysis Surveillance Network database and the National Surveillance System for Healthcare Workers database. The Dialysis Surveillance Network program was a voluntary national surveillance system that monitored BSIs and vascular infections in outpatient dialysis centers. The National Surveillance System for Healthcare Workers program collected information on exposures and infections among health care workers.

[52] Sections 304, 306, and 308(d) of the Public Health Service Act restrict the disclosure of information reported by hospitals.
[53] CDC officials reported that, as of December, 2007, 14 states had decided to use NHSN to collect data from hospitals on HAIs for state reporting programs that were either under way or under development. These states require or plan to require their hospitals to both enroll in the NHSN program and authorize CDC to release the hospitals' HAI data to the state.
[54] CDC officials told us that not all of the enrolled hospitals were reporting data to NHSN.
[55] States that mandate hospital participation in NHSN could also set their own requirements for the types of infections, hospital units, and procedures reported on, as well as number of months of HAI data required.
[56] The MPSMS sample is a subset of the random sample of patient records that CMS initially selects for the Hospital Payment Monitoring Program, which reviews patient records to estimate Medicare's payment error rate.
[57] We use the term abstractor to indicate persons who are trained to follow a detailed protocol in order to extract specified information in a consistent fashion from the medical records of patients.
[58] The algorithm calculates a rate of central-line-associated BSIs based on the number of patients with central line catheters who did not have an infection when they were admitted to the hospital and who subsequently tested positive for any of 16 designated BSI pathogens 2 or more days after the central line catheter was inserted.
[59] The Congress created the financial incentives that are implemented through the APU program as part of the Medicare Prescription Drug, Improvement, and Modernization Act of 2003. For more information on the collection and analysis of quality data under the APU program, see GAO, *Hospital Quality Data: CMS Needs More Rigorous Methods to Ensure Reliability of Publicly Released Data*, GAO-06-54 (Washington, D.C.: Jan. 31, 2006), and GAO, *Hospital Quality Data: HHS Should Specify Steps and Time Frame for Using Information Technology to Collect and Submit Data*, GAO-07-320 (Washington, D.C.: Apr. 25, 2007).
[60] Hospitals accredited by the Joint Commission are required to report quality-related data to the Joint Commission quarterly using third-party vendors, who also generally provide these data to CMS. Hospitals accredited by AOA are also required to submit these quality- related data to CMS.
[61] The Web site is http://www.hospitalcompare.hhs.gov.
[62] HCUP encompasses a set of related databases, one of which is the Nationwide Inpatient Sample, which AHRQ has used to generate national

estimates for its PSIs. According to AHRQ, the national sample approximates a 20 percent stratified sample of U.S. community hospitals. The sample is approximate because hospitals in the states that do not participate in HCUP are not included in the sample.

[63] The indicator is limited to patients undergoing elective surgeries to better capture patients for which sepsis is a potentially preventable complication and exclude patients that either had sepsis present on admission or had conditions predisposing them to sepsis.

[64] See K. M. McDonald et al., *Measures of Patient Safety Based on Hospital Administrative Data—The Patient Safety Indicators*, Technical Review 5, AHRQ Publication No. 02-0038 (Rockville, Md.: Agency for Healthcare Research and Quality, August 2002), 76–77.

[65] See http://www.hcupnet.ahrq.gov.

[66] FDA receives reports from manufacturers and hospitals regarding these adverse events, including concerns related to disinfection. FDA officials told us that they have received very few reports involving medical devices that might identify contaminated devices that would cause HAIs.

[67] Under the Patient Safety and Quality Improvement Act of 2005, Pub. L. No. 109-41, 119 Stat. 424, PSOs are entities that collect, aggregate, and analyze confidential information reported by health care providers in part to identify patterns of failures and propose measures to eliminate patient safety risks and hazards.

[68] AHRQ officials plan to release the first such reports once the PSOs become operational, which they expect could occur early in 2009.

[69] CDC officials estimate that approximately 22 percent of HAIs do not fall in the four types of infection currently addressed in whole or part by the four HHS databases—BSIs, UTIs, SSIs, and pneumonia. See R. M. Klevens et al., "Estimating Health Care-Associated Infections and Deaths in U.S. Hospitals, 2002," *Public Health Reports*, vol. 122 (2007): 160–166. These other infections include bone and joint infections; central nervous system infections; cardiovascular system infections; eye, ear, nose, throat, or mouth infections; skin and soft tissue infections; and gastrointestinal system infections

[70] When the National Quality Forum examined the application of the NHSN criteria for identifying patients with VAP, it found wide variations in the results obtained. According to the National Quality Forum, incidence could range from 4 to 48 percent, depending on which NHSN criteria were selected to diagnose VAP.

[71] Every quarter, CMS draws a sample of five patients for each hospital that submitted data for six or more patients in that quarter.

[72] Patient bills typically include one principal diagnosis code and multiple other diagnosis codes, which are used in determining the amount of payment that the hospital receives for treating that patient. After the patient has been discharged, hospital staff trained in medical record coding decide which ICD-9 diagnostic codes to enter on the patient's bill based on their review of the patient's medical record.

[73] The SCIP steering committee also includes representatives from the Joint Commission, the American College of Surgeons, and the American Hospital Association.

[74] See E. R. Sherman et al., "Administrative Data Fail to Accurately Identify Cases of Healthcare-Associated Infection," *Infection Control and Hospital Epidemiology*, vol. 27, no. 4 (2006): 332–337, and S. B. Wright et al., "Administrative Databases Provide Inaccurate Data for Surveillance of Long-term Central Venous Catheter-associated Infections," *Infection Control and Hospital Epidemiology*, vol. 24, no. 12 (2003): 946–949. In addition, HCUP's two HAI-related indicators do not correspond to the infection types usually tracked by hospital infection control programs. Postoperative sepsis would include some, but not all, central-line-associated BSIs, along with other BSIs not related to the insertion of central lines. Infections due to medical care would likewise include central-lineassociated BSIs as well as infections caused by other types of catheters and intravenous lines.

[75] Association for Professionals in Infection Control and Epidemiology, "National Prevalence Study of Methicillin-Resistant *Staphylococcus aureus* (MRSA) in U.S. Healthcare Facilities, Executive Summary," released June 25, 2007. See also W. R. Jarvis et al., "National Prevalence of Methicillin-Resistant *Staphylococcus aureus* in Inpatients at U.S. Health Care Facilities, 2006," *American Journal of Infection Control*, vol. 35, no. 10 (2007): 631–637. This figure represents the prevalence of MRSA on a given day in fall 2006, that is, all the known MRSA cases on that day in proportion to the total number of inpatients, across the 1,187 hospitals that responded to the survey.

[76] Another recent study using CDC's Active Bacterial Core Surveillance (ABCs) database found the national rate of invasive MRSA per 100,000 population to be 31.8 in 2005. However, the MRSA rates generated from the APIC survey and ABCs database are not comparable for several reasons. For example, the ABCs program collects data on invasive MRSA, which are cases found in a normally sterile site such as blood and are a subset of the cases of MRSA collected in the APIC survey. In addition, the ABCs database assesses the rate of infections with respect to populations residing in defined geographic areas, rather than at the provider level. The researchers noted that the

nine sites in the ABCs database are largely urban areas and that they had no information to establish that the MRSA incidence rates found in those sites reflected the incidence of MRSA in other parts of the United States. See R. M. Klevens et al., "Invasive Methicillin-Resistant *Staphylococcus aureus* Infections in the United States," *Journal of the American Medical Association*, vol. 298, no. 15 (2007): 1763–1771.

[77] According to AHRQ officials, the MPSMS data to be released in the next *National Healthcare Quality Report*, which AHRQ expects to issue in early 2008, will not include results on MRSA. Those may appear as early as the subsequent *National Healthcare Quality Report*, due in early 2009.

[78] R.M. Klevens et al., "Estimating Health Care-Associated Infections and Deaths in U.S. Hospitals, 2002," *Public Health Reports*, March–April 2007, vol. 122, 160–166.

[79] The proportion of NNIS hospitals reporting such comprehensive surveillance data dropped from about half in 1991 to none in 1998, when NNIS stopped collecting these data altogether.

[80] The mission of the National Center for Health Statistics is to collect health statistics in order to guide actions and policies to improve the health of the U.S. population. The National Hospital Discharge Survey is a national probability survey that collects information on the characteristics of inpatients discharged from nonfederal short-stay hospitals in the United States.

[81] VRE are bacteria that have become resistant to vancomycin, an antibiotic used to treat patients infected with bacterial pathogens. VRE can cause urinary tract infections, BSIs, and wound infections.

[82] Appendix A of the *State Operations Manual* is available at http://www.cms.hhs.gov/GuidanceforLawsAndRegulations/08_Hospitals.asp, downloaded on May 14, 2007.

[83] These revised guidelines are titled "Revisions to the Hospital Interpretive Guidelines for Infection Control" (memo number 08-04) and were effective immediately upon issuance. These revisions are available at http://www.cms.hhs.gov/SurveyCertificationGenInfo/PMSR, downloaded on November 29, 2007.

[84] The quality assessment and performance improvement COP states that the hospital must develop, implement, and maintain an effective, ongoing, hospitalwide, data-driven quality assessment and performance improvement program that reflects all of the hospital's departments and services.

In: Hospital-Acquired Infections
Editor: Julia B. Wilcox, pp. 295-347

ISBN: 978-1-60692-728-1
© 2009 Nova Science Publishers, Inc.

Chapter 3

HEALTH-CARE-ASSOCIATED INFECTIONS IN HOSPITALS: AN OVERVIEW OF STATE REPORTING PROGRAMS AND INDIVIDUAL HOSPITAL INITIATIVES TO REDUCE CERTAIN INFECTIONS[*]

United States Government Accountability Office

WHAT GAO FOUND

GAO identified 23 states that had established mandatory HAI public reporting systems through February 2008; most have used similar approaches to design their programs and address resource and technological challenges that affect their implementation. Most states have designed programs that focus on a few measures that were developed or endorsed by the CDC. Three states have chosen to collect information on hospital-associated MRSA infections. In addition, a majority of states have chosen to adopt the CDC's NHSN. Adopting NHSN allows states to minimize some of the resource and technological challenges that they confront in implementing HAI reporting systems including providing training for hospital staff in data collection and developing systems to collect HAI data that meet accepted infection control standards.

---

[*] This is an edited, excerpted and augmented edition of a United States Government Accountability Office publication, Report GAO-08-808, dated September 2008.

GAO reviewed a sample of 14 hospitals (including several hospital systems) with MRSA-reduction initiatives that were selected to provide variation in location, teaching status, and population of metropolitan area. GAO found all use routine testing for MRSA, although they chose different patient populations to test and used various testing methodologies. Three hospitals tested all patients for MRSA, while the other hospitals almost universally tested patients in adult or neonatal intensive care units. The hospitals reported changing their general infection control policies or practices as part of their initiatives—all 14 made changes for hand hygiene and more than half made changes to their contact precautions or disinfection of environmental surfaces. The hospitals GAO reviewed reported needing varying levels of funding and staff resources to implement and operate their initiatives, but all hospitals that tracked MRSA infection rates reported a decline in MRSA infections as a result of their initiatives.

Two hospital systems that GAO visited overcame a similar set of challenges in implementing MRSA-reduction programs. Both systems had to design and execute processes to put the elements of their MRSA-reduction initiatives into effect and promote compliance with those processes by hospital staff. In designing their systems, both hospital systems incorporated these processes as much as possible into the normal workflow of hospital staff and promoted staff compliance through a combination of concerted leadership and specific procedures designed to facilitate staff compliance reinforced through detailed feedback on their performance. However, the two hospital systems took different approaches in obtaining resources for their initiatives. One directed substantial financial resources into its MRSA-reduction initiative to implement the initiative simultaneously for all patients at all three of its hospitals, while the other relied largely on existing resources and implemented its initiative more incrementally at selected hospitals and in selected units.

GAO received technical comments from the Department of Health and Human Services and oral comments from the American Hospital Association on a draft of this chapter.

Why GAO Did this Study

Health-care-associated infections (HAI) are infections that patients acquire while receiving treatment for other conditions. Normally treated with antimicrobial drugs, HAIs are a growing concern as exposure to multidrug-resistant organisms (MDRO) becomes more common. Infections caused by MDROs, such as methicillinresistant *Staphylococcus aureus* (MRSA), lead to longer hospital stays, higher treatment costs, and higher mortality.

In response to demands for more public information on HAIs, some states began to establish HAI public reporting systems. The federal Centers for Disease Control and Prevention (CDC) developed a system—the National Healthcare Safety Network (NHSN)—to collect HAI data from hospitals and some states have chosen to use it for their programs. In addition, some hospitals have adopted initiatives to reduce MRSA by routinely testing some or all patients and isolating those who test positive for MRSA from contact with other patients.

GAO was asked to examine (1) the design and implementation of state HAI public reporting systems, (2) the initiatives hospitals have undertaken to reduce MRSA infections, and (3) the experience of certain early-adopting hospitals in overcoming challenges to implement such initiatives.

GAO interviewed state officials, reviewed documents, and surveyed or conducted site visits at hospitals with MRSA-reduction initiatives.

ABBREVIATIONS

AHA	American Hospital Association
AHRQ	Agency for Healthcare Research and Quality
AST	active surveillance testing
BSI	bloodstream infection
CDC	Centers for Disease Control and Prevention
CMS	Centers for Medicare & Medicaid Services
EMR	electronic medical record
ENH	Evanston Northwestern Healthcare
HAI	health-care-associated infection
HICPAC	Healthcare Infection Control Practices Advisory Committee
HHS	Department of Health and Human Services
ICP	infection control professional
ICU	intensive care unit
IHI	Institute for Healthcare Improvement
IPPS	inpatient prospective payment system
MDRO	multidrug-resistant organism
MRSA	methicillin-resistant *Staphylococcus aureus*
NHSN	National Healthcare Safety Network
NNIS	National Nosocomial Infections Surveillance
NQF	National Quality Forum
PCR	polymerase chain reaction

POA	present on admission
PSI	Patient Safety Indicator
SCIP	Surgical Care Improvement Project
SSI	surgical site infection
UPMC	University of Pittsburgh Medical Center
UTI	urinary tract infection
VAP	ventilator-associated pneumonia

September 5, 2008
The Honorable Henry Waxman
Chairman
Committee on Oversight and Government Reform
House of Representatives

Dear Mr. Chairman:

Health-care-associated infections (HAI) are one of the top 10 causes of death in the United States, according to estimates from the Centers for Disease Control and Prevention (CDC). Although patients can acquire HAIs in a wide variety of health care settings, including nursing homes and ambulatory surgery centers, hospital patients are especially vulnerable to HAIs. Normally treated with antimicrobial drugs, HAIs are a growing concern as multidrug-resistant organisms (MDRO) become more common.[1] Infections caused by MDROs lead to longer hospital stays, higher treatment costs, and higher mortality because they are more difficult to treat than infections caused by other organisms. A particular MDRO, methicillin-resistant *Staphylococcus aureus* (MRSA),[2] has gained attention recently. In 2003, it accounted for 64 percent of infections in intensive care units (ICU) caused by *Staphylococcus aureus*, one of the most common HAI pathogens, up from 36 percent in 1992.[3] Researchers estimate that the average cost of treating a MRSA infection exceeds $35,000.

In a separate report to you, we found that federal activities have not effectively addressed the HAI problem.[4] We also found that the extent of the problem, including the level of antimicrobial resistance, is uncertain because the data that CDC as well as other agencies of the Department of Health and Human Services (HHS)—such as the Centers for Medicare & Medicaid Services (CMS)—collect on HAIs are limited in scope and lack integration across multiple databases. CDC has created a data infrastructure that allows hospitals to voluntarily collect and input data using a uniform set of definitions on the incidence of selected HAIs in their own hospitals and to compare their rates with benchmarks derived from the data submitted by all participating hospitals. This began in the 1970s with the National Nosocomial Infections Surveillance (NNIS) system and continued with its replacement, the more sophisticated National Healthcare Safety Network (NHSN), introduced in 2005.

In response to demands for more public information on HAIs, some states have begun to develop and implement HAI public reporting systems— some using CDC's NHSN—to collect and disseminate HAI data from hospitals. Some states have also recently passed legislation relating specifically to MRSA, such as requiring specific actions for hospitals to prevent the spread of MRSA based in part on guidelines issued by CDC and collecting data from hospitals on MRSA cases that occur. In addition, some hospitals have implemented strategies for reducing MRSA by testing some or all patients and isolating those who test positive for MRSA from contact with other patients.

In response to your interest in these nonfederal efforts to address HAIs, including the role played by CDC's NHSN and its practice guidelines, we examined (1) the design and implementation of state HAI public reporting systems, (2) the initiatives hospitals have undertaken to reduce MRSA infections, and (3) the experience of certain early-adopting hospitals in overcoming challenges to implement such initiatives.

To describe the design and implementation of state HAI public reporting systems, we identified 23 states that were designing or had implemented state-mandated HAI public reporting systems through February 2008. We identified these programs through multiple sources, including resources maintained by organizations that track state infection control programs. We then collected information directly from each of those 23 states.

However, we did not independently verify that there were no state- mandated HAI public reporting programs planned or underway in any of the remaining states. We excluded from consideration programs in several states that collect limited data about HAIs, but do not report hospital- specific HAI data to the public.[5] For each of the 23 states, we reviewed the available legislation, administrative and departmental rules and regulations, advisory panel reports, and other documents for each system to compare the systems across states. However, the information that we collected does not provide a description or assessment of the legal requirements in any state regarding the collection and public reporting of data about HAIs or a comparison of the legal requirements among states regarding those requirements.

We also interviewed state officials and state hospital association representatives in 5 of the 23 states about the design, development, and implementation of their systems, including challenges they encountered, how they overcame those challenges, and how they validated the data from hospitals. We selected Missouri, New York, and Pennsylvania because each had relatively extensive experience in collecting HAI data, but used different data reporting systems. We selected Illinois and New Jersey because they had established mandatory reporting programs on MRSA infections designed to provide information on the performance of individual hospitals—as distinct from the communicable disease reporting systems that many state health department have operated for decades, which are designed primarily to provide an alert when new outbreaks of particular pathogens occur. What we learned about the challenges faced and implementation strategies adopted in those 5 states cannot be generalized to other states with HAI public reporting programs.

To describe the initiatives hospitals have undertaken to reduce MRSA infections, we consulted knowledgeable experts, and conducted a Web search to generate a list of hospitals or hospital systems[6] with MRSA reduction initiatives. From among those, we selected 17 that provided the greatest diversity in terms of location, teaching status, and population of metropolitan area. To obtain information about the hospitals' MRSA reduction initiatives, we visited 2 hospitals and sent surveys to officials at the remaining 15 hospitals, 12 of which responded. In total, we collected information from 14 hospitals with MRSA-reduction initiatives. Information on their characteristics is provided in appendix I. The information that we obtained from these 14 hospitals pertains specifically to those hospitals, and can not be generalized to other hospitals with MRSA-reduction initiatives.

To describe how early-adopting hospitals overcame challenges to implement MRSA-reduction initiatives, we visited Evanston Northwestern Healthcare (ENH) and the University of Pittsburgh Medical Center (UPMC). Both implemented MRSA-reduction initiatives several years ago and have published or otherwise publicly presented data on their outcomes. We interviewed key administrative and clinical personnel at each site to examine specific MRSA intervention options considered, challenges confronted, steps taken to overcome those challenges, and required financial and staff resources. Because these were case studies, what we found at these two hospitals can not be generalized to other hospitals with MRSA reduction initiatives.

We conducted this performance audit from October 2007 to September 2008 in accordance with generally accepted government auditing standards. Those standards require that we plan and perform the audit to obtain sufficient, appropriate evidence to provide a reasonable basis for our findings and conclusions based on our audit objectives. We believe that the evidence obtained provides a reasonable basis for our findings and conclusions based on our audit objectives.

RESULTS IN BRIEF

Most of the 23 states we reviewed with state-mandated HAI public reporting programs have used similar approaches to design their programs and address resource and technological challenges that affect their implementation. Most of these states have relied at least to some extent on advisory committees or technical advisors and designed programs that focus on a few measures that were developed or endorsed by CDC. Three states have chosen to collect information on hospital-associated MRSA infections. In addition, although some states developed their own data collection systems, a majority of the states we reviewed have chosen to use NHSN, the HAI data collection system developed by CDC. Adopting CDC-endorsed measures and the NHSN for data collection allowed states to minimize some of the resource and technological challenges that they confronted in implementing HAI reporting systems. These challenges included providing training for hospital staff in data collection as well as developing systems to collect HAI data that met accepted infection control standards and were user-friendly for those entering data.

The 14 hospitals with MRSA-reduction initiatives that we reviewed all conduct routine testing for MRSA, although they chose different patient populations to test and used various testing methodologies. Three hospitals tested all patients for MRSA, while the remaining hospitals almost universally tested patients in adult or neonatal intensive care units. The hospitals reported changing a number of general infection control policies or practices as part of their initiatives—all 14 made changes for hand hygiene and more than half made changes to their contact precautions or disinfection of environmental surfaces. The hospitals we reviewed reported needing varying levels of funding and staff resources to implement and operate their initiatives, but all hospitals that tracked MRSA infection rates reported a decline in MRSA infections as a result of their initiatives.

The two hospital systems that we visited overcame a similar set of challenges in implementing multifaceted MRSA-reduction initiatives. Both systems had to design and execute processes to put the elements of their MRSA-reduction initiatives into effect and promote compliance with those processes by hospital staff. In designing their MRSA-reduction initiatives, both hospital systems incorporated these processes as much as possible into the normal workflow of hospital staff and promoted staff compliance through a combination of concerted leadership on the part of the physicians who led their infection control programs and specific procedures designed to facilitate staff compliance reinforced through detailed feedback on their performance. However, the two hospital systems took different approaches to obtaining resources for their initiatives. One directed substantial financial resources into its MRSAreduction initiative to implement the initiative simultaneously for all patients at all three of its hospitals, while the other relied largely on existing resources and implemented its initiative more incrementally at selected hospitals and on selected units.

We obtained technical comments from HHS that we incorporated as appropriate. In addition, the department highlighted the scientific contributions that CDC has made pertaining to the detection, measurement, and prevention of HAIs and MRSA. The American Hospital Association (AHA) provided oral comments that underscored the importance of using HAI data to prevent and reduce infections and that raised serious concerns about using unvalidated NHSN data for public reporting of hospital performance on HAIs.

BACKGROUND

HAIs are infections that patients may acquire during the course of receiving medical treatment for other conditions.[7] HAIs occur as the result of patient exposure to a variety of pathogens and affect many different body systems. According to CDC estimates, urinary tract infections (UTI), surgical site infections (SSI), bloodstream infections (BSI), and pneumonia account for more than 80 percent of all HAIs. Frequently, an infectious pathogen is introduced by an invasive procedure, such as surgery or insertion of a urinary catheter, central line,[8] or ventilator. As a result, a subset of UTIs are identified as catheter-associated UTIs, a subset of BSIs are identified as central line-associated BSIs, and a subset of pneumonia HAIs are identified as ventilator-associated pneumonia (YAP).

Hospital Practices to Reduce HAIs

Any acute care hospital that participates in Medicare or Medicaid or is accredited through the Joint Commission must have an infection control program with a designated person in charge.[9] Infection control professionals (ICPs) receive specialized training to prepare them to lead and staff these programs. ICPs identify cases of HAI and promote infection control practices that help to reduce the occurrence and spread of HAIs. These practices include rigorous maintenance of hand hygiene standards as well as contact precautions, which involve the use of gloves, gowns, and sometimes masks worn by health care workers to prevent them from carrying the pathogen from an infected patient to other patients. One approach has focused on ensuring that each item on a short list of specific practices is consistently implemented. For example, the Institute for Healthcare Improvement (IHI)[10] has developed "bundles" or "components of care" designed to reduce the incidence of central line-associated BSIs, SSIs, VAP, and MRSA. Each of these bundles consists of four to six specific practices that research has shown affect the incidence of that type of infection. These practices include hand hygiene and contact precautions, where appropriate.

Strong clinical evidence indicates that contact precautions help to reduce the incidence of HAIs. However, for contact precautions to work, they have to be carefully and consistently followed. Hospitals need to closely monitor and reinforce staff compliance with these and related activities such as hand hygiene and environmental cleaning.[11] At the same time, some research suggests that patients placed under contact precautions may receive less attention from clinicians, receive lower quality care, and experience more adverse events such as falls or pressure ulcers.[12]

MRSA

MRSA is a particularly prevalent MDRO. It can cause virtually any type of HAI, including skin infections, BSIs, pneumonia, SSIs, and UTIs. MRSApositive patients may either have an active MRSA infection or be colonized with the organism. Colonized patients carry the bacteria in some part of their body, such as on their skin or in their nose, without showing any symptoms of infection themselves. Patients colonized with MRSA represent a primary source for transmission of the organism to other patients, often via the hands, clothing, or equipment of hospital staff. Individuals who acquire MRSA in a health care setting, such as a hospital, are referred to as having health-care-associated MRSA. Individuals who develop a MRSA infection outside of such settings and who do not have a history of recent hospitalization or surgery are referred to as having community-associated MRSA.

Because patients colonized with MRSA do not exhibit signs and symptoms of infection, the only way to identify them is through laboratory testing of specimens from asymptomatic patients. Specimens taken from a patient's nose can identify up to 80 percent of colonized patients and are therefore recommended for MRSA screening. Laboratory methods for MRSA testing use routine culture media, selective media, or polymerase chain reaction (PCR). Routine culture media require laboratory staff to culture specimens in a nutrient material, such as agar in a Petri dish, and then examine and test the organisms that grow in that medium. This process usually takes 2 to 5 days to produce results. Selective media are laboratory culture media that have been developed to identify the presence of specific organisms. Clinical specimens are swabbed onto culture plates containing selective media. The selective media allow certain organisms to grow while preventing other organisms from growing. In some cases, the selective media can also cause specific organisms to appear a certain color. MRSA test results using selective media are generally available within 24 hours. PCR is a highly sensitive, molecular testing technique that detects MRSAspecific DNA. PCR testing can identify a somewhat higher proportion of MRSA-positive patients than the alternative testing methods and it can generate results within 2 to 4 hours, but it is substantially more expensive than testing using routine or selective media. PCR screening costs $25 to $30 per test, while screening using selective media costs about $5 per test.[13]

Several European countries have largely eradicated transmission of MRSA to other patients by adopting procedures to identify and isolate MRSApositive patients on admission, demonstrating that hospitals can keep the MRSA infection rate low or nonexistent. In the United States, the consensus among experts is that hospitals should take measures to prevent the transmission of the MRSA organism from any patient known to be infected or colonized with MRSA to other patients in the hospital. CDC's guidelines for reducing the incidence of MDROs, including MRSA, emphasize the importance of implementing several recommended practices when treating MRSA-positive patients, including contact precautions, hand hygiene, and effective environmental cleaning.[14] The guidelines recommend placing MRSA-positive patients in private rooms or "cohorting" them by placing them in rooms with other MRSA-positive patients. In addition, the guidelines recommend that hospitals exercise antibiotic stewardship by implementing processes that encourage and facilitate judicious use of antimicrobial agents to maximize therapeutic impact while minimizing the development of antibiotic resistance.

Infection control experts differ as to the scope of routine MRSA testing, known as active surveillance testing (AST), they recommend to identify MRSA-positive patients. Some recommend as much routine testing as is necessary to identify all MRSA-positive patients in a hospital, which, depending on the prevalence of MRSA in that hospital or community, can mean testing all admitted patients—universal AST. Other experts, as well as CDC guidelines, recommend targeted AST—testing populations within a hospital who are more likely than others to be colonized with MRSA.

Populations targeted include patients in intensive care units, dialysis patients, and patients transferred from nursing homes or prisons. Targeted testing requires fewer resources than universal testing, but misses infected individuals outside of the targeted population.

Decolonization protocols have been developed to remove MRSA bacteria from a colonized patient's body, in order to reduce the likelihood that the patient will get an active infection or transmit the bacteria to someone else. Decolonization therapy can involve applying an antibiotic ointment in the nose for 5 days, bathing in chlorhexidine, or doing both. However, the clinical evidence supporting the effectiveness of these protocols in eradicating MRSA is limited, and researchers have reported that extensive use of this treatment can lead to increased MRSA resistance to the antibiotic in the nasal ointment. As a result, experts differ as to if and when to implement these protocols.

Federal Activities

CDC is the lead federal agency with respect to HAIs. It sets clinical definitions for identifying HAIs and has defined 13 categories of HAIs, including BSIs, SSIs, UTIs, and pneumonia. CDC's definitions and procedures for distinguishing HAIs from other infections, which rely on detailed clinical information obtained from patient medical records and direct observation, are widely accepted as the most appropriate technical standard by ICPs and others in the field.[15] CDC's Healthcare Infection Control Practices Advisory Committee (HICPAC) publishes guidelines that assemble and assess practices intended to reduce particular types of infections.[16]

Since the 1970s, CDC has managed systems to collect HAI data from hospitals on a strictly voluntary and confidential basis. Following the transition from the NNIS to the NHSN in 2005, participation in CDC's system has grown from approximately 300 hospitals to approximately 1,000 hospitals as of December 2007. Through the NHSN, CDC has established protocols for hospitals to report outcome data on central line-associated BSIs, SSIs, catheter-associated UTIs, VAP, and postprocedure pneumonia.[17] These protocols include questions about the organisms causing the reported infections and the results of any laboratory tests of their antibiotic susceptibility. NHSN also collects data that enable hospitals to risk adjust their HAI rates to take account of differences in the severity of illness of their patients and in the complexity of procedures they perform. The use of risk-adjusted rates allows hospitals to more accurately compare their own progress in infection prevention and control to that of other hospitals, as well as to their own rates in the past. Though participation in the NHSN remains voluntary and is free of charge, enrolling hospitals must agree to follow these protocols in collecting the data that they submit. As was true of the NNIS, CDC releases data from the NHSN only in the form of aggregate rates for different types of infections, with information on the individual participating hospitals legally protected from disclosure.

In contrast to the confidentiality guaranteed to hospitals participating in CDC's data systems, there has been a movement in recent years toward making information about the quality of care provided by individual hospitals publicly available. Several organizations have developed indicators to measure how often patients receive certain recommended processes of care for certain conditions (called process measures) and to measure how often adverse outcomes, such as infections, occur in certain patient populations (called outcome measures). For example, the Surgical Care Improvement Project (SCIP) has adopted a series of process measures to assess hospital compliance with practices designed to minimize SSIs, as well as other adverse events from surgery.[18] CMS routinely publishes the scores that hospitals receive for these SCIP measures on its Hospital Compare Web site, along with process and outcome measures for other medical conditions.[19]

STATES HAVE DESIGNED BROADLY SIMILAR MANDATORY HAI PUBLIC REPORTING SYSTEMS, WITH RESOURCE AND TECHNOLOGICAL CHALLENGES AFFECTING IMPLEMENTATION

Of the 23 states we reviewed that have state-mandated HAI public reporting programs, most have adopted similar approaches to address resource and technological challenges that affect their implementation. Most of these states have designed, and the early-adopting states have implemented, programs that focus on a few outcome and process measures that were developed or endorsed by CDC and are widely accepted by ICPs. Three states have decided to collect data on hospital-associated MRSA infections. In addition, after some early efforts by states to develop their own data collection systems, a majority of the states we reviewed have chosen to use NHSN, the HAI data collection system developed by CDC. Adopting CDC-endorsed measures and the NHSN for data collection allows states to minimize some of the resource and technological challenges that they confront in implementing HAI reporting systems.

States Have Designed HAT Public Reporting Systems with Most Using Similar Approaches

We reviewed 23 states that have state-mandated HAT public reporting systems (see table 1). By early 2008, 14 states had started to collect HAT data from hospitals. Most of the 23 states have adopted similar approaches involving (1) the use of advisory committees, (2) selection of many of the same measures, (3) decisions on systems for data collection, and (4) steps taken to validate the HAT data collected.

Table 1. States We Reviewed with HAI Public Reporting for Hospitals, by Date Data Collection Begins

State	Date data collection began or planned to begin
Pennsylvania	Jan 2004
Florida	April 2005
Missouri	Jul 2005
Vermont	Nov 2006
Maine	Jan 2007
New York	Jan 2007
Colorado	Jul 2007
Illinois	Jul 2007
South Carolina	Jul 2007
California	Jan 2008
Connecticut	Jan 2008
Delaware	Jan 2008
New Hampshire	Jan 2008
Tennessee	Jan 2008
Maryland	Jul 2008
Massachusetts	Jul 2008
Oklahoma	Jul 2008
Virginia	Jul 2008
Washington	Jul 2008
Minnesota	Jan 2009
New Jersey	Jan 2009
Oregon	Jan 2009
Texas	To be determined

Sources: State documents and communication with state government and hospital association officials.
Note: Some states have or will collect data on a pilot basis from the date listed above, but did not or will not publicly release data on hospitals until the pilot period, usually 6 months to a year, is completed.

Use of Advisory Committees

We identified 19 states that have instituted HAI advisory committees or use technical advisors. Many of these committee members and technical advisors are drawn from related occupations, organizations, or interests. These include clinicians such as physicians or nurses (13 states), consumers (10 states), hospital administrators or hospital association officials (11 states), and officials from the state health department (9 states). A few states also appoint advisory committee members who are academic researchers, technical specialists in microbiology or statistics, and representatives of health insurers, employers, and labor unions.

States seek input from their advisory committees or technical advisors on many of the same issues but differ in how extensively they rely on them. These issues include the initial selection of measures, data collection methods, the format of public reports, the selection of additional measures over time, data analysis techniques such as risk adjustment, and data validation methods. Several states have or plan to consult with advisory committees or technical advisors regarding all or nearly all these issues. Other states appear to restrict such consultation to as few as one or two of these issues.

Selection of HAI Measures

More state reporting systems have chosen to collect data on HAI outcomes, such as the rate at which certain types of HAIs occur, than collect data on compliance with processes intended to prevent HAIs. Twenty-one states have selected or are actively considering one or more outcome measures (see table 2) compared to 13 states that have selected or are actively considering one or more process measures (see table 3). Eleven states have selected or are considering both outcome and process measures.

For the most part, states have chosen to publicly report on a handful of measures relating to HAI outcomes and process that are well-established and clearly defined. For the states selecting HAI outcome measures, all but one have selected or are considering measures developed by CDC. Among the states that have selected process measures, most have emphasized the SCIP measures designed to prevent SSIs that both CDC and CMS helped develop.

The HAI outcome measures selected by the state reporting systems have largely focused on two types of infections as defined by CDC. Of the 18 states that have selected HAI outcome measures, 17 have chosen to collect rates of central line-associated BSIs, as defined by CDC and in accordance with NHSN collection protocols (see table 2). Three other states are actively considering this measure. Twelve states have chosen to collect rates of SSIs for specified procedures, as defined by CDC and in accordance with NHSN collection protocols, while 3 other states are actively considering this measure. Surgical procedures that states have selected for this outcome measure include coronary artery bypass grafts, hip replacements, knee replacements, and hysterectomies. All 12 states selecting the SSI measure were among the 17 that selected the central line- associated BSI measure. Both central line-associated BSIs and SSIs were recommended for use in public reporting by CDC's HICPAC and professional associations in infection control and epidemiology, and more recently by the National Quality Forum (NQF).[20]

Table 2. Outcome Measures by States We Reviewed with HAI Reporting, by Defining Entity

State[a]	HAI outcome measures				
	Central line-associated BSI[b]	SSI[c]	VAP	Catheter-associated UTI	HAI-related patient safety indicators[d]
Pennsylvania[e]	CDC	CDC	CDC	CDC	
Florida					AHRQ
Missouri	CDC	CDC			
Vermont	CDC	CDC			
Maine	CDC				
New York	CDC	CDC			
Colorado	CDC	CDC			
Illinois	CDC				
South Carolina	CDC	CDC			
California					
Connecticut	CDC				
Delaware	CDC	CDC			
New Hampshire	CDC	CDC	CDC		
Tennessee	CDC	CDC			
	HAI outcome measures				
Maryland	CDC	CDC			
Massachusetts	CDC	CDC			
Oklahoma	CDC			CDC	AHRQ
Virginia	CDC				
Washington	CDC	CDC	CDC		
Minnesota					
New Jersey	CDC	CDC			
Oregon	CDC	CDC			
Texas	CDC	CDC			

Sources: State documents and communication with state government and hospital association officials.

Notes:

CDC State has decided to collect data for this measure in accordance with CDC definitions and NHSN specifications.

CDC State is considering collection of data for this measure in accordance with CDC definitions and NHSN specifications.

AHRQ State has decided to collect data for "selected infections due to medical care" and "postoperative sepsis" in accordance with Agency for Healthcare Research and Quality (AHRQ) specifications.

[a] States listed in order of when they began collecting HAI data, as shown in table 1. [b] Most states have chosen to collect data on this measure for ICU patients only.

[c] Most states have chosen to collect data on this measure only for patients undergoing one or more selected procedures, such as coronary artery bypass surgery, hysterectomy, and hip and knee replacement.

[d] One patient safety indicator captures selected infections due to medical care, which includes many device-related infections such as central line-associated BSIs. Another indicator identifies cases of postoperative sepsis, which is aimed at certain infections in surgical patients but is distinct from surgical site infections.

[e] Pennsylvania collected data on these measures according to CDC definitions but not according to NHSN specifications between 2004 and 2007. In January 2008, the state began using NHSN specifications.

Table 3. Process Measures by States We Reviewed with HAI Reporting

State[a]	HAI process measures					
	Antibiotics administered prior to surgery[b]	Health care worker influenza vaccination	Central line insertion practices[c]	Central line bundle[d]	VAP prevention practices[e]	Ventilator bundle
Pennsylvania	f			f	f	
Florida	•					
Missouri					•[g]	
Vermont	•	o		•[h]		
Maine	•			•		•
New York						
Colorado						
Illinois	•					
South Carolina						
California	•	•	•			
Connecticut						
Delaware		o				
New Hampshire	•	•	•			
Tennessee						
Maryland	•	•				•
Massachusetts		o			o	
Oklahoma						
Virginia						
Washington						
Minnesota	•[i]					
New Jersey	•					
Oregon	•					
Texas						

Sources: State documents and communication with state government and hospital association officials.

Notes:

z State has decided to collect data for this measure.

0 State is considering collection of data for this measure.

[a] States listed in order of when they began collecting HAI data, as shown in table 1.

[b] Three measures, developed under the SCIP, are related to the routine administration of antibiotics to forestall SSIs: (1) the percentage of surgical patients who received an antibiotic within 1 hour prior to surgery, (2) the percentage of surgical patients who received the antibiotic recommended for their procedure, and (3) the percentage of surgical patients whose antibiotics were discontinued within 24 hours after the procedure's end time.

[c] Central line insertion practices is a set of process measures developed by CDC to monitor compliance with recommended practices outlined in CDC's guidelines for the prevention of intravascular catheter-related infections. They include occupation of the inserter, hand hygiene, use of sterile barrier precautions, type of skin preparation, location of insertion site, and type of central line inserted.

[d] Central line bundle was developed by IHI. It consists of five components: hand hygiene, using maximal sterile barrier precautions, chlorhexidine skin antisepsis, optimal catheter site selection, and prompt removal of lines that are no longer necessary. The bundle measure represents the percentage of patients for whom all five components of the bundle were complied with.
[e] VAP prevention practices include head-of-bed elevation and daily assessments of readiness to discontinue mechanical ventilation. These are two of the four components of the IHI ventilator bundle, which represents the percentage of patients for whom all four components of the bundle were complied with. The other two components of the ventilator bundle are medication to prevent peptic ulcer disease and medication or mechanical stimulation to prevent blood clots.
[f] Pennsylvania collects information on VAP prevention practices as well as some, but not all, items included in two of the other process measures: antibiotics administered prior to surgery and the central line bundle. However, it only collects these data for patients who develop SSIs, central line-associated BSIs, and VAP. It also collects similar information on patients who develop urinary tract infections. So Pennsylvania uses these data to help explain the infections that occur, rather than assess the extent to which hospitals comply with recommended infection prevention practices.
[g] Missouri hospitals report one VAP prevention measure, head-of-bed elevation, voluntarily.
[h] Vermont has hospitals self-report which components of the central line bundle they have adopted and whether they train their staff to perform those selected components and ensure that staff use them.
[i] Minnesota will also collect data for two additional SCIP infection prevention measures, one on controlling postoperative blood glucose levels for cardiac surgery patients and one on appropriate hair removal.

The states that have chosen to measure processes of care designed to prevent HAIs have focused on surgical measures (see table 3). Specifically, 10 states decided to track the routine administration of antibiotics to forestall SSIs. Three measures of this process were adopted under the SCIP program: antibiotic received within 1 hour of surgery, appropriate antibiotic selection, and antibiotics discontinued within 24 hours after the surgery end time. These are the same surgical measures that CMS reports on its Hospital Compare Web site, and they have also been recommended for use in public reporting by CDC's HICPAC committee.

A smaller number of states have selected HAI outcome and process measures for which there is less agreement in the infection control community. For example, among the outcome measures, VAP and catheter-associated UTI rates have not been recommended for public reporting by HICPAC or the professional associations, although both are among the HAI measures endorsed by NQF.[21] Several states have also selected influenza vaccination for health care workers as a process measure. While not endorsed by NQF, this measure has been recommended for public reporting by HICPAC, and CDC plans to include it in the NHSN.

Of the 23 states we reviewed, only 2 have selected HAI outcome measures that substantially diverge from CDC definitions and protocols. Florida and Oklahoma selected two measures developed by the Agency for Healthcare Research and Quality (AHRQ) as part of its Patient Safety Indicators (PSI).[22] One PSI measure identifies "selected infections due to medical care," which includes (but is not limited to) device-related infections such as central line-associated BSIs. In contrast to SSIs, which are infections at the site of the surgery, the second HAI-related PSI measure, postoperative sepsis, focuses on major, systemwide infections that occur following surgery. The two PSI measures are calculated by analyzing combinations of diagnosis and procedure codes in administrative billing records to identify certain adverse events using computer software. Both states have also selected at least one of the measures commonly selected by other states that accord with CDC definitions and protocols or guidance (see tables 2 and 3).[23]

Data Collection Systems

Table 4. Data Collection Systems,
by States We Reviewed with HAI Reporting

State[a]	Data collection system	
	NHSN	State developed
Pennsylvania[b]	●	
Florida		●
Missouri	●	●
Vermont		
Maine	●	●
New York	●	
Colorado	●	
Illinois	●	
South Carolina	●	
California	●	
Connecticut	●	
Delaware	●	
New Hampshire	●	
Tennessee	●	
Maryland	●	
Massachusetts	●	
Oklahoma	●	
Virginia	●	
Washington	●	
Minnesota	○	
New Jersey	○	
Oregon	●	
Texas	○	

Sources: GAO analysis of state documents and communication with state government and hospital association officials.

Notes:
z Data collection system selected.
0 Data collection system being considered.
A number of states that use the NHSN also use other data collection systems for measures that are not incorporated into the NHSN, such as those for antibiotics administered prior to surgery.
[a] States listed in order of when they began collecting HAI data, as shown in table 1. [b]From 2004 through 2007 Pennsylvania used its own state data collection system.

With respect to setting up systems for collecting HAI data from hospitals, states have increasingly relied on CDC's NHSN (see table 4). In January 2007, New York became the first state to begin collecting data for public reporting using the NHSN, and by June 2007, CDC had completed its development of the NHSN sufficiently to open enrollment in the system to hospitals in every state. Prior to that date, 4 states developed their own data collection mechanisms, beginning with Pennsylvania in 2004. Since CDC opened enrollment in NHSN to all hospitals, no state has chosen not to use NHSN to collect at least some of its HAI data.[24] In addition to New York, Colorado, South Carolina, and Vermont began collecting data through NHSN in 2007, and 13 other states have decided to use NHSN for their HAI public reporting programs.[25] Included in the latter group is Pennsylvania, which discontinued its original system in favor of NHSN starting in January 2008. Meanwhile Minnesota, New Jersey, and Texas are considering whether to use NHSN to collect HAI data for public reporting. Currently, only 3 states—Florida, Maine, and Missouri—use systems that do not rely on the NHSN to collect HAI data, though Maine and Missouri draw on CDC's definitions.

Data Validation

Data collection systems may or may not incorporate procedures to independently verify the accuracy of the data submitted to them. However, according to infection control experts as well as state officials responsible for HAI reporting programs, unless such procedures are in place, there is a substantial risk that the data provided by hospitals in a mandatory public reporting system will be misleading because some hospitals will provide data that are more accurate and complete than others. This variation in reporting accuracy and completeness can occur for several reasons. First, as New York health department officials found, hospitals can provide inconsistent information because they interpret the relevant definitions differently. Second, some hospitals are likely to have infection control programs that are more effective than others in identifying HAIs, which means that they detect a higher proportion of the HAIs that occur in their facilities. Finally, the act of publicly reporting infection rates as a guide for patients to use in selecting a hospital may encourage hospitals to be less rigorous in seeking to detect HAIs, since the fewer they find the better they look compared to their competitors.

Because the HAI data collection systems developed by CDC, including NHSN, were based on a model of voluntary participation by hospitals for purposes of internal quality improvement without public disclosure of the results, CDC systems did not incorporate processes for independent data validation. Voluntary participation without public disclosure was presumed to minimize any incentive for hospitals to submit inaccurate data. Consequently, CDC has not conducted an ongoing or systematic validation study of the data currently being submitted to NHSN,[26] though it has collaborated with states that adopt NHSN for mandatory public reporting to develop methods that the states can use to ensure the submitted data are accurate.

Of the 23 states we reviewed, 4 have plans to validate the accuracy of the data collected from hospitals, while several others indicated they may develop such plans in the future. New York has made the most progress on implementing a broad data validation process. It has hired five ICPs to review a systematic sample of infection reports submitted to the NHSN from each New York hospital and compare the reports with the hospitals' medical records. The ICPs review medical records of ICU patients with bloodstream infections from each hospital, as well as records of matched patients with similar surgeries for whom infections were and were not reported. After identifying which patient medical records showed HAIs that should have been reported, they compare them to the infection reports submitted by the hospitals. For any discrepancies, state officials meet with hospital staff to better ensure the accuracy of the data for the next reporting period.

Three other states—Pennsylvania, Missouri, and South Carolina—have undertaken less extensive efforts to validate data they receive from hospitals. Pennsylvania has conducted inspections of a limited number of hospitals selected on the basis of statistical anomalies in the HAI data that they submitted. However, Pennsylvania state officials have developed plans to emulate New York's approach and hire auditors to review a sample of patient medical records from each hospital. In addition, they plan to analyze utilization data obtained from insurance plans. In Missouri, health department officials conducting annual onsite inspections of licensed hospitals compare a hospital's HAI reports with a sample of patient medical records. This is one of many items covered during a licensing inspection and it is not designed to be a comprehensive data validation effort. South Carolina has initiated a pilot program with one hospital system to develop data validation methods based on linking NHSN data with hospital billing data from the state's hospital discharge data set.

Officials in other states have indicated similar concerns about the accuracy of data submitted to HAI public reporting programs, but have not yet acted on those concerns. Documents from seven states supported efforts to validate the data submitted by hospitals to ensure their accuracy.[27] However, most of these states are just beginning to implement their public reporting systems and have not yet begun to develop data validation methods.

Most States Do Not Require Hospitals to Track MRSA HAIs, though Some States Collect Limited MRSA Data through Public Reporting or Other Systems

States have generally not required MRSA-related outcome measures or process measures as a part of their public reporting programs, even though MRSA and other MDROs cause many HAIs. Three exceptions are Illinois, Maryland, and New Jersey. Illinois plans to collect data on the number of hospital patients with MRSA infections using diagnostic codes included in administrative data that hospitals routinely submit to the state. In January 2008, Illinois made two changes to its administrative data systems that will enhance its identification of hospital-associated MRSA infections. First, it required all hospitals to enter a code for each reported diagnosis to indicate if the condition was present when the patient was admitted.[28] The state also expanded the number of diagnosis codes that hospitals report to the state, from a maximum of 9 to 25, which will reduce the chances of undercounting the number of patients with MRSA infections for patients with more than 9 diagnoses.

New Jersey is also requiring hospitals to report on MRSA cases acquired in hospitals. Rather than rely on administrative data, New Jersey plans to use an MDRO module for the NHSN that CDC is developing and expects to release in the fall of 2008. Maryland has taken yet another approach by deciding to collect data on a MRSA-related process measure instead of outcomes. It will collect information from hospitals on the proportion of patients in ICUs who undergo AST for MRSA.

States also are able to obtain some data on HAIs caused by MRSA from the existing NHSN modules. Seventeen states have decided to use the NHSN to collect outcome measures on one or more types of HAIs for which there are NHSN protocols.[29] These protocols require hospitals to report available information about the pathogens causing the infections and the results of any antimicrobial susceptibility laboratory testing performed. However, these data are limited to the types of infections that the states require hospitals to report, and most states have opted not to require hospitals to report on all types of HAIs in hospitals for which NHSN has developed protocols. Moreover, the existing NHSN modules do not include community-associated MRSA, which can only be reported through NHSN as part of the MDRO module to be released in fall of 2008.

Although MRSA does not appear on CDC's list of nationally notifiable infectious diseases for 2008, we found 13 states that classify MRSA infections as a reportable disease under their state communicable disease programs.[30] These programs require hospitals, laboratories, or other providers to report some or all MRSA cases to the state or local departments of health periodically.[31] In all but one of these states, those reporting MRSA cases are not asked to distinguish between health-care- associated and community-associated infections.

Resource and Technological Challenges Influence How States Implement HAI Reporting Systems

State and state hospital association officials we interviewed mentioned a variety of resource and technology challenges they faced in implementing their HAI reporting systems. These challenges often limited the scope of their reporting systems and the timing of their implementation. Regarding resource challenges, officials in one state reported that they needed to train and provide technical assistance for hospital staff, some of whom struggled to implement the clinically sophisticated NHSN protocols for data collection. A status report issued by another state noted that the state resources dedicated to training hospital staff to use the NHSN prevented the state from conducting other program activities such as data validation. Officials in several states reported trouble hiring and retaining the staff they needed to initiate their HAI reporting systems, sometimes due to a lack of financial resources. State officials underscored their need for highly trained personnel to effectively implement these reporting systems. Hospital association and state officials in several states noted that hospitals did not have enough qualified ICPs, which has exacerbated implementation challenges. One state official indicated that although the health department had financial resources to hire staff, it did not have enough office space.

States also confronted technological challenges when implementing HAI reporting systems, especially if they developed their own data collection systems. Missouri officials, for example, found the system they developed had to balance competing technological demands to (1) collect all the necessary data elements for proper risk adjustment, (2) allow hospitals to extract the data using their existing computer systems, and (3) be user- friendly for those collecting and entering data. Pennsylvania also experienced technological challenges. For example, when it began collecting HAI data from hospitals using a data system that was developed for hospitals to report administrative data, it generated strong criticisms from hospital officials and clinicians who argued that this system did not collect the information needed to risk adjust the reported results as recommended by CDC.[32]

CDC had already dealt with such technological issues in developing the NHSN, building on its decades-long experience in operating the NNIS system. In June 2007, CDC opened enrollment in the NHSN to all U.S. hospitals. This made adoption of the NHSN an attractive option for state officials seeking to address these technological concerns. For example, New York officials reported to us that they considered developing their own data collection system tailored to the needs of the New York program before deciding to adopt the NHSN. Because New York's law required a reporting system that was functionally similar to the NHSN, these officials concluded that it made more sense to use the existing system than attempt to create a new system to perform the same functions.

These challenges, particularly with respect to resources, have affected the decisions states have made regarding timelines for implementation, measures to use, data collection mechanisms, and data validation processes. To ensure they have sufficient resources to adequately implement their reporting systems, some states have delayed the starting date for reporting or limited the number of measures to be collected. Frequently states restricted the measures that they selected to patients in certain units, such as ICUs, or those who underwent selected surgical procedures.

To avoid the resource and technological challenges of developing their own data collection systems, most states have decided to use the NHSN. State officials cited numerous reasons for adopting the NHSN, including that it is free to both the states and the hospitals, accessible on the Internet, requires no software development by the states or commercial software purchases by hospitals, uses professionally accepted definitions, and collects detailed data that hospitals can use for quality improvement. However, despite widespread recognition among state officials of the need to validate the data submitted by hospitals, only in a few states have officials determined how to accomplish data validation with the resources available to them.

HOSPITAL MRSA- REDUCTION INITIATIVES SHARE MULTIPLE COMPONENTS, BUT VARY IN SCOPE AND RESOURCE REQUIREMENTS

All the hospitals with MRSA-reduction initiatives that we reviewed use routine testing for MRSA as part of their initiative, although they chose different patient populations to test. These hospitals reported changing a number of general infection control policies or practices as part of their initiatives, and all included patient or health care staff decolonization as part of their initiative despite limited support for such practices among infection control experts. The hospitals we reviewed reported needing varying levels of funding and staff resources to operate their initiatives, but all hospitals that tracked MRSA infection rates reported a decline in MRSA infections as a result of their initiatives.

All Initiatives Use Routine Testing for MRSA but Vary in How Testing Is Targeted and Conducted

All 14 hospitals we reviewed reported that they conduct AST as part of their MRSA-reduction initiative. However, these hospitals vary in the patient populations tested (see table 5). Three hospitals conduct universal AST, testing all patients admitted. The remaining hospitals conduct targeted AST, screening select patient populations deemed to be at risk for MRSA colonization. Of the hospitals that conduct targeted AST, all but one screen patients in adult or neonatal intensive care units and 5 screen surgical patients.

The hospitals we reviewed divide fairly evenly in their choice of testing methods. Five of the hospitals conduct AST using selective media, which generally produces results in 24 hours at a cost of approximately $5 per test. All but one of the remaining hospitals reported using PCR testing, which provides results in only 2 to 4 hours but costs about $25 to $30 per test, and the one remaining hospital reported using routine culture media. Two hospitals reported using more than one testing method. One of these hospitals reported that PCR testing is used only when results are needed quickly because of limited staff availability to operate the equipment.

Hospitals Expanded Infection Control Activities and Information Systems to Reduce MRSA

In implementing their MRSA-reduction initiatives, all the hospitals we reviewed reported changing general infection control policies or practices. CDC guidelines for managing MDROs include recommended practices relating to hand hygiene adherence, contact precautions, environmental cleaning, and judicious use of antibiotics. All 14 hospitals made changes to their existing policies or practices for hand hygiene, while more than half of the hospitals made changes to their contact precautions or environmental cleaning policies (see table 6).[33] Fewer hospitals reported making changes to their antibiotic stewardship policies.

Table 5. Patient Populations Screened with Active Surveillance Testing, by Selected Hospital

	Targeted screening							
	All (Universal)	Adult intensive care unit	Neonatal intensive care unit	Surgical	Long-term care facility admissions	Jail or prison admissions	Dialysis	Other
Evanston Northwestern Healthcare	●	○	○	○	○	○	○	○
Medical University of South Carolina	●	○	○	○	○	○	○	○
Pitt County Memorial Hospital	●	○	○	○	○	○	○	○
Eastern Idaho Regional Medical Center		●	●	●[a]	●	●	●	●[b]
Centra, Lynchburg General and Virginia Baptist Hospitals		●		●[c]	●		●	●[d]
Wake Forest University Baptist Medical Center	●							●[e]
Mercy Medical Center					●			●[f]
Albany Medical Center		●	●					
Newark Beth Israel Medical Center	●	●						

	Targeted screening							
	All (Universal)	Adult intensive care unit	Neonatal intensive care unit	Surgical	Long-term care facility admissions	Jail or prison admissions	Dialysis	Other
Beth Israel Medical Center	●		●[g]					
Rochester General Hospital	●		●[h]					
University of Pittsburgh Medical Center	●							
Barnes-Jewish Hospital	●							
Pacific Hospital of Long Beach	●							

Source: GAO analysis of survey and site visit data.

Notes:

z Hospital screens patient population for MRSA.

0 Included in universal active surveillance testing where all admitted patients are tested.

[a] Screens patients admitted for open mediastinal procedures, total joint replacements, and open spine procedures.

[b] Screens patients admitted from another acute care hospital.

[c] Screens admissions to the surgical ICU.

[d] Screens patients who live in a household with a MRSA-positive individual or have been told in the past that they have an MDRO.

[e] Screens patients who have a length of stay in the hospital that is greater than 6 days and who have been given antibiotics; patients who have a length of stay greater than 21 days; patients known to have at least one MDRO; and patients transferred from other health care facilities.

[f] Screens patients with soft tissue or skin infections.

[g] Some surgical patients are screened.

[h] Screens cardiothoracic patients.

Table 6. Policy or Practice Changes Implemented by Selected Hospitals as Part of MRSA-Reduction Initiatives

	Hand hygiene	Contact precautions	Enhanced environmental cleaning	Antibiotic stewardship
Evanston Northwestern Healthcare	●	●		●
Medical University of South Carolina	●			
Pitt County Memorial Hospital	●		●	
Eastern Idaho Regional Medical Center	●	●	●	●
Centra, Lynchburg General and Virginia Baptist Hospitals	●	●		
Wake Forest University Baptist Medical Center	●	●	●	●
Mercy Medical Center	●		●	
Albany Medical Center	●	●	●	●
Newark Beth Israel Medical Center	●		●	●
Beth Israel Medical Center	●	●	●	
Rochester General Hospital	●	●	●	●
University of Pittsburgh Medical Center	●	●	●	
Barnes-Jewish Hospital	●	●		
Pacific Hospital of Long Beach	●	●	●	●

Source: GAO analysis of survey and site visit data.

- Hand hygiene—All of the hospitals we reviewed reported changing hand hygiene policies as part of their MRSA-reduction initiative. Eleven of the hospitals reported conducting observation audits to monitor compliance with hand hygiene protocols. Two of these hospitals noted that their audits are coupled with immediate feedback to staff who are noncompliant. More than half of the hospitals also reported increasing staff training or public awareness campaigns to increase compliance with hand hygiene among staff or hospital visitors, or both. Multiple hospitals have increased the use of alcohol-based gel hand sanitizers as part of their initiatives by providing more product dispensers in the hospital. In addition, 2 hospitals reported monitoring the consumption of hand hygiene products, such as hand sanitizer or soap, to gauge hand hygiene compliance. For more information on the changes hospitals made to hand hygiene polices, see appendix II, table 7.
- Contact precautions—Most hospitals reported making changes to their contact precautions as part of their MRSA-reduction initiatives, for example, by requiring health care workers to wear gowns and gloves when in contact with a MRSA-positive patient or with equipment used on a MRSA-positive patient. Two hospitals also began requiring health care workers to wear masks in addition to gowns and gloves when in contact with a MRSA-positive

patient.[34] Multiple hospitals use signs at room entrances of MRSA-positive patients to remind health care workers to follow contact precautions when entering those environments. Hospitals that changed their contact precautions also reported conducting audits to measure staff compliance with contact precaution procedures. For more information on the changes hospitals made to their contact precautions, see appendix II, table 8.
- Environmental cleaning—Most hospitals reported changing environmental cleaning procedures as part of their MRSA-reduction initiatives. Three hospitals reported that they disinfect patient equipment between uses or high-touch areas, such as keyboards and door knobs. Three hospitals implemented checklists for housekeeping staff to ensure that rooms are properly cleaned following the discharge of a MRSA-positive patient. One hospital began changing privacy curtains in patient rooms as part of its initiative because the curtains often become contaminated with MRSA. For more information on the changes hospitals made to environmental cleaning polices, see appendix II, table 9.
- Antibiotic stewardship—Half of the hospitals created new policies or revised their existing policies pertaining to antibiotic stewardship. These changes generally included tracking antibiotic prescriptions or restricting the use of certain antibiotics. For more information on the changes hospitals made to antibiotic stewardship policies, see appendix II, table 10.

In addition to changes in infection control practices, most of the hospitals we reviewed adapted their information systems to support their MRSAreduction initiatives. All but 1 of the 14 hospitals has a mechanism to identify previously colonized patients readmitted to their hospital. Most of these hospitals reported that they track patients' MRSA status in electronic medical records, using flags to identify a patient as MRSA-positive each time the patient's electronic medical record is accessed. This enables the staff to immediately implement contact precautions, without the cost or time needed for additional screening.

All 14 Hospitals Included Decolonization in Their MRSA-Reduction Initiatives

All the hospitals we reviewed included patient or health care staff decolonization as part of their MRSA-reduction initiatives, despite limited support for MRSA decolonization among infection control experts and in CDC's MDRO guidelines. Twelve hospitals reported decolonizing patients, with 6 of these hospitals decolonizing all MRSA-positive patients. Seven hospitals reported that they decolonize health care staff—

6 hospitals test health care staff for MRSA colonization during outbreaks and decolonize those found to be positive while the other hospital decolonizes staff found to be MRSA-positive during voluntary testing. For more information on these hospitals' approaches to decolonization, see appendix II, table 11.

Hospital MRSA Initiatives Reported Needing Varying Levels of Funding and Staff Resources

The hospitals we reviewed reported needing varying levels of funding and staff resources to implement and operate their MRSA-reduction initiatives. Half of the hospitals reported needing limited or no additional funding for these initiatives. However, the remaining hospitals reported that moderate to substantial additional funds were needed. Six of the seven hospitals that reported needing moderate to substantial additional funding use the more expensive PCR testing or screen all patients (see fig. 1). Several of the remaining hospitals that reported needing limited or no additional resources also use PCR testing, but all of them conduct AST on targeted patient populations. Eight hospitals reported needing additional staff to conduct patient testing, laboratory staff to process the tests, or both.

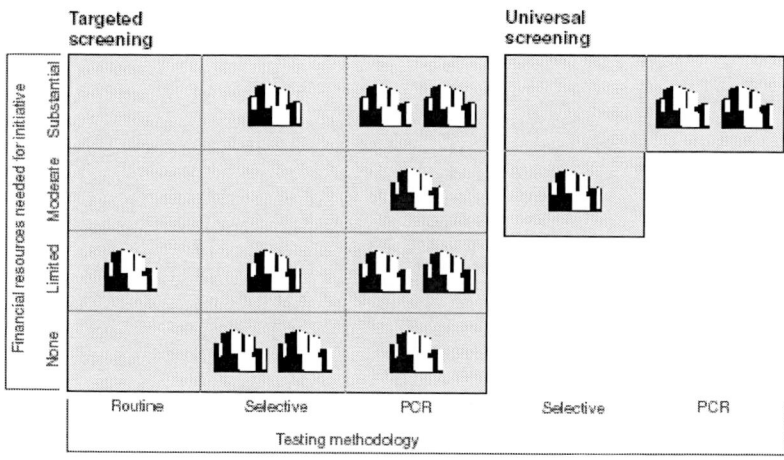

Source: GAO.

Note: Reporting hospitals characterized the level of additional resources needed for their MRSAreduction initiatives as none, limited, moderate, or substantial.

Figure 1: Selected Hospital-Reported Financial Resource Needs for MRSAReduction Initiative, by Type of Screening and Test Method.

Most hospitals reported that they place all or most MRSA-positive patients in private rooms as part of their initiative. However, several of these hospitals noted that the availability of single or semiprivate rooms was a factor in the approach or scope of their MRSA-reduction initiative. For example, at Newark Beth Israel, the first priority is to place all MRSApositive patients in single rooms. However, when single rooms are not available, a MRSA-positive patient is placed with another MRSA-positive patient. Eight hospitals reported at least some cohorting of MRSA-positive patients.

Hospitals with MRSA Initiatives Consistently Reported Reductions in MRSA Infection Rates

Of the 13 hospitals that tracked MRSA infection rates, all found a decline in MRSA infections as a result of their initiatives. Though some hospitals simply cited reductions or significant decreases in their MRSA infections, 5 hospitals provided estimates of the percentage by which their MRSA infection rates had declined. These estimates ranged from around 50 to 74 percent. Three hospitals assessed their reductions quantitatively, but in terms other than percentage or proportion. Two hospitals noted that infections from all organisms, not just MRSA, declined. Over half of the hospitals we reviewed reported that they have tracked MRSA colonization rates as part of their MRSA initiatives. Of the hospitals that reported tracking MRSA colonization rates, half reported an observed decrease in the incidence of MRSA colonization since implementing their initiatives.

TWO HOSPITAL SYSTEMS ADDRESSED SIMILAR CHALLENGES IN IMPLEMENTING MRSA- REDUCTION INITIATIVES

The two hospital systems that we visited overcame a similar set of challenges in implementing multifaceted MRSA-reduction programs. Both systems designed and executed processes to put the elements of their MRSA-reduction initiatives into effect and promote compliance with those processes by hospital staff. Both strove to facilitate the implementation of these processes by incorporating them as much as possible into the normal workflow of hospital staff. Both hospital systems promoted staff compliance with their MRSA-reduction initiatives through a combination of concerted leadership on the part of the physicians who led their infection control programs and specific procedures designed to facilitate staff compliance reinforced through detailed feedback on their performance. However, the two hospital systems took different approaches to marshalling resources for their initiatives. One directed substantial financial resources into its MRSA-reduction initiative to implement the initiative simultaneously for all patients at all of its hospitals, while the other relied largely on existing resources and implemented its initiative more incrementally at selected hospitals and on selected units.

The Two Systems Faced Process, Compliance, and Resource Challenges in Implementing Their MRSA Reduction Initiatives

The two hospital systems that we visited faced a similar set of challenges in implementing multifaceted MRSA-reduction programs over the past several years.[35] Evanston Northwestern Healthcare (ENH) and the University of Pittsburgh Medical Center (UPMC)—both multihospital systems[36]—each sought to reduce MRSA infections by instituting AST of patients for MRSA and ensuring consistent implementation of hospital procedures, such as hand hygiene procedures and contact precautions. To achieve these objectives, both systems had to overcome three challenges: (1) designing and executing processes to put the elements of their MRSA-reduction initiatives into effect, (2) promoting compliance with those processes by hospital staff, and (3) marshalling the required financial and staff resources to implement their initiatives.

The Two Systems Incorporated Processes to Implement Their MRSAReduction Initiatives into Routine Hospital Workflows

The two systems put processes in place to ensure that all eligible patients were tested for MRSA and that any positive results were quickly communicated to the clinical staff to alert them to initiate contact precautions for those patients. Both strove to facilitate the implementation of these processes by incorporating them as much as possible into the normal workflow of hospital staff. At ENH, the implementation of universal AST at admission meant that collecting specimens and submitting them to the laboratory became part of the routine admission procedure for every patient. Because all patients were tested, there were no target populations to identify. Although UPMC did not adopt universal AST, its strategy of screening every patient in selected hospital units had a similar advantage in terms of clearly identifying the patients to be tested.[37]

Both hospitals devised processes for easing access to the supplies that staff needed to conduct MRSA testing and to initiate contact precautions for the patients who tested positive. ENH developed a packet with all the supplies needed for testing a patient for MRSA. The housekeeping staff was responsible for leaving this packet on the bed as it finished preparing each room for the next patient. At ENH, supplies needed for contact precautions were stocked on isolation supply carts that were delivered to the room of each patient who tested positive for MRSA. To reduce the time of the arrival of that cart for patients undergoing contact precautions, ENH officials revised their procedure for ordering the carts. Instead of having the nursing staff order the cart once it had received notice of a patient's positive test result, ENH officials instructed the laboratory staff to order the cart directly for all patients with positive test results. According to ENH officials, this reduced the time from test result to initiation of isolation precautions by approximately 45 minutes. UPMC staff designed a special container to install at each patient room that was routinely kept stocked with the gloves, gowns, and other supplies needed whenever a patient was placed under contact precautions. Moreover, UPMC programmed its laboratory information system so that a positive MRSA test result automatically generated a notification by fax, e-mail, and pager to the clinical staff on that patient's hospital unit to initiate contact precautions.

Concerted Leadership and Monitoring of Staff Performance Fostered Compliance with MRSAReduction Initiatives

Both hospital systems promoted staff compliance with their MRSAreduction initiatives through a combination of concerted leadership on the part of the two physicians who led their respective infection control programs and specific procedures designed to facilitate staff compliance reinforced through detailed feedback on their performance. Much of the impetus for implementing MRSA-reduction programs at ENH and UPMC came from these two lead physicians, both of whom saw the potential to achieve substantial decreases in MRSA infection rates by putting a comprehensive program in place. These lead physicians worked extensively with hospital administrators and their fellow clinicians to build support for the MRSA-reduction initiative by documenting the extent of their existing problem with MRSA, laying out the steps that they could take to address the problem, and marshalling the evidence that the resulting initiative was producing positive results once implementation had begun. They also responded to any problems that arose during implementation or concerns expressed by the clinicians affected by the initiative by making adjustments in its operation. To identify emerging problems and find effective solutions, the lead physicians established internal working groups with representation across the affected hospital departments. At UPMC this group continued to meet regularly to review data on whether patients were being properly tested and isolated, to discuss any concerns raised by hospital staff, and to consider specific adjustments to the implementation of the initiative.

Both hospital systems relied heavily on information technology to facilitate compliance with the various components of the MRSA initiative. ENH made a number of specific adaptations to its electronic medical record (EMR) system.[38] For example, it added an orange banner on the medical record screen that highlighted any patient who had been admitted until staff entered a confirmation that the MRSA test had been performed.

ENH also created a prominent flag in its EMR for any patient who had been identified as MRSA-positive during a previous admission or outpatient encounter; all such patients were immediately placed under contact precautions. UPMC incorporated similar reminders into its EMR system and also implemented a flag to identify patients who had previously tested positive for MRSA so that they could be immediately placed under contact precautions at subsequent admissions.

In addition, ENH and UPMC monitored staff compliance with targeted hospital procedures. At ENH, hospital ICPs used their electronic record system to measure the length of time it took staff on various units to perform the MRSA test and to respond to positive test results by implementing contact precautions. They used these data to provide feedback to both units and individual staff members on their relative performance. At UPMC, the infection control department provided similar feedback at monthly meetings with staff in the individual hospital units, where they presented data on the proportion of patients who were tested at UPMC's designated time points.

UPMC also expanded its oversight of staff compliance with standard hand hygiene procedures in conjunction with its MRSA-reduction initiative. To obtain more accurate information on staff compliance with those procedures, UPMC implemented routine audits that used trained, anonymous observers to assess staff performance. UPMC officials sent formal letters to clinical staff, including physicians, who were observed not following hand hygiene procedures. Less formally, UPMC officials provided immediate, positive feedback to staff members who were observed complying with their hand hygiene procedures.

One Hospital System Marshalled Substantial Resources to Effect Systemwide Change while the Other Implemented Incremental Changes with Existing Resources

ENH directed substantial financial resources into its MRSA-reduction initiative to implement the initiative simultaneously for all patients at all three of its hospitals, while UPMC relied largely on existing resources and implemented its initiative more incrementally at selected hospitals and on selected units. For both hospital systems, one key resource challenge was paying for an increased number of MRSA tests. Ultimately, both systems conducted analyses indicating that the increased costs of their initiatives were more than compensated for by the reduced cost of treating a smaller number of patients with MRSA infections.

ENH officials made a key strategic decision to move expeditiously to implement MRSA screening for all patients admitted to ENH's three hospitals. To do this, they developed an implementation plan based on an analysis of clinical and financial data. Beginning in 2003, ENH piloted MRSA AST in one ICU. In 2004, it conducted a one-time prevalence survey[39] that determined that 8.5 percent of all patients were colonized with MRSA—most of them in units outside of the ICUs.[40] Based on this information and the ICU pilot experience, ENH officials developed a plan to implement universal AST within a year and budgeted $1 million per year in additional costs, mostly for the increased number of MRSA tests performed and additional laboratory staff. ENH officials conducted a cost-benefit analysis that concluded that the hospital system would save more from having fewer patients with MRSA infections needing treatment than it would spend for increased testing. Because ENH had collected detailed information on patient costs and charges over a number of years, these officials were able to develop their own estimates for the additional costs associated with an MRSA infection in the ENH hospitals.[41]

Administrators at ENH provisionally approved the MRSA-reduction initiative, pending confirmation during its first 2 years that it had the expected effect on the number of ENH patients who developed MRSA infections and had not increased overall costs. Ultimately, the number of MRSA cases at ENH decreased more rapidly than expected following implementation of the initiative, and the additional costs were less than expected—approximately $600,000 per year.

The cost-benefit analysis provided ENH officials with support for their choice of the more expensive PCR testing method. Under the plan, the projected cost savings from the anticipated reduction in MRSA infections were greater than the additional costs of the MRSA-reduction initiative, even using PCR to test every patient at admission. ENH officials were willing to pay approximately $25 per test to obtain two advantages offered by PCR testing—faster results and greater sensitivity in detecting patients with

MRSA. Getting results for most patients no later than 15 hours after testing reduces the amount of time that MRSA-positive patients spend in the hospital without contact precautions in place, which in turn reduces the chances that they will infect other patients.[42]

UMPC took a more incremental approach to implementing its MRSAreduction initiative and, as a result, did not need additional resources. It began its initiative in 2002 in one ICU at Presbyterian Hospital, and expanded it over 4 years to other ICUs in that hospital and then to all adult ICUs in the 19 other hospitals in the UPMC system. This measured pace of expansion restricted the number of additional patients who needed to undergo contact precautions at any one time, which eased potential logistical problems that stem from the predominance of semiprivate rooms in UPMC hospitals. UPMC officials told us that they expect to continue making such incremental decisions on where and when to expand their MRSA-reduction initiative in the future. They stated that this could eventually lead to screening of all inpatient admissions.

UPMC officials have relied, as did their counterparts at ENH, on their analysis of clinical and financial data in developing and expanding their MRSA-reduction initiative. UPMC officials selected the initial hospital unit from those that had the largest number of MRSA infections and, therefore, the greatest potential for improvement, with additional consideration given to the readiness of staff on the unit to fully support the initiative. On that basis, they began with the 20-bed medical ICU at Presbyterian Hospital. Once the initiative was implemented and the ICU's MRSA infection rate declined, they made the case for expanding the initiative to other units within Presbyterian and to other UPMC hospitals. As with the initial selection of the first ICU, UPMC officials selected the units for expansion of the initiative based on those with the highest MRSA rates, and they plan to continue expanding participation in the initiative on that basis.

Because UPMC began its MRSA-reduction initiative with just one unit, and monitored its progress for 3 years before expanding to other units, UPMC officials could implement their initiative with a relatively small upfront investment of resources. They hired no new staff for the initiative. Instead, to meet the demand for increased MRSA testing, they reallocated existing laboratory staff and financial resources. Other additional costs, such as for increased use of gowns, gloves, and masks to maintain contact precautions, were relatively minor.[43] In selecting which test to use for screening patients, UPMC officials chose the relatively inexpensive selective media test, which costs approximately $5 and requires only about 40 seconds of laboratory technician time to perform. Although using selective media did not produce results as quickly as PCR would, UPMC officials found that they could nonetheless identify 81 percent of MRSA-positive patients within 24 hours.

UPMC's MRSA-reduction initiative has achieved large reductions in the number of MRSA cases at a relatively low cost, resulting in a highly favorable ratio of benefits to costs. UPMC officials estimate that their savings in terms of the reduced costs to treat a smaller number of MRSA cases were 12 to 32 times greater than the costs they incurred to test patients for MRSA and implement contact precautions for those who test positive. To calculate those savings, they relied on estimates from the published literature for determining the difference in treatment costs for patients with and without MRSA infections,[44] and multiplied that figure by the reduction in the number of MRSA infections that have occurred in their targeted units. UPMC officials have used these estimates to build support for expanding the MRSA-reduction initiative into other units of the UPMC hospitals besides ICUs, including orthopedic units.

CONCLUDING OBSERVATIONS

Governmental initiatives to reduce HAIs involve a complicated mix of federal and state activities. The federal government, and in particular its lead agency for HAIs, CDC, have over the last few decades evolved a role that involves certain discrete activities. These include the development of guidelines that assess and recommend specific clinical practices for reducing HAIs. They also include the development and promulgation of procedures and definitions that enable ICPs to determine in a systematic and consistent way which patients have HAIs, and to measure their HAI rates over time. In addition, CDC has initiated and maintained data collection programs, such as NHSN, that provide a mechanism that hospitals can use to both collect information on their own HAIs and compare their experience with that of other hospitals using the same set of clinical definitions and data collection procedures. CDC provides these services to participating hospitals free of charge, and by law protects the confidentiality of the data that hospitals submit.

Meanwhile, at least 23 states have taken initiatives that seek to use comparable information about HAIs for a quite different purpose— informing consumers about the relative performance of specific hospitals. As the states have set up these programs, and confronted the challenges of implementing them with limited resources, many have found compelling advantages in drawing on CDC's procedures and data collection systems. CDC protocols for identifying HAIs are widely respected for their clinical sophistication, and are well known to the ICPs in individual hospitals who will most likely be the ones to report the data. NHSN not only incorporates those widely accepted definitions and procedures, it is also available at no cost to the hospitals that use it. Thus many states have chosen to implement their public reporting programs by mandating that hospitals in their states enroll in NHSN. Although CDC itself may not publicly release HAI data on individual hospitals enrolled in NHSN, hospitals can give access to the state agencies to view and analyze their data using the group feature of NHSN. The state agencies can then use those data for their public reporting programs.

The increasing number of states opting to use information obtained from this federal data collection system to publicly report on the relative performance of individual hospitals raises concerns about the lack of established mechanisms to check the completeness and accuracy of the data submitted by hospitals. When the data are released to the public in order to influence consumers to choose hospitals with lower rates of HAIs, hospitals may have an incentive to minimize the number of HAI cases that they identify and report if they believe either that the hospitals with which they compete for patients could be minimizing the number of HAIs they reported or that those hospitals have actually achieved lower rates of HAIs than their own hospital. NHSN was created under a completely different paradigm, in which hospitals voluntarily collected the data on HAIs to inform their own internal efforts to reduce HAIs, with a legal protection from public release. Because the data were intended strictly for internal use, CDC officials assumed that hospitals had an incentive to generate the most accurate and complete data possible. Consequently, the NHSN did not develop any process or mechanism to audit the accuracy and completeness of the data that hospitals submitted.

Both CDC and state officials have noted that converting NHSN to a source for publicly reported data on HAIs fundamentally changes the incentives for participating hospitals, and thereby creates a need for procedures to independently validate the data that hospitals submit. Specifically, CDC has collaborated with states using NHSN for public reporting to develop and implement data validation as part of their programs. However, few states have so far acted on this advice. Specific procedures for validating HAI data need to be developed and tested, and resources allocated to implement them. To some extent, New York has done the most to accomplish these tasks, but its experience indicates that systematic data validation requires substantial staff resources. Unless other states can marshal the resources needed to ensure the accuracy and completeness of the HAI data submitted by their hospitals, they are unlikely to make substantial progress in addressing this issue.

COMMENTS FROM HHS AND THE AMERICAN HOSPITAL ASSOCIATION AND OUR EVALUATION

We obtained written comments on our draft chapter from HHS, which were largely technical in nature. Overall, HHS commended GAO for developing a helpful chapter on an important topic. The department also highlighted the contributions that CDC has made, including its research into understanding the epidemiology of MRSA and HAIs. HHS noted that CDC's work in this area is reflected in a large number of scientific publications pertaining to the detection, measurement, and prevention of HAIs and MRSA. In addition, we incorporated the technical comments that HHS provided as appropriate.

The vice president of quality and patient safety policy for the American Hospital Association (AHA) provided oral comments on our draft chapter. The AHA appreciated that our chapter addressed state reporting programs for HAIs as a whole, along with a detailed review of hospital initiatives to reduce MRSA. It highlighted the technical and resource challenges described in our chapter that hospitals face in conducting HAI surveillance and prevention activities, which smaller hospitals in particular may have difficulty overcoming. Therefore, the AHA believes that it is important to link the collection of HAI data to achieving a reduction of HAIs including MRSA, and to acknowledge that different hospitals can use different approaches to accomplish this objective. In addition, the AHA expressed serious concern about public reporting of HAI data collected through NHSN. It noted that the NHSN data were not validated and that hospitals vary in how they collect the data submitted to NHSN. As a result, the AHA felt that the NHSN data do not provide a valid comparative assessment of hospital performance. The AHA also provided technical comments that we incorporated as appropriate.

We agree with HHS that CDC has played a central role in developing both the science and the data collection systems on which current efforts to assess and reduce HAIs rest. At the same time, we share AHA's concerns that to be viable in the long run, systems for collecting HAI data for public reporting need to produce data that are clinically accurate and that assist hospitals in their efforts to reduce HAIs. As evidenced by its widespread adoption, CDC's NHSN has made a substantial contribution in that direction, though questions remain regarding how best to ensure that the data it produces are accurate and complete.

Sincerely yours,
Cynthia A. Bascetta
Director, Health Care

APPENDIX I: CHARACTERISTICS OF SELECTED HOSPITALS WITH MRSA-REDUCTION INITIATIVES

	Location	Teaching Beds	Size of Metropolitan Area[b] Census region
Albany Medical Center	Albany, NY	599 Yes	2 Middle Atlantic
Barnes-Jewish Hospital	Saint Louis, MO	1,183 Yes	1 West North Central
Beth Israel Medical Center	New York, NY	794 Yes	1 Middle Atlantic
Centra, Lynchburg General and Virginia Baptist Hospitals	Lynchburg, VA	494 No	3 South Atlantic
Eastern Idaho Regional Medical Center	Idaho Falls, ID	289 No	3 Mountain
Evanston Northwestern Healthcare	Evanston, IL	629 Yes	1 East North Central
Pacific Hospital of Long Beach	Long Beach, CA	171 No	1 Pacific
Pitt County Memorial Hospital	Greenville, NC	761 Yes	3 South Atlantic
Medical University of South Carolina	Charleston, SC	596 Yes	2 South Atlantic
Mercy Medical Center	Cedar Rapids, IA	318 No	3 West North Central
Newark Beth Israel Medical Center	Newark, NJ	407 Yes	1 Middle Atlantic
Rochester General Hospital	Rochester, NY	492 No	1 Middle Atlantic
Wake Forest University Baptist Medical Center	Winston-Salem, NC	953 Yes	2 South Atlantic
University of Pittsburgh Medical Center	Pittsburgh, PA	1,492 Yes	1 Middle Atlantic

Sources: American Hospital Association, U.S. Census Bureau, Association of American Medical Colleges, U.S. Department of Agriculture.

[a] Hospitals were designated as teaching hospitals if they were members of the Association of American Medical Colleges' Council of Teaching Hospitals and Health Systems.

[b] All hospitals were located in metropolitan counties according to the Economic Research Service of the U.S. Department of Agriculture, using the rural-urban continuum codes defined by the U.S. Census Bureau. The codes break down as follows: 1= Counties in metropolitan areas of 1 million population or more; 2= Counties in metropolitan areas of 250,000 to 1 million population; and 3= Counties in metropolitan areas of fewer than 250,000 population.

APPENDIX II: CHANGES MADE BY SELECTED HOSPITALS WITH MRSA-REDUCTION INITIATIVES

Table 7. Hand Hygiene Changes by Selected Hospitals with MRSA-Reduction Initiatives

	Hand hygiene compliance audits	Enhanced staff training or public education campaigns	Increased number of dispensers of alcohol-based hand sanitizer	Monitor consumption of hand hygiene products
Albany Medical Center	●		●	
Barnes-Jewish Hospital	●	●		
Beth Israel Medical Center	●	●		
Centra, Lynchburg General and Virginia Baptist Hospitals	●			
Eastern Idaho Regional Medical Center	●	●	●	●
Evanston Northwestern Healthcare	●	●		
Pacific Hospital of Long Beach	●			
Pitt County Memorial Hospital	●	●		
Medical University of South Carolina	●			
Mercy Medical Center	●			
Newark Beth Israel Medical Center	●		●	
Rochester General Hospital		●	●	●
Wake Forest University Baptist Medical Center	●			
University of Pittsburgh Medical Center	●	●	●	

Source: GAO analysis of survey and site visit data.

Table 8. Contact Precaution Changes by Selected Hospitals with MRSA-Reduction Initiatives

	Required gown & gloves for contact with MRSA-positive patients and their environment	Isolation cart/supply holder	Mask required when in contact with MRSA-positive patient	Room entrance signs or checklists to remind staff of MDRO patient	Enhanced staff training or public awareness campaigns	MRSA-positive patients in private rooms or cohorted	Contact precaution compliance audits
Albany Medical Center	●						
Barnes-Jewish Hospital		●				●	●
Beth-Israel Medical Center				●	●	●	●
Centra, Lynchburg General and Virginia Baptist Hospitals					●	●	●
Eastern Idaho Regional Medical Center	●		●			●	
Evanston Northwestern Healthcare		●		●	●	●	
Pacific Hospital of Long Beach						●	
Pitt County Memorial Hospital						●	
Medical University of South Carolina						●	
Mercy Medical Center						●	

Table 8. (Continued).

	Required gown & gloves for contact with MRSA-positive patients and their environment	Isolation cart/supply holder	Mask required when in contact with MRSA-positive patient	Room entrance signs or checklists to remind staff of MDRO patient	Enhanced staff training or public awareness campaigns	MRSA-positive patients in private rooms or cohorted	Contact precaution compliance audits
Newark Beth Israel Medical Center							
Rochester General Hospital					●	●	●
Wake Forest University Baptist Medical Center	●					●	●
University of Pittsburgh Medical Center	●	●	●	●	●	●	●

Source: GAO analysis of survey and site visit data.

Table 9. Environmental Cleaning Changes by Selected Hospitals with MRSA-Reduction Initiatives

	Checklist or electronic notification system for housekeeping staff	Environmental cleaning compliance audits	Enhanced training	Change curtains	Enhanced cleaning of hospital environment or patient equipment	Dedicated equipment for MRSA-positive patients
Albany Medical Center	●					
Barnes-Jewish Hospital						
Beth Israel Medical Center	●	●	●		●	
Centra, Lynchburg General and Virginia Baptist Hospitals						
Eastern Idaho Regional Medical Center		●	●			
Evanston Northwestern Healthcare						
Pacific Hospital of Long Beach			●			
Pitt County Memorial Hospital						
Medical University of South Carolina						
Mercy Medical Center		●				
Newark Beth Israel Medical Center					●	
Rochester General Hospital					●	●
Wake Forest University Baptist Medical Center		●			●	
University of Pittsburgh Medical Center	●			●	●	

Source: GAO analysis of survey and site visit data.

Table 10. Antibiotic Stewardship Changes by Selected Hospitals with MRSA-Reduction Initiatives

	Description
Albany Medical Center	• Antibiotic stewardship team • Electronic system to track antibiotic usage and evaluate microorganism combinations • Reduced usage of certain antibiotics
Barnes-Jewish Hospital	
Beth Israel Medical Center	
Centra, Lynchburg General and Virginia Baptist	
Eastern Idaho Regional Medical Center	
Evanston Northwestern Healthcare	• Tracking of mupirocin resistance • Removal by pharmacy of mupirocin ointment from authorized use for anything other than decolonization to keep resistance under control • Tracking of utilization of vancomycin
Pacific Hospital of Long Beach	• Education • Implementation of the hospital antibiogram, which tests for the sensitivity of isolated bacterial strains to different antibiotics
Pitt County Memorial Hospital	
Medical University of South Carolina	
Mercy Medical Center	
Newark Beth Israel Medical Center	• Development of an antibiotic deescalation program • Introduction of an antibiotic substitution policy • Institution of antibiotic restriction requiring approval by an infectious diseases specialist
Rochester General Hospital	• Monitor drug selection and duration and make recommendations based on this review • In process of implementing an electronic surveillance system with antibiotic monitoring capabilities
Wake Forest University Baptist Medical Center	• Two pharmacy positions dedicated to antibiotic stewardship • Physician dedicated to the prudent use of antibiotics
University of Pittsburgh Medical Center	

Source: GAO analysis of survey and site visit data.

Table 11. Decolonization Characteristics by Selected Hospitals with MRSA-Reduction Initiatives

	All MRSA-positive patients identified through screening	Orthopedic surgery patients	Cardiothoracic surgery patients	Other	Health care workers
Albany Medical Center	●	○	○	○	
Barnes-Jewish Hospital					●[f]
Beth Israel Medical Center		●	●		●[f]
Centra, Lynchburg General and Virginia Baptist Hospitals				●[b]	
Eastern Idaho Regional Medical Center	●	○	○	○	●[fg]
Evanston Northwestern Healthcare	●	○	○	○	
Medical University of South Carolina					●[f]
Mercy Medical Center		●			
Newark Beth Israel Medical Center	●	○	○	○	●[f]
Pacific Hospital of Long Beach	●	○	○	○[c]	
Pitt County Memorial Hospital	●	○	○	○	●[h]
Rochester General Hospital			●[a]		
Wake Forest University Baptist Medical Center				●[d]	
University of Pittsburgh Medical Center				●[e]	●[f]

Source: GAO analysis of survey and site visit data.

Notes:
● Hospital decolonizes these individuals.
○ Included within "All MRSA-positive patients" category.

[a] All cardiothoracic surgery patients, including those who have not tested positive for MRSA, receive decolonization therapy. Mupirocin ointment is also applied to chest tube sites when removing chest tubes.
[b] MRSA-positive patients scheduled to undergo implant procedures are decolonized.
[c] All patients admitted to hospital undergo skin decolonization plus daily cleansing.
[d] Newly colonized patients are decolonized. Patients with a history of MRSA are decolonized at a physician's request.
[e] Patients are decolonized only if they request it and if the physician believes that decolonization is reasonable.
[f] Health care workers are decolonized if identified as MRSA-positive as part of an outbreak investigation.
[g] All newly hired health care workers are screened and decolonized if positive.
[h] Health care workers are provided voluntary MRSA screening at annual physical, and MRSA decolonization is offered at no charge for those who test positive.

REFERENCES

[1] MDROs develop resistance to antimicrobial drugs when bacteria change or adapt in a way that allows them to survive in the presence of antibiotics designed to kill them. In some cases, bacteria become resistant to all available antibiotics.

[2] Although named for its resistance to methicillin, MRSA is also resistant to a large group of commonly prescribed antibiotics.

[3] R.M. Klevens et al., "Changes in the Epidemiology of Methicillin-Resistant Staphylococcus aureus in Intensive Care Units in US Hospitals, 1992–2003," *Clinical Infectious Diseases,* 2006, 42:389–91. These trends are based on data from 1,268 ICUs in 337 U.S. hospitals.

[4] GAO, Health-Care-Associated Infections in Hospitals: Leadership Needed from HHS to Prioritize Prevention Practices and Improve Data on These Infections, GAO-08-283 (Washington, D.C.: Mar. 31, 2008).

[5] The HAI public reporting system in Arkansas does not require hospitals to report data to the state and will report only aggregate data on HAIs to the public. Nevada and Nebraska will not report any HAI data publicly. Utah has begun to collect HAI data from hospitals, but has not yet decided whether it will report these data to the public. Ohio requires hospitals to report quality data publicly, but did not include HAI measures in its initial set of measures. An advisory committee convened to consider and possibly recommend HAI measures for inclusion. Its final report was expected in August 2008.

[6] In several instances, including the two site visits we conducted, the MRSA-reduction initiative applied to multiple hospitals that belonged to the same hospital system. Because our analysis of MRSA-reduction initiatives examined the variation across the different initiatives, we use the term hospital in the following discussion to refer to the single or multiple facilities that adopted a particular MRSA-reduction initiative.

[7] The term HAI is often used synonymously with hospital-acquired infection and nosocomial infection. HAIs are distinct from community-acquired infections, which are infections that were transmitted to patients prior to their admission to a hospital or other health care facility.

[8] Central lines are intravenous lines inserted into a large vein typically in the neck or near the heart.

[9] To be eligible for payment under the Medicare and Medicaid programs, hospitals must comply with HHS-established health and safety standards, known as conditions of participation (COP), which include a COP for infection

control. Many hospitals meet this requirement through accreditation by the Joint Commission.
[10] IHI is an independent, nonprofit organization that works to improve the quality of health care.
[11] Hand hygiene is a general term that applies to handwashing, antiseptic handwash, antiseptic hand rub, or surgical hand antisepsis. Environmental cleaning refers to the disinfection of environmental surfaces and equipment for infection control efforts in hospitals.
[12] H.T. Stelfox et al., "Safety of Patients Isolated for Infection Control," *Journal of the American Medical Association* (Oct. 8, 2003) 290:14, 1899-1905; see also K.B. Kirkland & J.M. Weinstein, "Adverse effects of contact isolation" (Oct. 2, 1999) *The Lancet*, 354, 1177- 1178; S. Saint et al., "Do physicians examine patients in contact isolation less frequently? A brief report," *American Journal of Infection Control*, 31:6 (October 2003) 354-356.
[13] These costs do not include laboratory overhead and personnel costs.
[14] J.D. Siegel et al., *Management of Multidrug-Resistant Organisms in Healthcare Settings, 2006*, downloaded from www.cdc.gov/ncidod/dhqp/guidelines.html on Jun. 5, 2007.
[15] See, CDC/NHSN Surveillance Definition of Health Care-Associated Infection and Criteria for Specific Types of Infections in the Acute Care Setting (www.cdc.gov/ncidod/dhqp/nhsn_documents.html) and CDC, The National Healthcare Safety Network (NHSN) Manual: Patient Safety Component Protocol, Division of Healthcare Quality Promotion, National Center for Infectious Diseases (Atlanta, Ga.: updated January 2008).
[16] See GAO-08-283 for a description of this process.
[17] The NHSN allows hospitals to identify and report HAIs that fall into any of the other 13 categories of HAIs for which CDC has developed definitions but without specific data collection protocols.
[18] he CMS and CDC are represented on the SCIP steering committee, along with such groups as the American College of Surgeons, the American Hospital Association, the American Society of Anesthesiologists, the Institute for Healthcare Improvement, and the Joint Commission.
[19] This Web site can be accessed at www.hospitalcompare.hhs.gov . Since 2004, hospitals' submission of data for a series of process measures has been part of the Medicare hospital inpatient prospective payment system (IPPS). In addition, CMS issued a final rule stating that, effective October 1, 2008, hospitals would no longer receive higher payment under IPPS for eight

preventable outcomes, including three HAIs. See 72 *Fed. Reg.* 47200, 472 17-8 (Aug. 22, 2007).

[20] NQF, "National Voluntary Consensus Standards for the Reporting of Healthcare- Associated Infection Data" (Washington, D.C.: 2008). NQF is a voluntary standard-setting, consensus-building organization representing providers, consumers, purchasers, and researchers.

[21] NQF recently requested that CDC consider revising its definitions for these two measures. See NQF, "National Voluntary Consensus Standards for the Reporting of Healthcare- Associated Infection Data," p. 12.

[22] AHRQ is an HHS agency that conducts and funds research to promote more effective and higher quality care.

[23] Florida selected the antibiotics administered prior to surgery process measures, and Oklahoma selected rates for central line-associated BSIs and VAP.

[24] A number of these states use other systems to collect data for measures not incorporated into NHSN, such as the SCIP measures on antibiotics administered prior to surgery.

[25] Although participation in the NHSN is, from a federal perspective, voluntary on the part of hospitals, and the confidentiality of the data they submit is protected by law, the mandatory state reporting programs require hospitals in those states to enroll in the NHSN and to authorize access to their data by state officials through the group feature in NHSN

[26] CDC researchers did conduct one pilot study in the mid-1990s that examined the accuracy of HAI reporting at nine hospitals participating in the voluntary NNIS system that preceded NHSN. In general they found that the patients that the hospitals reported as having HAIs did have them, but that an additional number of patients had HAIs that were not reported to NNIS. The extent of underreporting varied by type of infection, lower for BSIs and higher for UTIs, for example. The researchers concluded that "Data integrity is essential and can be accomplished only when an ongoing and objective method to assess the quality of the data is included as an integral part of the surveillance system." See T.G. Emori et al., "Accuracy of Reporting Nosocomial Infections in Intensive-Care-Unit Patients to the National Nosocomial Infections Surveillance System: A Pilot Study," *Infection Control and Hospital Epidemiology,* 19 (May 1998) 308-3 16.

[27] The seven states are Colorado, Connecticut, Maryland, New Hampshire, Oregon, Texas, and Washington.

[28] CMS developed this "present on admission" (POA) indicator to identify hospital-acquired conditions. All hospitals paid under Medicare's IPPS must

attach this indicator to the diagnosis codes that they submit with their claims. Certain hospitals that Medicare pays outside of the IPPS, such as critical access hospitals, are not subject to this CMS requirement, but Illinois requires all hospitals to report the POA code.

[29] There are NHSN protocols for central line-associated BSIs, VAP, catheter-associated UTIs, SSIs, and postprocedure pneumonia.

[30] Several other states require hospitals and other providers to report only suspected cases of community-associated MRSA.

[31] Some states focus their reporting requirement on cases of invasive MRSA. The frequency of reporting varies from within 12 hours of identification in Connecticut to semiannually in Maine.

[32] Pennsylvania's original data collection system recorded each instance where hospitals found a patient had an HAI. However, it did not collect information on the number of patients at risk of developing comparable HAIs, information which the NHSN collects in order to risk adjust its results. In 2007 the Pennsylvania legislature passed a law that mandated adoption of NHSN for HAI data collection.

[33] We do not know the extent to which hospitals already had in place extensive policies for contact precautions, environmental cleaning, or antibiotic stewardship. We asked hospitals to report changes they made to these policies for their MRSA-reduction initiatives.

[34] One of these hospitals reported that it included the use of masks because their use may help prevent health care staff from being colonized with MRSA in their nasal passages, a common site of MRSA colonization. However, a hospital official noted that the use of masks has not been adequately studied.

[35] UPMC and ENH began implementing their MRSA-reduction initiatives in January 2002 and February 2003, respectively.

[36] ENH is a 3-hospital system located on separate campuses in Chicago's northern suburbs. All 3 hospitals primarily function as community hospitals with many surgical and long-term care patients and relatively few ICU patients. UPMC is a 20-hospital system, largely located in the Pittsburgh metropolitan area but with some hospitals scattered across Western Pennsylvania. One of the UPMC hospitals is Presbyterian Hospital, a large academic medical center with a substantial number of ICUs and ICU patients. Some of the other hospitals in the UPMC system function more as community hospitals.

[37] In addition to testing patients for MRSA on admission to the selected units, UPMC tested them again (unless they had already tested positive) once a week while on the unit and at the time of discharge from the unit. UPMC made it easier to ensure that patients were tested weekly by testing all patients in the

unit on the same day of the week, rather than counting 7 days from each patient's admission date.

[38] In 2003, ENH converted all its patient medical records to an EMR system. Paper records received from other facilities were scanned and converted into electronic documents, allowing ENH to become a completely "paperless" facility.

[39] The prevalence survey determined the number of patients across all units of the three ENH hospitals who were colonized with MRSA at a particular point in time.

[40] This contrasted with a report published the previous year that 2.7 percent of patients admitted to Emory University Hospital were MRSA-positive. J.A. Jernigan et al., "Prevalence of and Risk Factors for Colonization with Methicillin-Resistant Staphylococcus Aureus at the Time of Hospital Admission," *Infection Control and Hospital Epidemiology*, 24:6 (June 2003) 409-14.

[41] Financial experts at ENH constructed an internal database that recorded actual costs associated with individual chargable items and procedures going back to fiscal year 2005. They used these data to assess the net costs of treating patients with MRSA infections, after taking account of any higher payments received, compared to the costs of treating comparable patients who did not have MRSA infections. These analyses found that ENH absorbed a net cost of approximately $10,000 for each patient with a MRSA-related respiratory infection and a net cost of $19,000 for each patient with a MRSA-related bloodstream infection.

[42] Individual PCR tests require only about 2 to 4 hours to produce a result, but it takes additional time to transport specimens to the laboratory site and it is more efficient to conduct the tests in batches.

[43] UPMC officials estimated that the total cost, including testing, for the first year of the initiative was just over $62,000.

[44] P.W. Stone et al., "A Systematic Audit of Economic Evidence Linking Nosociomial Infections and Infection Control Interventions: 1990-2000," *American Journal of Infection Control*, 30 (2002) 145-52.

In: Hospital-Acquired Infections
Editor: Julia B. Wilcox, pp. 349-361

ISBN: 978-1-60692-728-1
© 2009 Nova Science Publishers, Inc.

Chapter 4

HEALTH-CARE-ASSOCIATED INFECTIONS IN HOSPITALS: NUMBER ASSOCIATED WITH MEDICAL DEVICES UNKNOWN, BUT EXPERTS REPORT PROVIDER PRACTICES AS A SIGNIFICANT FACTOR[*]

United States Government Accountability Office

September 26, 2008

The Honorable Edward M. Kennedy
Chairman

The Honorable Michael B. Enzi
Ranking Member
Committee on Health, Education, Labor, and Pensions United States Senate

The Honorable John D. Dingell
Chairman

---

[*] This is an edited, excerpted and augmented edition of a United States Government Accountability Office publication, Report GAO-08-1091R.

The Honorable Joe Barton
Ranking Member
Committee on Energy and Commerce
House of Representatives

Health-care-associated infections (HAI) in hospitals can be expensive to treat and, according to the Department of Health and Human Services' (HHS) Centers for Disease Control and Prevention (CDC), HAIs are estimated to be one of the top 10 causes of death in the United States. HAIs can be caused by bacteria or viruses, which may be introduced to a patient through the use of a device used to treat them, such as a needle or tube to deliver medicine, fluids, or blood. Common HAIs that are often associated with the use of medical devices are urinary tract infections (UTI), surgical site infections (SSI), pneumonia, and bloodstream infections (B SI). A number of federal agencies within HHS, including CDC and the Agency for Healthcare Research and Quality (AHRQ), currently collect HAI-related data for a variety of purposes. Nearly half of the states also require public reporting of hospital HAI rates, according to a summary report of these state laws.[1]

The Food and Drug Administration Amendments Act of 2007[2] requires us to conduct work on HAIs in hospitals associated with medical devices.[3] The act defines these infections as those that are acquired while an individual is a patient at a hospital and were neither present nor incubating prior to the patient's receiving services in the hospital. Specifically, the act requires us to report on the number of HAIs in hospitals attributable to new and reused medical devices and on the causes of such infections. As agreed with the committees of jurisdiction, in this chapter we examine two questions: (1) What is known from available federal and state data about the number of HAIs in hospitals associated with the use of medical devices? (2) What factors affect the occurrence of HAIs in hospitals associated with the use of medical devices?

To obtain information about the number of HAIs in hospitals associated with the use of medical devices, we identified available federal data sources at four HHS agencies—AHRQ, CDC, the Centers for Medicare & Medicaid Services (CMS), and the Food and Drug Administration (FDA)—and reviewed a summary report of available state data sources.[4] We interviewed relevant officials responsible for these federal data sets to determine the extent to which they included information specifically on HAIs in hospitals associated with the use of medical devices, how these data were collected, and whether the data were nationally representative. To identify the factors affecting the occurrence of HAIs in hospitals associated with the use of medical devices, we conducted a literature review and interviewed infection control experts. For the literature review, we identified 38 relevant articles from nearly 200 peer-reviewed scientific studies and medical literature published since 2000 and examined them to determine the significant risk factors and how these factors varied for different HAIs in hospitals. In addition, on the basis of our literature review and recommendations from officials at several federal agencies, professional associations, and advocacy groups, we identified 11 experts to interview about factors that affect the occurrence of HAIs in hospitals. When interviewing these experts, we asked them to identify causes of HAIs in hospitals from among those listed in the mandate and to identify any additional known causes.[5] We further relied on the literature review and these interviews to identify related prevention strategies. We conducted this performance audit from March 2008 through August 2008, in accordance with generally accepted government auditing standards. Those standards require that we plan and perform the audit to obtain sufficient, appropriate evidence to provide a reasonable basis for our findings and conclusions based on our audit objectives. We believe that the evidence obtained provides a reasonable basis for our findings and conclusions based on our audit objectives.

In summary, multiple federal programs and states collect data on HAIs in hospitals, but none of the data sources we identified provide a national estimate of the number of all HAIs in hospitals associated with medical devices. At the federal level, three HHS agencies, AHRQ, CDC, and CMS, specifically collect or have collected HAI-related data in databases maintained by separate programs, such as CDC's National Healthcare Safety Network (NHSN) program and CMS's Medicare Patient Safety Monitoring System (MPSMS). However, limitations in the scope and collection methods for these databases preclude them from developing a national estimate of HAIs in hospitals associated with medical devices. For example, CDC's NHSN data are not drawn from a representative sample of hospitals nationwide. Similarly, the infection rates included in the MPSMS are based on the experiences of a representative sample of Medicare fee-for-service beneficiaries and are not representative of the experiences of other Medicare or non-Medicare patients. Also, because the HAI-related information in two of these federal databases is gleaned from patient discharge and other medical records, the quality of the data is dependent on the accuracy with which the information was documented. Finally, although a Consumers Union summary report indicates that nearly half of the states mandate public reporting of hospital HAI rates, a number of factors limit the generalizability and usefulness of the state-reported rates.

Improper patient examination and treatment practices by health care professionals, such as the improper insertion of urinary catheters, are the most significant factor affecting the occurrence of HAIs in hospitals associated with medical devices, according to most medical experts we interviewed. Certain in-hospital sterilization techniques and improper handling of sterilized medical devices were also commonly identified as significant causes of such infections, as was the inherent risk of using medical devices, which can introduce bacteria into the body. Our review of medical literature corroborated many of the risk factors cited by the experts and identified additional factors. For example, patient characteristics such as old age, diabetes, or compromised immune systems were frequently cited in the literature as risk factors. In terms of preventing HAIs, improved hygiene, such as appropriate hand-washing, and the use of barrier precautions, such as caps and gloves, were commonly identified strategies.

In commenting on a draft of this chapter, HHS suggested that the chapter would be enhanced by providing a more detailed discussion of HAIs caused by reusable medical devices but acknowledged the difficulties in doing so. HHS also provided technical comments, which we incorporated as appropriate. HHS's comments are reprinted in the enclosure.

BACKGROUND

Within HHS, three agencies currently collect or have collected data on HAIs in hospitals associated with medical devices in databases maintained by separate programs: AHRQ's Healthcare Cost and Utilization Project (HCUP), CDC's NHSN, and CMS's MPSMS.[6] In addition, FDA's Manufacturer and User Facility Device Experience Database (MAUDE) collects reports of deaths or serious injuries related to the use of medical devices, a small number of which may involve HAIs. In addition to the data collection efforts of these federal agencies, nearly half of the states require public reporting of HAI rates.

Among the federal agencies, CDC's NHSN collects information from hospitals that voluntarily report data on five HAIs associated with medical devices: central-line-associated bloodstream infections (CLABSI), ventilator-associated pneumonia (YAP), catheter-related UTIs, SSIs, and postprocedure pneumonia.[7] In its 2006 annual report, NHSN calculated national rates for three of these HAIs—CLABSI, VAP, and catheter-related UTI—and reported the rates by hospital unit, including various types of intensive care units (e.g., burn, surgical, medical).[8] For example, NHSN reported a rate of 2.9 CLABSIs per 1,000 central line days in medical intensive care units.[9] CMS's MPSMS includes information on the rates of HAIs in hospitals associated with three medical devices, including catheter-related UTIs, catheter-related bloodstream infections, and VAP. To calculate these rates, a CMS contractor extracted information from the medical records of a representative sample of certain fee-for-service Medicare beneficiaries. AHRQ's HCUP database collects discharge data from all the community hospitals in 39 participating states. The states voluntarily report these data, which include information on the number of infections associated with certain medical devices, including CLABSI and catheter-associated UTI.[10] Collected data are categorized either as the principal condition or complication a patient had during his or her hospitalization or as one of several conditions or complications. Finally, FDA's MAUDE includes reported incidents of serious injuries and deaths that medical devices have or may have caused or contributed to, which manufacturers, importers, and user facilities are required to report to FDA.[11] MAUDE also includes reports of adverse events voluntarily submitted to FDA.[12]

AVAILABLE FEDERAL AND STATE DATA DO NOT PROVIDE A NATIONAL ESTIMATE OF HAIs IN HOSPITALS ASSOCIATED WITH MEDICAL DEVICES

Although multiple federal agencies and states collect data on HAIs in hospitals, limitations in the scope of the information they collect in their databases or their collection methods have precluded the development of national estimates of all HAIs in hospitals associated with medical devices. Among the federal data sources, CDC's NHSN database provides the most clinically detailed information about HAIs in hospitals, and its procedures for identifying patients with these HAIs draw on the wider range of clinical information available while patients are still in the hospital, as opposed to retrospective reviews of patient medical records after discharge. However, the utility of its data in developing a nationwide estimate has been limited for at least two reasons, specifically its limited scope and its use of a nonrepresentative sample. For example, the NHSN does not collect information on all HAIs in hospitals associated with medical devices; however, in its 2006 annual report, it calculated national rates by hospital unit for three such HAIs—CLABSI, VAP, and catheter-related UTI.[13] In addition, the sample of hospitals used in the 2006 annual report was not necessarily representative of hospitals nationwide, as a random sample would be. The sample included 211 hospitals, which voluntarily submitted data to NHSN. Further, hospitals that reported to NHSN may vary in the scope of their data collection efforts. For example, hospitals can collect data on different infections and monitor HAIs in different units within their hospitals.[14,15]

In addition, limitations in the scope and collection methods for CMS's MPSMS and AHRQ's HCUP databases have precluded the use of their data in developing a national estimate of HAIs in hospitals associated with medical devices. For example, in 2006 MPSMS reported rates of infection for three HAIs in hospitals: 5.35 percent of reviewed medical charts showed evidence of catheter-related UTIs, 2.80 percent showed evidence of catheter-related bloodstream infections, and 9.02 percent showed evidence of VAP infections. However, these rates were based on the experiences of a representative sample of Medicare fee-for-service beneficiaries and did not include other Medicare or non-Medicare patients. Further, because MPSMS data were extracted from medical records, the quality of the data depended on the accuracy with which the patient information was documented, according to a CMS official. Similarly, AHRQ's HCUP database relies on patient discharge records to collect information on the number of HAIs in hospitals associated with certain medical devices, including CLABSI and UTI. For example, data from 2006 showed an estimated 45,879 instances of catheter-associated UTI as one of several complications or conditions patients experienced and an estimated 21,123 instances as the principal complication or reason for admission. However, differences in how hospital staff assign discharge codes may result in inconsistent reporting of HAIs. Further, prior to 2008, the HCUP database did not include information about whether an infection was present on admission. As a result, the number of HAIs in the hospital could have been overstated in previous years as it may have included patients who were infected prior to their hospital stay, according to an AHRQ official. Finally, although a small portion of the incidents reported to FDA's MAUDE database may involve HAIs in hospitals, the principal purpose of the database is to identify devices whose safety and effectiveness warrant closer scrutiny and not to determine the frequency of HAIs in hospitals.

Over 20 states mandate public reporting of hospital HAI rates, according to Consumers Union, and variation exists in the types of data they require hospitals to report.[16] For example, Missouri requires hospitals to report data on CLABSI, SSI, and VAP, while as of July 2008, Washington requires hospitals to collect data only on CLABSI. Because of the variation among state reporting requirements, data from individual states cannot be generalized, thereby limiting the usefulness of state data in determining a national estimate of HAIs in hospitals associated with medical devices.

PATIENT EXAMINATION AND TREATMENT PRACTICES CITED AS THE MOST SIGNIFICANT FACTOR AFFECTING THE OCCURRENCE OF HAIs IN HOSPITALS

The most significant factor affecting the occurrence of multiple types of HAIs in hospitals from among possible causes listed in the mandate is health care professionals' improper patient examination and treatment practices, according to the experts we interviewed. All 11 experts we interviewed identified health care professionals' improper patient examination and treatment practices as a factor, with 7 of the 11 medical experts identifying it as one of the most significant factors affecting the occurrence of HAIs in hospitals associated with medical devices. As a specific example of such practices, experts cited the improper insertion and maintenance of medical devices such as urinary catheters and central lines. In addition, about half of the medical experts identified certain in-hospital sterilization processes and improper handling of sterilized devices as potential causes of such infections. Specifically, the experts cited the inadequate preparation of a device for sterilization and the improper storage of sterile devices, which may result in their contamination, as examples of potential causes. Although the use of reprocessed single-use devices is on the list of potential causes included in the mandate, none of the experts we interviewed cited the use of reprocessed single-use devices as a factor contributing to HAIs in hospitals.[17] Beyond the list of potential causes included in the mandate, the medical experts we interviewed referred to other risk factors for developing HAIs in hospitals. For example, 8 of the 11 experts identified the intrinsic risk of using medical devices, including the inability to completely disinfect the area where a device is inserted, as a factor affecting the occurrence of HAIs in hospitals.

Our literature review largely corroborated many of the risk factors cited by the experts and identified additional risk factors. For example, similar to the examples cited above, a number of articles identified health care professionals' improper patient examination and treatment practices and handling of sterilized medical devices as causes of HAIs in hospitals. In addition, half of the articles we reviewed referred to the inherent risk of using medical devices, which can introduce bacteria into the body. The increased risk of infection based on patient characteristics such as old age, diabetes, or compromised immune systems was also cited in more than one-third of the reviewed articles. Other risk factors cited in articles were specific to certain HAIs in hospitals. For example, risk factors specific to CLABSI included the design of the device, such as the materials a catheter is made from and the location on a patient's body where a catheter is inserted, and risk factors specific to VAP included the prolonged duration of mechanical ventilation.

The medical experts and literature highlighted a variety of strategies to prevent the occurrence of HAIs in hospitals associated with the use of medical devices. Three specific prevention strategies—barrier precautions, such as caps, gowns, and gloves; general hygiene measures, such as appropriate hand washing technique; and the use of antimicrobial-coated or antimicrobial-impregnated devices—were the strategies most frequently identified through our expert interviews and our literature review. Other strategies, such as the use of disinfectants, particularly chlorhexidine gluconate, and reducing unnecessary use of medical devices, were also often identified. Finally, bundling prevention strategies, a practice whereby a number of prevention strategies are implemented together, was identified as an additional strategy to prevent the occurrence of HAIs in hospitals. For example, some of the bundled prevention strategies for VAP cited in the literature included elements related to bed elevation and oral hygiene. Although a number of effective prevention strategies exist, the need for evidence-based research on effective prevention techniques for HAIs in hospitals associated with medical devices was identified by several medical experts and studies. In addition, to help reduce HAIs in hospitals, we previously recommended that HHS identify priorities among effective evidence-based practices for infection control and prevention.[18]

AGENCY COMMENTS AND OUR EVALUATION

In its written comments, HHS stated that the chapter correctly points out the extent of surveillance conducted for single-use, disposable devices, such as urinary catheters. HHS also said a limitation is that the chapter combines single-use devices and reusable devices and that the chapter would be improved by clarifying the distinction between these types of devices. HHS further suggested that the chapter would be enhanced by including a more detailed discussion of HAIs caused by reusable medical devices. However, HHS acknowledged, and we agree, that very little is known about infections caused by reusable devices. Therefore, it was not feasible to discuss reusable devices separately because no data sources focused on or explicitly included these devices. Nevertheless, HHS's point is important in that it highlights another area in which knowledge is lacking about medical devices and HAIs.

HHS also provided technical comments, which we incorporated as appropriate. HHS's comments are reprinted in the enclosure.

Cynthia A. Bascetta
Director, Health Care

Enclosure:
Comments from the Department of Health and Human Services

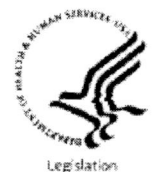

DEPARTMENT OF HEALTH & HUMAN SERVICES OFFICE OF THE SECRETARY

Assistant Secretary for
Legislation
Washington, DC 20201

SEP 1 1 2008

Cynthia Bascetta
Director, Health Care
U.S. Government Accountability Office
441 G Street N.W.
Washington, DC 20548

Dear Ms. Bascetta:

Enclosed are comments on the U.S. Government Accountability Office's (GAO) report entitled: "Health-Care-Associated Infections in Hospitals: Number Associated with Medical Devices Unknown, but Experts Report Provider Practices as a Significant Factor" (GAO 08-1091R).

The Department appreciates the opportunity to review this report before its publication.

Sincerely,

Vincent J. Ventimiglia, Jr.
Assistant Secretary for Legislation

Attachment

COMMENTS OF THE DEPPARTMENT OF HEALTH AND HUMAN SERVICES (HHS) ON THE U.S. GOVERNMENT ACCOUNTABILITY OFFICE'S (GAO) DRAFT REPORT ENTITLED: HEALTH-CARE-ASSOCIATED INFECTIONS IN HOSPITALS" (GAO-08-1091R)

General Comments:

Thank you for the opportunity to review and comment on the GAO report, Health-Care-Associated Infections in Hospitals: Number Associated with Medical Devices Unknown, but Experts Report Provider Practices as a Significant Factor (GAO-08-1091R).

Single Use Versus Reusable Devises

A limitation of this report is that it combines, and hence equates, two very different types of medical devices. The report focuses on infections due to urinary catheters, vascular catheters and ventilators, and is correct in pointing out that there is quite a bit of surveillance conducted for these types of infections. However, the report does not point out that these devices are exclusively single use, disposable devices (in the case of the ventilator, the portions that contact the patient are single use and disposed or between patients) that are left in patients for prolonged periods of time. These devices are very different from other devices such as colonoscopes and surgical instruments that are used for time limited procedures (i.e. they are not left in patients for long periods of time), re-used on multiple patients and are cleaned and disinfected between uses.

We believe the report would be improved by providing more clarity on the different types of devices and discussing each type separately. In addition, the top paragraph on page 2 makes a distinction between "new and used medical devices." We suggest considering instead explaining the difference between disposable, single use devices and reusable devices.

Identification of Infections from Reusable Devices

Much is known about both the numbers of, and risk factors for, infections associated with the disposable devices and we would agree that there are surveillance systems in place that do provide some estimates about how often these occur. However, very little is known about infections caused by the reusable devices. The report highlights the availability of the FDA's MAUDE system, but points out various limitations in the ability of this system to provide information on healthcare associated infections. To these, we would add the important fact that often times healthcare providers do not know when a particular infection is associated with a device and thus would be unable to report this information through a surveillance system.

Special investigative efforts are often needed to associate a HAI with a particular reusable device. Public health officials at state and federal levels have been involved in investigations of outbreaks of healthcare associated infections of unknown etiology which turned out to be caused by contaminated, reusable medical devices. These infections were not reported as device-associated infections, because the etiology was not known until after the investigation occurred. Published investigations have shown that

COMMENTS OF THE DEPPARTMENT OF HEALTH AND HUMAN SERVICES (HHS) ON THE U.S. GOVERNMENT ACCOUNTABILITY OFFICE'S (GAO) DRAFT REPORT ENTITLED: HEALTH-CARE-ASSOCIATED INFECTIONS IN HOSPITALS" (GAO-08-1091R)

these types of infections can be due not only to problems with the handling, cleaning and disinfection of the devices, as is mentioned in the report, but also to defects in the devices themselves.

We believe that the report would be enhanced by including a more detailed discussion of the issues of infections caused by reusable medical devices. It should be noted that investigations of these infections have led to a variety of improvements, not just in the handling, cleaning and disinfection devices in healthcare, but also in device design. The investigation of these types of device-associated infections remains an important part of improving the overall safety of medical devices.

REFERENCES

[1] Consumers Union, "State Hospital Infection Disclosure Laws," available at http://www.stophospitalinfections.org/learn.html (accessed July 30, 2008).
[2] Pub. L. No. 110-85, § 229, 121 Stat. 823, 858.
[3] The act uses the term nosocomial infections instead of HAIs. However, for consistency with our previous work, we use the term HAIs in hospitals. See GAO, *Health-Care-Associated Infections in Hospitals: Leadership Needed from HHS to Prioritize Prevention Practices and Improve Data on These Infections*, GAO-08-283 (Washington, D.C.: Mar. 31, 2008).
[4] Consumers Union, "State Hospital Infection Disclosure Laws," available at http://www.stophospitalinfections.org/learn.html (accessed July 30, 2008).
[5] The Food and Drug Administration Amendments Act of 2007 included the following possible causes: reprocessed single-use devices, handling of sterilized medical devices, in-hospital sterilization of medical devices, health care professionals' practices for patient examination and treatment, hospital-based policies and procedures for infection control and prevention, hospital-based practices for handling of medical waste, and other causes.
[6] For additional information regarding these three databases and their limitations, see GAO-08-283. According to a CMS official, data on HAIs in hospitals associated with medical devices were collected from 2002 through 2007.

[7] Hospitals submit data to the NHSN database using a uniform set of definitions.
[8] According to a CDC official, the agency will update these HAI rates in NHSN's 2007 annual report, which the agency plans to publish at the end of 2008, based on data submitted by 621 hospitals. The increased participation is largely due to recent state mandates that require hospitals to report HAI data to NHSN. For example, although hospitals may continue to join NHSN voluntarily, 89 percent of the facilities that joined NHSN in 2007 and 2008 were in states that required participation through a mandate.
[9] Jonathan R. Edwards et al., "National Healthcare Safety Network (NHSN) Report, Data Summary for 2006, issued June 2007," *American Journal of Infection Control*, vol. 35, 290-301 (2007). The rate of 2.9 CLABSIs per 1,000 central line days was calculated by dividing the aggregate number of reported instances of CLABSI (489) by the total number of days central lines were used (170,719) for all hospitals reporting such data, and multiplying this number by 1,000.
[10] HCUP encompasses a set of related databases, one of which is the Nationwide Inpatient Sample (NIS). NIS contains data from 5 million to 8 million hospital stays from about 1,000 hospitals. According to an AHRQ official, NIS approximates a 20-percent stratified sample of U.S. community hospitals drawn from the participating states, which represent 90 percent of hospital discharges across the United States.
[11] Manufacturers and importers are also required to report device malfunctions to FDA.
[12] Medical device user facilities, manufacturers, importers, and distributors must all maintain records of adverse events.
[13] Edwards et al., "National Healthcare Safety Network (NHSN) Report, Data Summary for 2006, issued June 2007." NHSN reports national rates for other HAIs, including SSI and postprocedure pneumonia. However, SSI and postprocedure pneumonia rates were not calculated for the 2006 annual report due to insufficient data, but will be reported in NHSN's 2007 annual report, according to a CDC official.
[14] Despite these limitations, data from the National Nosocomial Infections Surveillance System—the predecessor to NHSN—were used, along with data from CDC's National Hospital Discharge Survey and the American Hospital Association Survey, to calculate the 2002 nationwide estimate of 1.7 million HAIs in hospitals. CDC officials estimated that over half of these infections were associated with the use of certain medical devices. CDC has no specific plans to update this number using a comparable methodology; however, the

agency is exploring the feasibility of developing a national estimate of HAIs in the future using an alternative methodology that has been successful in other countries, according to a CDC official.

[15] Despite this flexibility, voluntary participation in NHSN involves fulfilling a number of requirements, including submitting a monthly reporting plan, adhering to the NHSN reporting protocol, and using NHSN surveillance methods.

[16] Consumers Union, "State Hospital Infection Disclosure Laws," available at http://www.stophospitalinfections.org/learn.html (accessed July 30, 2008).

[17] Further, one of our recent reports found that available data, while limited, did not indicate that reprocessed single-use medical devices present elevated health risks to patients. See *Reprocessed Single-Use Medical Devices: FDA Oversight Has Increased, and Available Information Does Not Indicate That Use Presents an Elevated Health Risk*, GAO-08-147 (Washington, D.C.: Jan. 31, 2008).

[18] GAO-08-283, 41.

INDEX

A

abdominal cramps, 27
abnormalities, 132
academic, 196, 257, 283, 303, 339
ACC, 32
access, 26, 45, 47, 91, 185, 207, 220, 239, 281, 322, 327, 338, 339
accessibility, 47
accidental, 168
accountability, 193, 221
accounting, 20
accreditation, 146, 240, 250, 251, 252, 280, 281, 285, 337
accuracy, 207, 263, 309, 310, 327, 338, 343, 346
achievement, 41
acid, 11, 35, 123, 223
Acinetobacter, 19, 143, 158, 174, 175, 177, 209, 210, 212, 213, 216, 223, 225
acne, 55
acquired immunity, 58
acquired immunodeficiency syndrome, 154, 212
acute, 1, 2, 9, 19, 20, 27, 33, 35, 37, 38, 43, 45, 48, 69, 80, 92, 93, 94, 95, 96, 98, 100, 105, 106, 110, 115, 118, 120, 122, 126, 130, 132, 134, 136, 144, 147, 150, 151, 156, 157, 159, 160, 161, 168, 169, 171, 178, 187, 191, 192, 196, 206, 211, 216, 225, 239, 267, 298, 316
acute lymphoblastic leukemia, 187
acute myeloid leukemia, 187
adaptation, 38
adenovirus, 14, 34, 36, 61, 77, 88, 131, 178, 184, 228, 230
adenoviruses, 33, 40
adjustment, 49, 304, 312
administration, 26, 27, 43, 69, 74, 91, 149, 258, 261, 306, 307
administrative, 3, 4, 5, 20, 21, 42, 57, 64, 69, 81, 248, 295, 296, 308, 311, 312
administrators, 3, 8, 42, 81, 84, 303, 322
adolescents, 69, 212
adult, 15, 31, 33, 69, 84, 129, 146, 153, 158, 159, 175, 177, 189, 194, 215, 216, 218, 230, 292, 297, 314, 325
adult learning, 84
adult population, 218
adults, 24, 37, 40, 69, 116, 119, 131, 175, 181, 217
adverse event, 22, 40, 76, 124, 136, 166, 233, 240, 244, 258, 259, 271, 287, 299, 302, 308, 345, 352
advisory body, 238, 242, 283
advisory committees, 297, 302, 303
advocacy, 343
aerosol, 3, 13, 15, 16, 17, 25, 30, 58, 59, 87, 97, 120, 126, 129, 130, 132, 133, 134, 135, 138, 160, 173

aerosols, 15, 16, 29, 30, 59, 66, 90, 135, 138, 142, 158, 175
aetiology, 168
afebrile, 74
Africa, 26
agar, 299
age, 11, 23, 25, 31, 35, 60, 63, 69, 104, 105, 110, 111, 155, 189, 344, 347
agent, 2, 5, 10, 11, 12, 13, 15, 16, 19, 20, 21, 23, 28, 54, 58, 60, 61, 62, 71, 78, 87, 89, 92, 98, 101, 102, 115, 118, 126, 143, 149, 162, 165, 167, 173, 211
aggregation, 49
aid, 158, 338
AIDS, 218
air, 6, 14, 15, 16, 32, 57, 64, 67, 73, 77, 80, 90, 96, 97, 99, 100, 136, 139, 142, 143, 145, 147, 148, 149, 158, 175, 226, 280
air embolism, 280
air quality, 80
airborne particles, 14
airways, 52
alcohol, 20, 28, 51, 85, 88, 102, 103, 108, 109, 133, 144, 172, 222, 242, 253, 317
alcoholism, 38
alcohols, 86
algorithm, 286
allergic rhinitis, 74
allergy, 205
allogeneic, 2, 4, 9, 10, 17, 39, 71, 80, 99, 139, 144, 145, 147, 219
allogeneic HSCT, 10, 17, 39, 71, 80, 145
allograft, 190
allografts, 190
alternative, 56, 59, 96, 98, 147, 300, 353
alternatives, 95
ambulance, 64
amebiasis, 227
American Academy of Pediatrics, 212, 214
anaerobe, 162
anaerobic, 19
anaesthesia, 218
angina, 123, 125

animals, 23, 26, 27, 28, 29, 132, 136
anthrax, 17, 21, 22, 214
antibacterial, 68
antibacterial agents, 68
antibiotic, 19, 20, 37, 45, 122, 135, 136, 150, 154, 180, 182, 183, 192, 195, 196, 219, 249, 260, 271, 283, 289, 300, 301, 306, 307, 314, 318, 334, 339
antibiotic ointment, 300
antibiotic resistance, 45, 150, 195, 196, 300
antibiotics, 108, 236, 242, 258, 261, 306, 307, 308, 314, 316, 318, 334, 336, 338
antibody, 69, 134, 145, 190
antigen, 28, 79, 116, 119, 134, 161, 216
antigenicity, 11
antimicrobial therapy, 35, 77, 79, 129, 131, 176
antineoplastic, 11
antineoplastic agents, 11
antiviral, 68, 195, 225
antiviral therapy, 225
anxiety, 76
apparel, 53
appendix, 264, 269, 296, 317, 318, 319
application, 4, 19, 20, 39, 63, 72, 76, 84, 128, 146, 171, 218, 224, 259, 287
Arkansas, 336
ARS, 2, 9, 14, 17, 106, 120, 130
arterial blood gas, 47
artery, 237, 262, 304, 305
arthritis, 187
arthroplasty, 262
ascites, 132
aseptic, 36, 74, 75, 90
ash, 118
aspergillosis, 99, 161, 162, 177, 220
Aspergillus terreus, 80, 220
aspirate, 132, 134
aspiration, 182
aspiration pneumonia, 182
assessment, 42, 43, 45, 48, 50, 115, 134, 162, 168, 180, 181, 196, 256, 272, 281, 283, 289, 295, 328
assignment, 8, 16, 50, 82

Index 357

assumptions, 234, 241, 256, 266
asthma, 74
asymptomatic, 10, 11, 36, 63, 111, 153, 299
Atlantic, 329
atmosphere, 34
attachment, 55
attacks, 2, 43
attitudes, 199, 202
atypical, 24, 115, 117, 131, 169
atypical pneumonia, 24, 117
auditing, 239, 296, 343
authority, 82, 146, 281
autologous bone, 206
autologous bone marrow transplant, 206
autopsy, 24, 30, 168
availability, 26, 45, 46, 77, 82, 149, 234, 241, 256, 265, 314, 320
avian influenza, 16, 58, 95, 112, 130, 142, 163
Avian influenza, 2, 103
awareness, 23, 42, 44, 317

B

B19 infection, 219
babesiosis, 41, 190
babies, 32
bacilli, 6, 20, 35, 51, 53, 123, 136, 143, 147, 154, 164, 183
bacillus, 19, 51
Bacillus, 86, 161, 162, 223
bacteremia, 48, 154, 164, 222, 231
bacteria, 10, 11, 13, 20, 31, 33, 34, 45, 48, 134, 135, 136, 142, 146, 177, 180, 183, 188, 195, 221, 222, 223, 224, 236, 289, 299, 300, 336, 342, 344, 347
bacterial, vii, 13, 31, 39, 75, 105, 114, 117, 118, 125, 136, 149, 154, 159, 162, 178, 188, 189, 191, 196, 218, 222, 285, 289, 334
bacterial contamination, 188, 218
bacterial infection, 39, 118, 125
bacterial strains, 334
bacterium, 136, 236

barrier, 3, 29, 32, 46, 52, 53, 71, 80, 126, 129, 134, 136, 198, 199, 205, 218, 306, 307, 344, 347
barriers, 38, 52, 64, 147, 148, 205
behavior, 14, 42, 47, 198, 202, 222, 256
behavioral change, 249, 270
Beijing, 169
benchmark, 237, 257
benchmarking, 180
benchmarks, 295
benefits, 46, 196, 215, 265, 270, 326
benign, 104
bioaerosols, 3, 143
bioassays, 133
biocontainment, 173
biological weapons, 166
biopsies, 132
biopsy, 132, 168
biosafety, 136
bioterrorism, 4, 18, 21, 22, 26, 45, 126
bioweapon, 30, 134
birth, 68, 84
birth weight, 68
birthweight, 32
bleeding, 28, 134
blepharitis, 136
blood, 12, 13, 24, 28, 29, 37, 46, 47, 52, 53, 54, 55, 58, 59, 65, 66, 67, 72, 85, 86, 87, 89, 93, 101, 102, 111, 122, 126, 128, 129, 132, 134, 136, 137, 144, 149, 156, 168, 172, 185, 188, 197, 199, 201, 205, 206, 208, 222, 223, 230, 236, 280, 288, 307, 342
blood and body fluids, 46, 52, 59, 126, 134
blood clot, 307
blood glucose, 156, 307
blood group, 28, 172
blood pressure, 66, 86, 93
blood safety, 24
blood sampling, 156
blood stream, 222
blood supply, 24
blood transfusion, 24, 122, 168
blood vessels, 280

bloodstream, 32, 37, 42, 44, 152, 155, 174, 175, 176, 177, 185, 194, 200, 203, 220, 235, 236, 261, 271, 293, 298, 310, 340, 342, 344, 346
body fluid, 12, 13, 29, 46, 52, 53, 54, 55, 56, 58, 59, 62, 65, 66, 72, 85, 86, 87, 89, 101, 126, 129, 134, 136, 137, 149, 199, 201, 202
bone marrow, 144, 153, 162, 187, 188, 221
bone marrow transplant, 153, 162, 187, 188, 221
botulinum, 22, 104
botulism, 21
bovine, 23, 168
bovine spongiform encephalopathy, 23, 168
breaches, 26, 74, 75
bronchiolitis, 62, 131, 211
bronchopulmonary dysplasia, 231
bronchoscopy, 30, 55, 58, 59, 87, 157
brucellosis, 228
bundling, 347
Burkholderia, 18, 36, 39, 143, 157, 185, 188, 189
burn, 18, 31, 32, 121, 154, 162, 175, 176, 177, 193, 213, 216, 264, 266, 344
burns, 32, 177
bypass, 11, 237, 260, 262, 264, 304, 305

C

campaigns, 69, 281, 317, 330, 331, 332
Canada, 19, 23, 151, 161, 192, 212, 222
cancer, 145, 187, 216
candida, 31
Candida, 31, 174, 175, 176, 204
candidates, 69
capacity, 77, 82
capillary, 156
caps, 32, 344, 347
cardiac surgery, 153, 262, 307
cardiology, 50
cardiopulmonary, 13, 16, 157
cardiopulmonary resuscitation, 13, 16, 157

cardiovascular system, 262, 287
caregiver, 12, 44, 59, 142
caregivers, 111, 115, 120, 125
carrier, 153, 154
cataract, 271
cataract surgery, 271
category a, 5, 101
catheter, 32, 37, 42, 75, 91, 124, 155, 182, 185, 194, 196, 197, 200, 203, 220, 222, 240, 245, 249, 253, 257, 258, 260, 261, 262, 286, 298, 301, 306, 307, 339, 344, 345, 346, 347
catheterization, 249, 283
catheters, 11, 31, 32, 35, 60, 73, 75, 87, 155, 194, 222, 237, 259, 262, 286, 288, 343, 347, 348
cattle, 23
causality, 147
CD8+, 167
CDR, 212
cell, 4, 6, 9, 27, 39, 99, 116, 139, 144, 145, 147, 151, 219, 225
cell culture, 27
Census, 329
Census Bureau, 329
Centers for Disease Control, 4, 6, 160, 162, 190, 234, 235, 236, 271, 293, 294, 342
central nervous system, 287
cephalosporin, 35, 177
cerebrospinal fluid, 75, 136, 196
certification, 192, 240, 250, 251
Chagas disease, 41
chancre, 104
changing environment, 318
chemicals, 52, 279
chemotherapeutic agent, 52
chemotherapy, 35, 39, 75, 144, 145, 206
child care centers, 33, 179
childhood, 39, 69, 70, 187, 216
children, 24, 26, 32, 33, 37, 40, 60, 62, 63, 69, 70, 104, 106, 107, 109, 110, 114, 116, 117, 118, 119, 121, 123, 126, 129, 131, 153, 169, 175, 176, 177, 178, 179,

189, 195, 207, 211, 212, 216, 219, 227, 229
China, 24
Chlamydia trachomatis, 104
chlorine, 28, 65
Cholera, 104, 108
choriomeningitis, 41, 113, 190
chronic disease, 35, 116, 145, 146
chronic diseases, 35, 145
chronic illness, 38
Cincinnati, 153
ciprofloxacin, 103, 133
circulation, 142
civilian, 22, 166
classes, 11, 19, 20, 65, 146
classification, 16, 147
classroom, 158
cleaning, 13, 20, 25, 28, 33, 35, 53, 61, 64, 65, 66, 67, 80, 87, 89, 90, 94, 108, 109, 126, 137, 140, 147, 172, 209, 210, 212, 213, 223, 271, 299, 300, 314, 317, 318, 333, 337, 339
clients, 185
clinical diagnosis, 61, 62
clinical judgment, 131
clinical presentation, 7, 62, 78, 96, 228
clinical symptoms, 145
clinical syndrome, 4, 62, 71, 78, 123, 128
clinical trial, 188
clinical trials, 188
clinician, 131, 195, 249
clinics, 33, 35, 37, 38, 43, 62, 63, 69, 73, 83, 88, 90, 105, 142, 148
clonality, 195
clusters, 3, 18, 36, 48, 49
coccidioidomycosis, 228
Cochrane, 178
codes, 259, 261, 263, 265, 288, 308, 311, 329, 339, 346
coding, 263, 269, 288
codon, 168
cohort, 92, 94, 96, 112, 143, 154, 211
colds, 158
colitis, 103, 206
colon, 260, 262, 264

colonization, 5, 11, 31, 32, 33, 35, 54, 66, 68, 79, 91, 92, 115, 117, 118, 143, 146, 152, 154, 175, 177, 182, 188, 189, 206, 210, 212, 214, 219, 222, 223, 314, 319, 320, 339
colonoscopy, 156
Colorado, 103, 105, 190, 303, 305, 306, 308, 309, 338
Colorado tick fever, 103, 105
Committee on Oversight and Government Reform, 236, 294
communication, 20, 43, 44, 47, 146, 149, 264, 303, 305, 306, 308
communication systems, 20
communities, 88
community, 2, 20, 25, 27, 30, 32, 33, 34, 35, 36, 44, 62, 70, 82, 85, 88, 105, 115, 131, 146, 153, 154, 170, 179, 182, 195, 198, 203, 210, 222, 239, 262, 279, 285, 287, 299, 300, 307, 311, 336, 339, 344, 352
comorbidity, 280
compatibility, 235, 241, 264, 269
competency, 50, 83
complexity, 42, 43, 81, 250, 301
compliance, 159, 192, 198, 199, 201, 202, 203, 221, 224, 234, 235, 237, 238, 241, 242, 243, 244, 250, 251, 252, 254, 255, 265, 270, 284, 292, 297, 299, 302, 304, 306, 317, 318, 320, 321, 322, 323, 330, 331, 332, 333
complications, 32, 175, 193, 271, 280, 345, 346
components, 2, 3, 4, 7, 10, 39, 42, 57, 68, 146, 147, 148, 234, 240, 243, 250, 251, 299, 307, 323
composition, 2, 44, 82, 194
computer software, 308
computer systems, 312
concrete, 270
confidence, 147
confidentiality, 301, 326, 338
conflict, 149
confounding variables, 8
congestive heart failure, 31

conjunctiva, 29, 206
conjunctivitis, 34, 105, 110, 124, 136, 181, 228
Connecticut, 285, 303, 305, 306, 308, 338, 339
connective tissue, 280
consciousness, 35
consensus, 32, 40, 81, 182, 191, 246, 269, 300, 338
consolidation, 45
construction, 9, 17, 32, 42, 43, 67, 77, 80, 82, 96, 100, 139, 142, 146, 220
consultants, 45
consulting, 184
consumers, 303, 326, 327, 338
consumption, 23, 317, 330
contact time, 65
contaminated food, 17, 27, 28
contamination, 5, 19, 27, 28, 36, 51, 52, 53, 54, 59, 61, 64, 66, 74, 75, 76, 85, 86, 87, 89, 90, 148, 156, 157, 160, 161, 170, 172, 188, 204, 205, 209, 213, 214, 218, 219, 220, 221, 223, 224, 229, 230, 347
controlled trials, 8
cooling, 143
coordination, 240, 250
COP, 235, 237, 238, 240, 243, 251, 252, 268, 269, 272, 283, 285, 289, 336
corneal transplant, 23, 106, 167, 229, 231
coronary artery bypass graft, 237, 262, 304
coronary bypass surgery, 264
coronavirus, 2, 9, 14, 24, 157, 160, 168, 169
correlation, 8
corticosteroids, 11, 145
cost effectiveness, 32
cost saving, 324
cost-benefit analysis, 324
costs, 19, 34, 62, 181, 215, 237, 240, 268, 292, 294, 300, 314, 324, 325, 326, 337, 340
cough, 13, 62, 73, 74, 94, 126, 129, 131, 132, 134, 136, 138, 149

coughing, 54, 73, 74, 88, 94, 138, 142, 143, 148, 159
coverage, 54
covering, 73, 147, 148, 167, 265
CPR, 158
Creutzfeldt-Jakob disease, 22, 106, 167, 168
critical care units, 260
critically ill, 196, 198, 225
cryptococcosis, 229
CSF, 75, 132, 136
culture, 2, 4, 22, 42, 46, 48, 78, 79, 127, 132, 134, 135, 148, 181, 196, 197, 219, 249, 299, 314
culture media, 299, 314
cystic fibrosis, 37, 39, 51, 63, 151, 156, 157, 185, 188, 189, 212
cytomegalovirus, 40
cytotoxic, 145
Cytotoxic, 167

D

daily living, 35, 37, 60
data analysis, 304
data collection, 37, 234, 239, 241, 252, 256, 257, 262, 263, 264, 266, 269, 291, 297, 302, 303, 304, 308, 309, 312, 313, 326, 327, 328, 337, 339, 344, 345
data set, 180, 259, 310, 342
database, 256, 257, 258, 259, 260, 261, 263, 265, 266, 285, 288, 340, 344, 345, 346, 352
death, 23, 27, 234, 236, 250, 252, 255, 267, 268, 284, 294, 342
deaths, 162, 179, 259, 266, 344, 345
debridement, 17
decision making, 150
decisions, 30, 42, 45, 46, 51, 60, 82, 88, 92, 94, 95, 302, 313, 325
decolonization, 5, 20, 68, 79, 313, 318, 334, 335
decontamination, 32, 40, 85, 103, 109, 133, 222, 253
decontamination procedures, 222

Index

decubitus ulcer, 118
defects, 13, 39
defense, 145
defense mechanisms, 145
defenses, 11
deficiency, 11, 145
Deficit Reduction Act, 235, 237
deficits, 146
definition, 3
dehydration, 27
delivery, 1, 6, 7, 8, 9, 35, 38, 49, 85, 90, 99, 125, 135, 144, 179, 191, 283
Delphi, 43, 191
demand, 325
demographics, 161, 259
demography, 192
dengue, 103
density, 14, 194
Department of Agriculture, 329
Department of Defense, 22
Department of Health and Human Services, 142, 232, 234, 235, 237, 292, 293, 294, 342
depression, 76, 218
dermatitis, 55, 85
dermatology, 183, 225
desiccation, 14
destruction, 145
detection, 24, 25, 27, 28, 34, 45, 79, 83, 134, 135, 161, 170, 173, 195, 196, 219, 271, 298, 328
detergents, 64, 67
developed countries, 29
developmental delay, 60
diabetes, 11, 145, 154, 344, 347
diabetes mellitus, 145
diabetic patients, 154, 156
dialysis, 35, 37, 44, 64, 142, 144, 183, 194, 215, 285, 300
diarrhea, 19, 27, 61, 62, 101, 129, 132, 133, 156, 162, 163, 206, 209, 210, 223
diarrhoea, 210
dietary, 83, 144
diphtheria, 78
diplopia, 133

direct observation, 234, 241, 251, 301
disability, 250
disabled, 33, 34, 146, 280
discharges, 76, 258, 267, 352
disclosure, 286, 301, 309
diseases, 23, 26, 31, 38, 57, 69, 70, 76, 78, 79, 97, 100, 126, 183, 253, 272
disinfection, 13, 20, 28, 51, 64, 65, 66, 89, 90, 94, 106, 108, 109, 120, 137, 168, 172, 212, 213, 223, 246, 287, 292, 297, 337
diskitis, 204
disorder, 22
dispersion, 66, 90, 142
disposables, 156
disseminate, 259, 295
distribution, 45, 157
diversity, 296
dizziness, 133
DNA, 27, 28, 156, 162, 226, 229, 300
dogs, 26
donor, 40, 144, 167, 188, 190
doors, 103, 113, 139
draft, 149, 241, 242, 246, 269, 270, 281, 292, 328, 344
drainage, 64, 76, 88, 92, 97, 102, 103, 104, 105, 107, 118, 121, 123, 124, 125, 126, 132
dressings, 22, 64, 85, 115, 167
drinking, 67
drug resistance, 164
drug use, 38
drug-resistant, 164, 175, 266
drugs, 11, 35, 236, 279, 292, 294, 336
drying, 51, 222
duplication, 268
dura mater, 23, 167
durability, 86
duration, 5, 23, 39, 78, 79, 91, 107, 108, 109, 110, 111, 112, 116, 119, 121, 125, 127, 143, 158, 334, 347
dust, 17, 32, 64, 67, 80, 100, 140, 142, 146, 147, 148
duties, 86, 220
dysarthria, 133

dysphagia, 35, 133
dysplasia, 231
dyspnea, 132, 134, 136

E

eating, 34, 67
Ebola, 28, 29, 106, 126, 129, 172, 173
Economic Research Service, 329
eczema, 22, 136
edema, 132
effusion, 132
elderly, 27, 34, 109, 152, 171, 179, 181, 182, 194, 215, 280
elective surgery, 259
electrodes, 23
electroencephalogram, 23
electronic surveillance, 334
ELISA, 132
elk, 23
emergency departments, 36, 62, 73, 77, 83, 88, 138, 148
emphysema, 145
employees, 57, 143, 153, 201, 208, 226, 253, 256
employers, 57, 68, 303
employment, 57
encephalitis, 103, 124
encephalomyelitis, 103, 107
encephalopathy, 23, 123, 168
endoscope, 156
endoscopy, 74
endotracheal intubation, 13, 16, 25, 30, 59, 87, 137
endotracheal suctioning, 55
England, 19, 163
enrollment, 258, 309, 312
enterococci, 7, 31, 143, 152, 153, 156, 157, 175, 176, 180, 197, 203, 206, 209, 210, 211, 216, 219, 220, 224, 225, 236, 261, 271
enterocolitis, 115, 230
enterovirus, 105, 196, 228
enteroviruses, 46

environment, 10, 16, 17, 20, 21, 28, 38, 39, 50, 52, 54, 67, 72, 76, 78, 87, 89, 93, 96, 99, 103, 127, 137, 138, 147, 148, 149, 158, 175, 184, 209, 210, 213, 272, 331, 332, 333
environmental contamination, 19, 54, 61, 64, 76, 160, 161, 170, 213, 223, 224
environmental control, 2, 80
environmental factors, 14, 173, 196
environmental protection, 39
Environmental Protection Agency, 214
EPA, 64, 89, 140, 224
epidemic, 9, 23, 36, 127, 153, 160, 162, 163, 167, 171, 172, 175, 184, 185, 186, 208, 209, 210, 222, 228, 229
epidemics, 33, 174
epidemiologic studies, 32, 81, 246, 282
epidemiology, 10, 17, 21, 28, 30, 32, 44, 49, 61, 85, 112, 134, 144, 145, 150, 154, 158, 162, 177, 182, 187, 188, 191, 193, 201, 206, 209, 220, 228, 230, 231, 283, 304, 328
epiglottitis, 107
Epstein-Barr virus, 107
equipment, 4, 5, 7, 13, 20, 21, 32, 36, 37, 39, 42, 46, 47, 50, 52, 53, 55, 56, 57, 61, 64, 65, 66, 67, 72, 74, 82, 83, 86, 87, 89, 90, 93, 94, 95, 98, 105, 128, 137, 139, 145, 147, 149, 176, 188, 196, 199, 212, 213, 242, 254, 299, 314, 317, 318, 333, 337
erythema multiforme, 125
Escherichia coli, 107, 108, 131, 183, 204
esophagus, 280
estimating, 266
etiologic agent, 71, 107, 131
etiology, 7, 26, 71, 106, 122
etiquette, 73, 74, 138
Europe, 23, 160, 163
evidence-based practices, 348
evolution, 4
exanthem subitum, 119
excision, 32
exclusion, 70
excretion, 229

exercise, 300
experimental condition, 15
experimental design, 8, 147
exposure, 2, 9, 11, 12, 14, 17, 19, 22, 23, 24, 25, 26, 27, 28, 29, 30, 31, 32, 33, 39, 43, 52, 54, 55, 56, 57, 59, 62, 63, 68, 69, 70, 72, 82, 91, 96, 97, 98, 99, 101, 102, 103, 104, 110, 111, 113, 114, 116, 117, 120, 121, 125, 128, 129, 133, 135, 147, 148, 149, 152, 157, 163, 172, 173, 178, 197, 201, 205, 208, 215, 226, 292, 298
exposure, 58, 59, 98, 133
expulsion, 143
eye contact, 56
eyes, 54, 55, 56, 59, 87

F

fabric, 219
failure, 2, 9, 31, 36, 53, 65, 75, 113, 145, 226, 228, 285
falciparum malaria, 230
familial, 23
family, 24, 27, 33, 49, 50, 60, 62, 63, 70, 73, 79, 102, 114, 123, 143, 148, 169, 172, 227, 231, 252, 255
family members, 33, 49, 50, 62, 63, 70, 73, 79, 114, 123, 148, 172, 252, 255
farms, 163
fax, 322
FDA, 6, 24, 52, 55, 207, 235, 238, 239, 259, 281, 287, 342, 344, 345, 346, 352, 353
feces, 109, 128
federal government, 326
federal law, 146
Federal Register, 205, 243
fee, 343, 344, 346
feedback, 42, 47, 49, 50, 83, 145, 149, 203, 221, 222, 292, 297, 317, 321, 322, 323
feeding, 32, 33, 35, 71, 182
feet, 14, 15, 28, 62, 73, 76, 77, 88, 92, 95, 138, 148

fetal, 22
fever, 3, 18, 22, 24, 28, 30, 74, 87, 104, 106, 118, 119, 120, 121, 124, 126, 129, 130, 132, 134, 136, 144, 166, 172, 173
fibrosis, 6, 37, 39, 51, 63, 151, 156, 157, 185, 188, 189, 212
Fibrosis, 10, 39, 40
Filoviridae, 28
filters, 96, 97, 99, 101, 139, 140, 145, 148
filtration, 6, 31, 32, 55, 56, 77, 80, 101, 139, 147, 149, 227
financial resources, 292, 297, 312, 321, 324, 325
financial support, 249
fingerprinting, 156, 229
fixation, 223
flammability, 149
flexibility, 257, 353
flight, 29, 160
float, 44
flora, vii, 2, 10, 11, 35, 75, 144, 153, 162, 176, 189, 204
flow, 32, 80, 139, 142, 145, 147
flow rate, 142, 145
fluid, 29, 53, 54, 55, 72, 75, 91, 101, 124, 126, 129, 132, 134, 135, 136, 149, 196, 199, 201, 202
fluoroquinolones, 19
foams, 51
focusing, 8, 59
food, 16, 17, 27, 28, 133, 135, 172
Food and Drug Administration, 6, 147, 149, 235, 238, 342, 351
Food and Drug Administration (FDA), 238, 342
Ford, 157, 177, 179, 210
Fox, 224
fractures, 280
France, 211
fulfillment, 41
funding, 249, 292, 297, 313, 319
funds, 240, 319, 338
fungal, 2, 17, 31, 39, 67, 80, 99, 142, 162
fungal infection, 2, 80, 99, 162
fungal spores, 67, 80, 142

G

fungi, 9, 11, 17, 39, 99, 147, 148, 220
furniture, 140, 219

gallbladder, 264
gangrene, 105
GAO, 233, 234, 235, 245, 248, 261, 281, 285, 286, 291, 292, 293, 308, 316, 317, 319, 328, 330, 332, 333, 334, 335, 336, 337, 351, 353
gas, 47, 107
gas gangrene, 107
gastric, 11, 35
gastroenteritis, 27, 28, 102, 104, 106, 107, 108, 110, 115, 119, 120, 124, 125, 126, 160, 161, 171
gastrointestinal, 10, 15, 27, 31, 60, 67, 88, 136, 194, 219, 223, 262, 287
gastrointestinal bleeding, 31
gastrointestinal tract, 10, 60, 67, 136, 223
Gastrostomy, 182
gauge, 99, 139, 237, 317
gel, 19, 317
gels, 51
gender, 60
gene, 2, 40, 163, 164, 189
gene therapy, 2, 40, 189
general anesthesia, 224
general surgery, 201
generalizability, 343
generation, 19
genes, 45, 195
Geneva, 136, 281
genotype, 222
Georgia, 162
geriatric, 171, 180, 219
German measles, 110, 120
Germany, 160, 173
gestation, 33
GH, 181, 207
Gibbs, 167, 231
gland, 280
glasses, 56, 67
globulin, 69
gloves, 4, 12, 29, 32, 52, 53, 54, 56, 59, 71, 72, 75, 76, 83, 86, 87, 89, 93, 100, 112, 113, 124, 126, 134, 137, 138, 139, 147, 149, 157, 204, 205, 206, 223, 225, 230, 298, 317, 322, 325, 331, 332, 344, 347
glucose, 13, 156, 307
glutaraldehyde, 223
glycoprotein, 23
goals, 30, 42, 243, 254
goggles, 30, 54, 55, 56, 72, 87, 120, 126, 134, 137, 147, 207
gonadotropin, 23
gonorrhea, 38
Gore, 156
government, 238, 239, 242, 281, 296, 303, 305, 306, 308, 326, 343
Government Accountability Office, v, 233, 291, 341
grafting, 32
grafts, 23, 167, 304
graft-versus-host disease, 9, 39, 188
gram negative, 51, 143
gram-negative bacteria, 31, 116, 188
Gram-positive, 183
grouping, 61, 143
groups, 39, 47, 51, 69, 86, 249, 271, 280, 283, 323, 337, 343
growth, 23, 167
growth hormone, 23, 167
guidance, 1, 4, 10, 21, 35, 38, 46, 59, 66, 99, 102, 112, 113, 115, 142, 146, 149, 169, 207, 238, 241, 242, 251, 252, 269, 282, 308
guidelines, 2, 3, 4, 9, 18, 30, 35, 37, 39, 45, 48, 66, 73, 79, 81, 96, 99, 163, 169, 183, 195, 200, 214, 217, 220, 233, 234, 235, 237, 238, 239, 240, 242, 244, 245, 246, 248, 249, 251, 253, 267, 268, 270, 271, 272, 281, 282, 284, 289, 295, 300, 301, 306, 314, 318, 326, 337

H

H5N1, 112

H7N7, 163
handicapped, 230
handling, 14, 15, 24, 29, 52, 53, 66, 67, 77, 89, 96, 102, 105, 126, 128, 134, 145, 149, 198, 344, 347, 351
hands, 12, 20, 28, 36, 51, 52, 53, 56, 59, 72, 85, 86, 87, 88, 138, 144, 155, 156, 166, 204, 222, 223, 224, 240, 244, 254, 299
hazards, 40, 59, 190, 208, 287
HBV, 6, 12, 38, 52, 58, 68, 74, 208
HBV infection, 68
headache, 24, 132, 133, 134, 135
Health and Human Services, 142, 234, 235, 237, 273, 292, 293, 294, 342, 349
Health and Human Services (HHS), 234, 237, 294
health care professionals, 215, 343, 346, 347, 351
health care system, 35
health care workers, 169, 170, 197, 198, 199, 204, 205, 215, 231, 239, 240, 242, 244, 251, 254, 256, 285, 298, 307, 317, 335
Health care workers, 335
health clinics, 33, 35, 142
health insurance, 280
health services, 33, 43, 146
heart, 31, 190, 259, 280, 336
heart valves, 259
Helicobacter pylori, 110
hematemesis, 132
hematologic, 80
hematology, 39, 74, 210, 225
hematopoietic, 2, 4, 83, 99, 144, 151, 225
hematopoietic stem cell, 4, 99, 144, 151, 225
Hematopoietic stem cell, 144
hematopoietic stem cells, 144
hematopoietic stem-cell transplant, 2
hemodialysis, 31, 36, 69, 110, 183, 216
hemoptysis, 134
hemorrhage, 126, 133
hepatic failure, 31

hepatitis, 2, 12, 36, 38, 40, 44, 67, 68, 69, 74, 101, 110, 131, 152, 155, 156, 183, 184, 190, 194, 206, 208, 215, 222, 224, 225, 229
hepatitis A, 229
hepatitis B, 2, 12, 36, 68, 69, 101, 110, 156, 183, 184, 208, 215, 222, 224
Hepatitis B, 6
hepatitis c, 74
hepatitis C, 2, 40, 44, 155, 156, 190, 194, 206, 224, 225
Hepatitis C virus, 6
herpes, 96, 98, 126, 129, 226, 229
herpes simplex, 129
herpes zoster, 96, 98, 126, 226
herpetic whitlow, 12
heterogeneity, 158
HHS, v, 232, 233, 234, 235, 237, 238, 239, 240, 241, 242, 244, 250, 256, 257, 258, 259, 260, 261, 263, 264, 265, 266, 267, 268, 269, 270, 280, 281, 283, 286, 287, 293, 294, 298, 328, 336, 338, 342, 343, 344, 348, 351
high risk, 25, 26, 29, 31, 51, 65, 69, 70, 74, 78, 86, 87, 130, 136, 168, 187
higher quality, 338
high-risk, 2, 22, 49, 51, 54, 69, 82, 83, 84, 97, 98, 112, 115, 174, 178, 199
high-risk populations, 49, 84
hip, 262, 304, 305
hip arthroplasty, 262
hip replacement, 304
hiring, 312
histology, 24
HIV, 6, 11, 12, 36, 38, 52, 58, 68, 127, 130, 145, 154, 155, 160, 184, 187, 188, 198, 208, 214, 218
HIV infection, 130, 198
HIV/AIDS, 11, 127
Holland, 184
home care services, 94
home-care, 185
homeless, 34, 186
Hong Kong, 24, 25, 158, 201, 212
hormone, 23, 167

hormones, 167
hospice, 7, 145
hospital stays, 280, 292, 294, 352
hospitalization, vii, 110, 116, 218, 237, 269, 299, 345
hospitalizations, 79, 116, 119, 211
hospitalized, 31, 32, 33, 35, 153, 155, 169, 178, 209, 211, 212, 218, 229, 258, 260
host, 9, 10, 11, 23, 39, 125, 129, 143, 144, 145, 188, 190, 209
host tissue, 145
hot water, 67
hotels, 27
House, 236, 294, 342
household, 10, 50, 63, 65, 70, 114, 116, 162, 316
households, 29, 212
housing, 187
HSCT, 6, 9, 10, 17, 39, 70, 71, 80, 83, 87, 99, 139, 144, 145, 147
human, 10, 11, 23, 24, 26, 27, 33, 41, 42, 62, 81, 82, 101, 102, 112, 130, 143, 145, 154, 157, 159, 163, 167, 168, 170, 187, 190, 206, 208, 213, 216, 228, 231
human immunodeficiency virus, 11, 101, 130, 145, 154, 159, 187, 206, 208
human resources, 42, 81
human subjects, 157
humans, 2, 17, 22, 23, 26, 28, 29, 41, 105, 132, 168, 170
humidity, 14
hurricane, 27, 171
hydatidosis, 106
hygiene, 3, 13, 20, 25, 29, 42, 44, 46, 47, 50, 51, 52, 53, 56, 61, 64, 67, 72, 73, 74, 83, 84, 85, 87, 88, 92, 93, 95, 103, 124, 126, 133, 134, 135, 136, 137, 138, 139, 144, 149, 192, 194, 199, 203, 204, 217, 223, 238, 240, 244, 250, 252, 253, 254, 255, 272, 284, 292, 297, 298, 299, 300, 306, 307, 314, 317, 321, 323, 330, 337, 344, 347
hygienic, 66
hypotension, 133
hysterectomy, 262, 305

I

iatrogenic, 217
IBD, 188
ICD, 235, 259, 261, 263, 288
ICU, 6, 17, 31, 32, 51, 87, 145, 154, 177, 191, 203, 283, 293, 294, 305, 310, 316, 324, 325, 339
Idaho, 315, 317, 329, 330, 331, 333, 334, 335
identification, 3, 20, 26, 36, 45, 49, 133, 146, 171, 195, 196, 209, 311, 339
identity, 54
idiopathic, 187
Illinois, 206, 223, 296, 303, 305, 306, 308, 311, 339
imaging, 142
immune function, 35, 219
immune globulin, 98, 113
immune response, 143
immune system, 33, 39, 111, 145, 147, 344, 347
immunity, 33, 34, 58, 69, 98, 208, 219
immunization, 36, 69, 82, 166, 202, 216, 227, 241, 254
immunocompromised, 2, 9, 17, 31, 39, 63, 67, 79, 80, 83, 92, 95, 96, 97, 98, 100, 109, 111, 112, 116, 117, 119, 125, 145, 187, 209, 219
immunodeficiency, 6, 102, 111
immunodeficient, 219, 225
immunofluorescence, 211
immunohistochemical, 173
immunohistochemistry, 134
immunosuppression, 60, 144, 145
immunosuppressive, 11, 39, 145
immunosuppressive drugs, 11
immunosuppressive therapies, 39
impetigo, 37
implants, 11
implementation, 6, 25, 34, 36, 43, 44, 46, 49, 59, 73, 81, 82, 85, 122, 146, 209, 233, 234, 237, 238, 240, 244, 246, 247, 248, 249, 251, 253, 263, 267, 268, 270,

Index 367

272, 282, 291, 293, 295, 297, 302, 312, 313, 320, 321, 322, 324
in vitro, 172
in vivo, 40, 172, 216
inactivation, 172
inactive, 103, 133
incentive, 258, 309, 327
incentives, 47, 286, 327
incidence, 3, 5, 19, 20, 22, 37, 51, 68, 74, 84, 85, 156, 163, 170, 185, 210, 213, 241, 256, 258, 265, 266, 271, 285, 287, 289, 294, 299, 300, 320
inclusion, 42, 336
incompatibility, 281
incubation, 10, 23, 24, 27, 111
incubation period, 10, 23, 24, 27
index case, 27, 29
India, 228
indicators, 96, 99, 259, 288, 301
indices, 75
induction, 13, 149
industrial, 101, 139
industry, 38, 57, 270
inert, 143
infants, 32, 33, 60, 62, 68, 69, 88, 101, 102, 104, 106, 110, 111, 114, 116, 119, 121, 123, 129, 131, 162, 178, 210
Infants, 107, 117, 118, 126
infectious disease, 10, 19, 30, 41, 45, 60, 62, 70, 78, 100, 101, 118, 126, 136, 142, 143, 150, 154, 183, 186, 191, 241, 254, 311, 334
infectious diseases, 41, 45, 60, 62, 70, 78, 150, 154, 183, 186, 191, 241, 254, 311, 334
infectious mononucleosis, 107
infestations, 37
inflammation, 271, 280
inflammatory, 39
inflammatory bowel disease, 39
infliximab, 187
influenza, 9, 11, 14, 15, 16, 17, 18, 26, 33, 34, 37, 39, 43, 46, 48, 49, 50, 58, 60, 62, 68, 69, 70, 74, 77, 85, 88, 95, 103, 112, 130, 131, 142, 144, 151, 152, 160, 163, 178, 181, 195, 202, 211, 215, 219, 221, 240, 242, 245, 251, 254, 284, 306, 307
influenza a, 16, 26, 34, 39, 160
influenza vaccine, 69, 202, 215
information systems, 271, 314, 318
information technology, 323
Information Technology, 286
infrastructure, 34, 41, 182, 191, 294
ingestion, 132
inhalation, 16, 55, 56, 57, 80, 100, 105, 132, 148, 149, 160, 188, 228
initiation, 127, 135, 136, 322
injection, 2, 29, 36, 38, 72, 73, 74, 75, 90, 224
injections, 2, 224
injuries, 58, 134, 175, 196, 208, 259, 280, 344, 345
injury, iv, 31, 58, 59, 133, 143, 176, 205, 243, 284
inmates, 187
inoculation, 29, 104, 136, 158
insertion, 73, 262, 283, 288, 298, 306, 343, 347
inspection, 310
inspections, 310
institutions, 34, 146, 223, 283
instructional materials, 84
instruments, 13, 23, 24, 65, 89, 93, 105, 106, 271
insurance, 280, 310
integration, 46, 234, 235, 241, 264, 294
integrity, 53, 55, 205, 338
intensity, 30, 64, 144
intensive care unit, 7, 32, 33, 54, 83, 151, 152, 153, 154, 155, 161, 164, 174, 175, 177, 178, 193, 194, 196, 197, 200, 203, 204, 206, 207, 210, 211, 212, 213, 216, 222, 223, 224, 225, 228, 229, 231, 249, 253, 257, 264, 266, 292, 293, 294, 297, 300, 314, 315, 316, 344
interaction, 4, 11, 30, 52, 53, 71, 72, 86, 159
interactions, 9, 72, 76, 100
interdisciplinary, 191

interleukin, 187
International Classification of Diseases, 235, 259, 261
Internet, 260, 313
interpretation, 16, 45, 48, 150, 281
interval, 79
intervention, 8, 44, 47, 48, 144, 147, 180, 186, 192, 203, 249, 296
interview, 343
interviews, 343, 347
intestinal tract, 61, 64, 77, 154
intraocular, 271
intraoperative, 208
intravascular, 31, 185, 306
intravenous, 17, 36, 43, 65, 74, 90, 91, 185, 196, 220, 259, 261, 288, 336
intravenous fluids, 17
intrinsic, 11, 347
invasive, 11, 18, 29, 31, 33, 35, 55, 58, 79, 80, 85, 122, 131, 161, 162, 207, 222, 231, 288, 298, 339
investment, 325
irrigation, 97, 143
isoforms, 23
isolation, 2, 3, 4, 5, 6, 7, 13, 16, 17, 18, 32, 50, 53, 54, 55, 58, 60, 77, 83, 115, 127, 128, 142, 143, 149, 150, 159, 162, 167, 177, 182, 184, 197, 199, 207, 209, 214, 218, 221, 226, 228, 232, 242, 245, 322, 337
Israel, 315, 316, 317, 320, 329, 330, 331, 332, 333, 334, 335

J

jails, 34, 186, 187
JAMA, 133, 156, 160, 161, 164, 165, 166, 179, 183, 185, 190, 191, 192, 196, 202, 205, 207, 215, 217
Japan, 23, 167
jewelry, 51
joints, 139
Jordan, 154
jurisdiction, 342
juvenile idiopathic arthritis, 187

K

Katrina, 171
Kentucky, 153
keratoconjunctivitis, 36, 61, 184, 210, 229
kidney, 190
kidney transplant, 190
kidney transplantation, 190
killing, 89
knee arthroplasty, 262
knee replacement, 304, 305

L

labor, 303
lamina, 32, 80
laminar, 32, 80
language, 50, 73, 84
large-scale, 171
laser, 149
Lassa fever, 29, 112, 172, 173
late-onset, 188
latex, 52, 205
laundering, 66, 67
laundry, 66, 67, 83, 90, 126, 137, 214
law, 59, 146, 312, 326, 338, 339
laws, 79, 238, 342
lead, 31, 34, 237, 280, 285, 292, 294, 298, 301, 322, 325, 326
leadership, 42, 48, 191, 241, 268, 271, 292, 297, 320, 322
League of Nations, 136
leakage, 57, 139, 147
learning, 50, 192, 202, 284
left ventricular, 31, 174
legal protection, 327
Legionella, 17, 18, 117, 143
legislation, 49, 295
legislative, 59
lenses, 55
Leprosy, 110, 112
lesions, 26, 63, 64, 97, 98, 102, 105, 111, 114, 115, 117, 122, 124, 125, 127, 132, 135, 136, 149

lettuce, 172
leukemia, 39, 162, 187
Liberia, 172
lice, 37, 113, 116
licensing, 146, 310
life-threatening, 31
likelihood, 33, 49, 78, 92, 123, 300
limitation, 176, 348
limitations, 234, 241, 263, 266, 343, 345, 351, 352
linen, 54, 214, 224
linkage, 169
Listeria monocytogenes, 114, 230
location, 52, 66, 130, 144, 292, 296, 306, 347
London, 226
long distance, 14, 15, 16, 77
longitudinal study, 181
long-term, 1, 7, 8, 33, 35, 40, 47, 60, 83, 92, 93, 95, 96, 98, 156, 162, 165, 171, 179, 180, 181, 182, 183, 192, 194, 198, 200, 211, 215, 219, 339
Los Angeles, 156, 163, 184
low birthweight, 178
low risk, 101, 130, 205
lower respiratory tract infection, 181
lumbar, 73, 75, 91, 217
lumbar puncture, 73, 75, 91, 217
lumen, 52
lung, 74, 105, 130
lung disease, 74
lungs, 280
lymph, 134, 216
lymph node, 134
lymphadenopathy, 216
lymphocytes, 167
lymphogranuloma venereum, 104
lymphoid, 24
lymphoid tissue, 24

M

mad cow disease, 23
Maine, 186, 271, 303, 305, 306, 308, 309, 339

Mainland China, 24
maintenance, 50, 57, 83, 144, 148, 298, 347
malaise, 132, 133, 135, 136
malaria, 41, 190, 230
malignancy, 11
malnutrition, 35, 145
Malta, 104
management, 21, 22, 30, 46, 66, 67, 68, 79, 82, 83, 98, 115, 120, 146, 148, 152, 162, 165, 166, 173, 180, 191, 196, 201, 214, 216
mandates, 257, 352
manufacturer, 55, 64, 89, 91, 259
manufacturing, 13, 53, 157
market, 271
marrow, 144
Marx, 153, 171
Maryland, 171, 285, 303, 305, 306, 308, 311, 338
mask, 2, 4, 14, 25, 54, 55, 56, 62, 64, 70, 72, 74, 75, 77, 78, 87, 91, 95, 96, 97, 98, 103, 104, 111, 112, 113, 119, 120, 125, 129, 133, 138, 139, 148, 149, 207
masking, 78
Massachusetts, 303, 305, 306, 308
MDR, 20, 61, 65, 79
measles, 15, 16, 33, 36, 49, 58, 62, 69, 77, 96, 97, 98, 120, 129, 152, 226, 227
measurement, 298, 328
measures, 2, 5, 8, 9, 10, 18, 20, 26, 32, 34, 36, 38, 40, 41, 43, 46, 48, 58, 59, 61, 62, 68, 71, 73, 74, 83, 85, 88, 94, 105, 136, 146, 148, 166, 173, 197, 203, 207, 210, 217, 230, 244, 258, 262, 263, 265, 269, 271, 287, 291, 297, 300, 301, 302, 304, 305, 306, 307, 308, 311, 313, 336, 337, 338, 347
meat, 23
mechanical ventilation, 157, 307, 347
mechanical ventilator, 31
media, 75, 136, 299, 314, 325
median, 23
mediastinitis, 237

Medicaid, 35, 180, 234, 235, 237, 271, 272, 281, 293, 294, 298, 336, 342
medical care, 148, 259, 261, 288, 305, 307
medical products, 43
medical student, 158, 201, 203
Medicare, 35, 180, 234, 235, 236, 237, 241, 257, 258, 260, 263, 265, 266, 269, 271, 272, 280, 281, 284, 286, 293, 294, 298, 336, 337, 338, 342, 343, 344, 346
medication, 74, 75, 91, 136, 145, 149, 307
medications, 11, 17, 26, 74, 90, 91
medicine, 190, 236, 342
Mediterranean, 104
membranes, 59, 111
meningitis, 2, 75, 114, 123, 132, 217, 218
meningococcemia, 157, 159
meta-analysis, 215
methicillin-resistant, 20, 151, 152, 153, 154, 157, 165, 176, 179, 187, 188, 193, 194, 203, 210, 219, 220, 222, 224, 225, 236, 261, 271, 293, 294
metropolitan area, 285, 292, 296, 329, 339
microbes, 279
microbial, 155, 195, 204
microorganism, 93, 143, 334
microorganisms, 10, 11, 12, 18, 20, 34, 53, 60, 66, 76, 82, 137, 143, 145, 149
microscopy, 135
military, 22, 166, 217, 228
Minnesota, 179, 198, 285, 303, 305, 306, 307, 308, 309
misleading, 309
Mississippi, 156, 187
Missouri, 295, 303, 305, 306, 307, 308, 309, 310, 312, 346
mites, 12, 142
mobile device, 90
modalities, 31
models, 57
modules, 311
monkeys, 173
monoclonal, 69, 145
monoclonal antibodies, 145
monoclonal antibody, 69
mononucleosis, 112

Monroe, 229
mood, 76
morbidity, 19, 21, 31, 34, 40, 48, 163, 178, 181
morning, 123
morphology, 134
mortality, 19, 21, 25, 28, 29, 31, 34, 40, 48, 152, 163, 175, 177, 178, 181, 215, 292, 294
mosquitoes, 17
mothers, 33
mouse, 136
mouth, 13, 25, 29, 54, 55, 56, 59, 73, 87, 110, 123, 125, 133, 137, 138, 146, 147, 148, 149, 287
movement, 93, 95, 98, 301
MRSA, 2, 7, 13, 18, 19, 20, 32, 33, 35, 36, 38, 48, 51, 52, 53, 61, 65, 68, 69, 79, 85, 107, 115, 117, 130, 131, 147, 150, 182, 186, 206, 209, 211, 214, 223, 224, 236, 260, 261, 262, 266, 271, 285, 288, 289, 291, 292, 293, 294, 295, 296, 297, 298, 299, 300, 302, 311, 313, 314, 316, 317, 318, 319, 320, 321, 322, 323, 324, 325, 326, 328, 329, 330, 331, 332, 333, 334, 335, 336, 339, 340
mucormycosis, 126
mucosa, 13
mucous membrane, 12, 52, 55, 59, 72, 77, 85, 86, 87, 118, 122, 128, 133, 137, 147, 149
mucous membranes, 52, 55, 59, 72, 85, 86, 87, 133, 137, 147, 149
multidisciplinary, 46, 146, 178
multidrug-resistant tuberculosis, 197, 212
mumps, 227
musculoskeletal, 190
myalgia, 24
Mycobacterium, 9, 10, 15, 56, 99, 150, 155, 156, 159, 160, 184, 206, 207, 208, 212, 227, 245
Mycoplasma pneumoniae infection, 158
myelogram, 73, 75
myeloid, 187
myocardial infarction, 31

N

nation, 6, 34, 263
national, 20, 30, 44, 115, 178, 185, 192, 195, 208, 234, 237, 241, 253, 256, 258, 259, 261, 265, 266, 268, 269, 271, 280, 285, 286, 288, 289, 343, 344, 345, 346, 352, 353
National Hospital Discharge Survey, 267, 289, 352
National Institute for Occupational Safety and Health, 7, 148
National Institutes of Health, 142, 281
natural, 15, 16, 32, 33, 58, 78, 86, 134, 135, 204, 205, 226
nausea, 27, 132
Nebraska, 184, 336
neck, 54, 336
needles, 58, 74, 90, 128, 137
negative consequences, 250
neonatal, 33, 105, 113, 122, 151, 152, 178, 193, 203, 204, 206, 210, 216, 228, 229, 230, 231, 292, 297, 314
neonatal intensive care unit, 151, 152, 178, 193, 203, 204, 206, 210, 216, 228, 229, 231, 292, 297, 314
neonates, 19, 84, 106, 114, 131, 178, 211, 230
Netherlands, 19, 163, 227
neural tissue, 106
neutralization, 133
neutropenia, 39
Nevada, 336
New England, 283
New Jersey, 296, 303, 305, 306, 308, 309, 311
New York, 136, 156, 184, 194, 221, 285, 295, 303, 305, 306, 308, 309, 310, 312, 327, 329
NICU, 7, 31, 33, 68, 70, 87, 119, 121, 200
Nile, 40, 103, 189, 228
NIS, 352
normal, 11, 35, 143, 145, 227, 292, 297, 320, 321
norms, 46

North America, 19, 23, 103, 163
North Carolina, 156
nosocomial pneumonia, 175
not-for-profit, 272
nuclei, 14, 15, 120, 142, 143, 148, 149, 157, 159
nurse, 2, 4, 20, 42, 44, 82, 186, 193, 194, 206, 220, 231
nurses, 3, 4, 44, 47, 82, 145, 157, 186, 196, 197, 201, 202, 211, 303
nursing, 27, 33, 34, 38, 44, 50, 77, 83, 145, 146, 155, 156, 171, 177, 180, 181, 182, 183, 192, 194, 200, 206, 211, 212, 219, 223, 228, 231, 272, 281, 294, 300, 322
nursing home, 27, 33, 34, 77, 146, 155, 171, 180, 181, 182, 183, 192, 194, 200, 211, 212, 219, 228, 231, 281, 294, 300
nutrient, 299
nutrition, 38

O

obligate, 16
observations, 2, 9, 28, 182, 214, 225, 254
obstructive lung disease, 74
occupational, 26, 33, 37, 41, 42, 47, 50, 56, 68, 81, 82, 128, 145, 155, 169, 197, 214
occupational groups, 47
occupational health, 33, 42, 82
occupational therapy, 37, 145
Office of Management and Budget, 281
Ohio, 156, 336
oil, 230
Oklahoma, 184, 303, 305, 306, 307, 308, 338
old age, 344, 347
older adults, 181
oncology, 33, 39, 51, 74, 83, 156, 185, 210, 212, 225
online, 9, 84
on-line, 202
onychomycosis, 153, 204
oral, 12, 59, 67, 75, 111, 137, 173, 292, 298, 328, 348

oral hygiene, 348
Oregon, 153, 285, 303, 305, 306, 308, 338
organ, 11, 31, 80, 103, 118, 155, 188, 189, 190, 228
organic, 65, 89
organism, 6, 11, 18, 61, 85, 125, 136, 145, 218, 236, 261, 262, 293, 299, 300
organization, 41, 42, 45, 46, 48, 81, 83, 84, 142, 143, 146, 238, 239, 243, 272, 337, 338
organizations, 41, 45, 82, 196, 200, 234, 237, 238, 240, 242, 243, 249, 250, 253, 254, 267, 270, 283, 295, 301, 303
orientation, 50, 83
osteomyelitis, 204
otitis externa, 152
outpatient, 35, 36, 37, 62, 73, 83, 88, 142, 146, 183, 184, 285, 323
outpatients, 225
oversight, 43, 46, 75, 83, 146, 246, 281, 323
oxygenation, 31, 174
oxyuriasis, 107

P

pacemakers, 31
Pacific, 316, 317, 329, 330, 331, 333, 334, 335
pain, 74, 224
pain clinic, 74
palivizumab, 216
pandemic, 9, 16, 26, 43, 58, 60, 62, 70, 95, 112
Parainfluenza, 116, 225
paralysis, 133
parasites, 11, 113
parenteral, 74, 91
parenting, 178
Paris, 178, 203
parotitis, 115
particles, 14, 15, 16, 25, 28, 29, 55, 56, 99, 100, 139, 142, 143, 145, 148, 149, 227
partnership, 271
passive, 70

pathogenesis, 14, 145, 175, 187
pathogenic, 10, 11, 13, 51, 66, 162
pathogens, 2, 3, 4, 7, 8, 11, 12, 13, 14, 15, 17, 18, 20, 31, 33, 34, 35, 36, 37, 40, 41, 45, 48, 51, 52, 61, 65, 66, 67, 71, 74, 76, 77, 78, 82, 85, 87, 88, 89, 91, 94, 101, 128, 129, 131, 142, 143, 148, 151, 154, 155, 164, 169, 182, 194, 197, 201, 205, 208, 213, 220, 221, 223, 261, 285, 286, 289, 294, 296, 298, 311
Pathologists, 168
patient care, 7, 9, 20, 29, 37, 44, 46, 51, 52, 53, 54, 58, 59, 66, 72, 74, 82, 83, 86, 87, 89, 90, 111, 113, 117, 144, 147, 204, 213, 254, 263
patient management, 46, 196, 201
PCR, 19, 22, 25, 116, 132, 134, 135, 136, 195, 223, 293, 299, 314, 319, 324, 325, 340
PDAs, 66
pediatric, 13, 31, 32, 33, 34, 35, 58, 64, 70, 90, 105, 112, 116, 153, 154, 155, 156, 159, 176, 177, 178, 179, 185, 193, 194, 195, 198, 202, 203, 208, 210, 211, 217, 222, 223, 228
pediatric patients, 13, 33, 58, 70, 90, 155, 177, 202
pediatrician, 155
peer, 343
penicillin, 20, 227
Pennsylvania, 153, 164, 189, 237, 280, 283, 296, 303, 305, 306, 307, 308, 309, 310, 312, 339
peptic ulcer, 307
peptic ulcer disease, 307
perception, 180
perceptions, 48, 76, 148, 202
performance, 20, 42, 47, 55, 58, 59, 83, 146, 192, 207, 237, 239, 243, 244, 251, 252, 253, 255, 258, 272, 283, 289, 292, 296, 297, 298, 321, 322, 323, 326, 327, 328, 343
performance indicator, 83
perinatal, 214
periodic, 45, 50, 57, 242

peripheral blood, 144, 188
peritoneal, 37
permit, 90
personal, 4, 5, 13, 21, 22, 26, 37, 47, 50, 54, 55, 60, 66, 67, 83, 93, 95, 98, 124, 128, 148, 199
personal hygiene, 60, 67
personnel costs, 337
pertussis, 11, 14, 33, 34, 46, 49, 62, 68, 69, 70, 74, 77, 85, 126, 131, 153, 158, 181, 195, 201, 211, 214, 215
Pharyngeal, 106
phenolic, 28
Philadelphia, 154, 171, 188, 213, 221, 227, 229
PHS, 231
physical therapy, 142
physicians, 19, 47, 62, 145, 197, 202, 218, 297, 303, 320, 322, 323, 337
physiotherapy, 13, 40, 157
pilot study, 214, 338
pituitary, 23, 167
placental, 144
plague, 21, 22, 134, 136, 166
planning, 9, 18, 26, 43, 46, 60, 82, 146
plants, 80, 100, 140, 147, 220
Plasmodium falciparum, 230
plastic, 32, 66, 88, 94
play, 33, 90, 204
pleural, 132
pleural effusion, 132
pneumococcus, 164
pneumonia, 44, 48, 102, 114, 115, 117, 125, 131, 136, 152, 154, 174, 175, 181, 201, 203, 209, 230, 231, 236, 246, 249, 257, 260, 261, 264, 283, 287, 294, 298, 299, 301, 339, 342, 344, 352
poisoning, 105, 107
polio, 107
polymerase, 136, 196, 211, 293, 299
polymerase chain reaction, 136, 196, 211, 293, 299
polymorphism, 159
poor, 35, 38, 60, 86, 194, 254

population, 23, 30, 31, 32, 34, 43, 46, 73, 81, 84, 154, 176, 181, 186, 208, 218, 227, 245, 261, 263, 264, 265, 266, 288, 289, 292, 296, 300, 316, 329
pores, 17
pork, 122
ports, 139
positive feedback, 323
postoperative, 154, 177, 200, 259, 260, 261, 262, 305, 307
postpartum, 153, 162
poultry, 163
powder, 103, 132, 133
preclinical, 199, 202
predictors, 11, 196
pregnant, 99, 106, 120, 125
pregnant women, 99, 125
prehospital, 198
premature infant, 231
preparedness, 18, 21, 43, 146, 150, 165
Prescription Drug, Improvement, and Modernization Act, 286
president, 328
pressure, 5, 16, 58, 66, 77, 80, 86, 93, 96, 99, 100, 118, 139, 142, 148, 149, 152, 162, 181, 208, 280, 299
pressure gauge, 139
pressure sore, 118
preterm infants, 229
prevention of infection, 35, 39
preventive, 18, 84, 155, 158, 214, 283
primary care, 49
primary caregivers, 49
primates, 29, 132
prion diseases, 23, 168
prions, 3, 11, 18, 23, 24
priorities, 30, 60, 235, 268, 348
prisons, 34, 186, 300
privacy, 92, 95, 318
private, 40, 60, 74, 78, 117, 145, 184, 209, 237, 238, 242, 265, 267, 271, 283, 300, 320, 331, 332
probability, 289
process control, 49, 200, 222

production, 11, 19, 62, 65, 73, 94, 136, 163
professions, 50
profit, 272
program, 5, 22, 34, 42, 43, 46, 51, 57, 59, 68, 77, 81, 84, 115, 144, 146, 167, 180, 193, 195, 197, 198, 199, 201, 203, 234, 240, 241, 249, 250, 251, 252, 253, 257, 258, 263, 264, 265, 266, 269, 272, 280, 281, 283, 284, 285, 286, 288, 289, 298, 307, 310, 312, 322, 334, 343
proliferation, 145
promote, 44, 64, 72, 222, 233, 234, 238, 240, 243, 244, 249, 267, 268, 270, 292, 297, 298, 320, 338
property, iv, 83
prophylactic, 32
prophylaxis, 39, 69, 103, 104, 116, 118, 122, 125, 133, 135, 176, 199, 214, 215, 249, 283
prostration, 136
protection, 13, 15, 25, 28, 29, 39, 43, 48, 52, 54, 55, 56, 57, 58, 72, 73, 75, 77, 79, 80, 83, 87, 91, 95, 97, 98, 100, 111, 113, 120, 125, 126, 129, 130, 134, 137, 138, 139, 149, 150, 186, 205, 207, 208, 227, 327
protective clothing, 103, 133, 206
protein, 23
protocol, 32, 286, 353
protocols, 40, 66, 257, 258, 262, 272, 300, 301, 304, 307, 311, 312, 317, 326, 337, 339
pseudomembranous colitis, 19
Pseudomonas, 13, 18, 37, 61, 143, 152, 153, 154, 156, 157, 175, 176, 177, 185, 188, 189, 204, 212, 221
Pseudomonas aeruginosa, 13, 18, 37, 61, 143, 152, 154, 156, 157, 175, 177, 185, 188, 204, 212
PSI, 236, 259, 294, 307
psychiatric hospitals, 146
psychological injury, 284
psychosocial factors, 60
Pub Med, 8
public, 4, 21, 22, 23, 26, 35, 43, 46, 48, 49, 70, 126, 142, 147, 165, 166, 168, 169, 186, 193, 198, 201, 237, 238, 243, 261, 265, 271, 281, 291, 293, 295, 296, 297, 298, 302, 304, 307, 309, 310, 311, 317, 326, 327, 328, 330, 331, 332, 336, 342, 343, 344, 346
public awareness, 317, 331, 332
public education, 330
public health, 21, 22, 23, 26, 35, 46, 48, 126, 142, 147, 165, 166, 168, 169, 186
Public Health Service, 41, 190, 208, 214, 232, 281, 286
Puerto Rico, 228
pulse, 86
pumps, 65
pyelonephritis, 124

Q

Q fever, 118
quality assurance, 193, 272
quality control, 46
quality improvement, 191, 192, 259, 271, 309, 313
Quebec, 163
questionnaire, 70

R

Rabies, 118, 231
rabies virus, 190, 231
race, 185
radiation, 11, 145
radiation therapy, 11
radiological, 260
rain, 26
rain forest, 26
random, 162, 258, 264, 286, 345
random amplified polymorphic DNA, 162
range, 14, 15, 23, 34, 145, 227, 258, 263, 264, 287, 345
rash, 28, 62, 113, 120, 135
rat, 121

Index

rats, 17, 26
reading, 84
reaffirmation, 2
receptacle, 138, 148
reception, 62, 73, 88, 138, 148
recognition, 18, 26, 57, 158, 313
recombination, 40
recovery, 158
recurrence, 284
reduction, 60, 268, 292, 293, 296, 297, 313, 314, 317, 318, 319, 320, 321, 322, 323, 324, 325, 326, 328, 336, 339
reflection, 14
refractory, 187
regional, 30, 85, 115, 153, 197, 203, 220
regression, 8, 150
regular, 44, 90, 243, 255
regulation, 81, 146, 237, 280
regulations, 35, 59, 66, 67, 79, 295
rehabilitation, 33, 35, 43, 119, 142, 145, 146, 203, 231
reimbursement, 60
reinforcement, 72
relationship, 60, 182, 192, 197
relationships, 44, 139
relevance, 164, 225
reliability, 234, 241, 256, 263, 265, 266
remediation, 224
renal, 31, 219
renal failure, 31
replication, 40
reprocessing, 13, 24, 66, 94, 221
Republic of the Congo, 170, 172, 173
research, 38, 43, 146, 186, 200, 240, 242, 270, 271, 299, 328, 338, 348
researchers, 249, 288, 300, 303, 338
reservoir, 5, 10, 17, 32, 33, 35, 37, 60, 64, 154, 225
reservoirs, 10, 26, 65, 212, 213, 220
residential, 34, 61, 63, 70, 92, 93, 95, 98, 146, 155, 228
resistance, 18, 19, 20, 28, 33, 35, 37, 45, 89, 149, 150, 155, 163, 164, 165, 174, 180, 181, 191, 192, 194, 195, 196, 205, 212, 261, 271, 279, 294, 300, 301, 334, 336
resolution, 120
resources, 21, 30, 42, 45, 49, 67, 78, 81, 82, 88, 171, 209, 292, 295, 296, 297, 300, 312, 313, 319, 321, 324, 325, 326, 327
respirator, 15, 25, 56, 57, 58, 59, 77, 78, 80, 97, 98, 100, 103, 111, 113, 125, 136, 138, 139, 148, 207
respiratory failure, 31, 133
respiratory syncytial virus, 11, 13, 14, 18, 144, 152, 153, 156, 158, 159, 181, 196, 201, 207, 209, 210, 211, 231
respiratory therapist, 145
responsibilities, 42
restaurant, 161
restriction fragment length polymorphis, 159
resuscitation, 47, 59, 137, 198, 199
retention, 45
retirement, 146
retroviruses, 40
rheumatoid arthritis, 187
rhinorrhea, 73
ringworm, 122, 231
risk assessment, 43, 82, 145
risk factors, 11, 35, 84, 92, 155, 172, 179, 181, 182, 184, 185, 187, 189, 209, 210, 216, 219, 225, 229, 231, 343, 344, 347
RNA, 25
rotavirus, 15, 18, 33, 61, 62, 65, 89, 131, 144, 153, 160, 178, 210, 211, 213, 219, 223, 225, 230
RSV infection, 207
rubber, 205
rubella, 69, 105, 110, 120, 227
rubeola, 15, 33, 36, 77, 97, 98, 113
rural, 43, 170, 193, 329

S

safety, 2, 4, 5, 6, 41, 42, 46, 48, 59, 67, 81, 91, 96, 126, 129, 134, 137, 148, 168, 190, 191, 196, 197, 208, 222, 237, 243,

249, 250, 259, 269, 281, 287, 305, 328, 336, 346
saline, 74, 230
saliva, 118
Salmonella, 109, 124
sample, 42, 241, 256, 258, 259, 260, 261, 263, 264, 265, 267, 286, 287, 292, 310, 343, 344, 345, 346, 352
sampling, 156
SARS, 2, 3, 7, 9, 14, 16, 18, 24, 25, 26, 43, 48, 49, 57, 60, 61, 62, 63, 70, 72, 73, 76, 77, 87, 95, 106, 120, 130, 138, 142, 148, 151, 157, 158, 159, 160, 169, 201, 211, 212
SARS-CoV, 2, 9, 14, 16, 18, 25, 26, 60, 72, 77, 106, 142, 148
savings, 326
scabies, 12, 37, 38, 155
scheduling, 64
Schmid, 226
school, 27, 34, 88, 158, 161
scores, 302
search, 8, 296
seasonality, 213
segregation, 40, 63, 185
selecting, 49, 52, 57, 242, 258, 261, 304, 309, 325
self-assessment, 244
self-care, 146
self-monitoring, 156
self-report, 47, 307
sensing, 96
sensitivity, 46, 52, 324, 334
sensors, 221
sensory symptoms, 23
separation, 25, 36, 73, 76, 77, 88, 138, 148
sepsis, 48, 114, 121, 154, 259, 262, 287, 288, 305, 308
septicemia, 134, 193
series, 7, 26, 271, 302, 337
serologic test, 98
serology, 132, 133, 134, 136
serum, 136
services, 33, 37, 43, 45, 46, 94, 144, 145, 146, 272, 284, 289, 326, 342

severe acute respiratory syndrome, 2, 106, 130, 150, 151, 157, 159, 160, 161, 168, 169, 211, 225
severity, 11, 18, 19, 26, 145, 163, 255, 301
sexual contact, 104, 113
shape, 58
sharing, 26, 76, 89
sheep, 23
shelter, 38, 186
Shigella, 109, 131
shingles, 111
shock, 121, 122, 132, 133
short supply, 92, 94
sibling, 32, 70
siblings, 40, 70, 227
signs, 9, 24, 68, 70, 73, 74, 78, 83, 88, 94, 96, 131, 132, 260, 299, 318, 331, 332
Singapore, 24, 169
sinusitis, 152
sites, 1, 21, 22, 30, 38, 53, 55, 61, 124, 143, 167, 255, 285, 289, 335
skills, 199
skin, 11, 12, 28, 29, 33, 35, 37, 51, 52, 54, 55, 59, 62, 64, 68, 72, 75, 85, 86, 87, 93, 97, 98, 102, 111, 117, 119, 120, 121, 133, 135, 137, 147, 149, 173, 178, 184, 187, 226, 231, 236, 262, 287, 299, 306, 307, 316, 335
smallpox, 14, 15, 17, 21, 22, 26, 27, 43, 57, 69, 78, 97, 98, 99, 114, 125, 129, 148, 158, 160, 165, 166, 167, 227, 246
smoke, 96, 99, 139
social services, 145
socialization, 46
sodium, 65
software, 49, 313
solid waste, 67
solutions, 36, 96, 108, 109, 323
sorting, 161
South Carolina, 158, 303, 305, 306, 308, 309, 310, 315, 317, 329, 330, 331, 333, 334, 335
spatial, 73, 76, 138, 148
species, 36, 75, 107, 108, 109, 162, 165, 174, 186, 188, 204, 223

specificity, 46, 241, 269
spectrum, 2, 6, 11, 20, 35, 147, 152, 177, 204
speculation, 29, 75
speech, 145
sperm, 228
spermatozoa, 104
spills, 65
spinal anesthesia, 75
spinal tap, 218
spine, 316
sporadic, 19, 23, 209
spore, 19, 65, 80, 103, 133
sports, 22
sputum, 94, 123, 128, 134, 136, 149
SSI, 236, 258, 260, 261, 294, 298, 304, 342, 346, 352
St. Louis, 175
staffing, 2, 4, 20, 26, 42, 43, 44, 60, 61, 64, 82, 191, 193, 194, 196, 220
stages, 126
stakeholders, 270
standardized testing, 149
standards, 77, 142, 195, 205, 234, 237, 238, 239, 240, 242, 243, 248, 250, 251, 252, 253, 254, 255, 267, 268, 269, 270, 281, 282, 284, 291, 296, 297, 298, 336, 343
Standards, 6, 7, 45, 195, 242, 243, 250, 251, 254, 338
staphylococcal, 107, 119, 120, 122, 193, 231
staphylococci, 165, 222
Staphylococcus aureus, 7, 11, 20, 31, 61, 117, 131, 143, 151, 152, 153, 154, 157, 159, 163, 164, 165, 176, 179, 182, 183, 186, 187, 188, 193, 194, 203, 206, 210, 215, 216, 218, 219, 220, 222, 224, 225, 236, 261, 271, 288, 289, 292, 293, 294, 336
state laws, 79, 342
state legislatures, 238
statistical analysis, 49
statistics, 289, 303
STD, 186

stem cell transplantation, 219
sterile, 54, 74, 75, 90, 91, 288, 306, 307, 347
sterilization, 13, 65, 89, 106, 168, 212, 242, 246, 254, 344, 347, 351
stethoscope, 66, 94
stigma, 76
stock, 53
stool culture, 79
stool cultures, 79
storage, 66, 222, 347
strain, 18, 19, 27, 156, 162, 163, 165, 168, 171, 173, 185
strains, 20, 27, 40, 80, 112, 153, 165, 167, 334
strategic, 88, 165, 324
strategies, 17, 34, 44, 49, 50, 80, 84, 85, 99, 146, 155, 158, 174, 192, 203, 215, 227, 242, 249, 270, 271, 283, 295, 296, 343, 344, 347
strength, 67, 127, 233, 240, 244, 246, 250, 268, 282
streptococci, 162, 217
strokes, 31
students, 50, 83, 158, 198, 199, 201, 202, 203, 217
subgroups, 12
substance abuse, 142
substances, 109, 128
substitution, 334
suburbs, 339
suffering, 267, 268
summaries, 71
summer, 189
supervisors, 149
supply, 91, 99, 139, 264, 322, 331, 332
support services, 37
suppression, 39
surface area, 31
surgeries, 262, 287, 310
surgery, 29, 43, 153, 168, 196, 199, 201, 204, 237, 242, 254, 258, 260, 261, 262, 264, 265, 280, 294, 298, 299, 302, 305, 306, 307, 308, 335, 338

surgical, 13, 24, 35, 42, 46, 48, 50, 52, 55, 57, 58, 62, 69, 73, 91, 97, 98, 105, 111, 120, 125, 138, 144, 146, 147, 148, 149, 153, 174, 184, 194, 199, 200, 209, 215, 217, 218, 225, 228, 236, 249, 253, 257, 258, 261, 264, 265, 266, 268, 271, 283, 294, 298, 305, 306, 307, 313, 314, 316, 337, 339, 342, 344
surgical intervention, 144
surveillance, 3, 4, 5, 19, 20, 23, 24, 34, 37, 40, 42, 43, 45, 48, 49, 82, 84, 146, 161, 173, 179, 180, 183, 185, 186, 192, 193, 194, 200, 208, 211, 220, 242, 252, 253, 271, 281, 284, 285, 289, 293, 300, 316, 328, 334, 338, 348, 353
survey design, 267
survival, 181, 182
susceptibility, 11, 30, 31, 34, 45, 63, 82, 145, 163, 164, 195, 196, 301, 311
sweat, 29, 72, 128, 149
swelling, 115
Switzerland, 158, 170, 281
symptoms, 2, 9, 23, 24, 25, 62, 70, 74, 78, 83, 88, 94, 96, 110, 112, 120, 131, 132, 145, 148, 260, 299
syndrome, 7, 11, 30, 102, 110, 112, 119, 120, 121, 122, 158, 169, 216, 227, 231
syphilis, 38, 122
systems, 11, 15, 17, 41, 42, 45, 49, 70, 82, 83, 90, 97, 127, 131, 145, 179, 212, 220, 254, 261, 270, 271, 283, 284, 291, 292, 293, 295, 296, 297, 298, 301, 302, 304, 308, 309, 310, 311, 312, 313, 318, 320, 321, 322, 323, 324, 326, 328, 338

T

Taiwan, 216
target population, 321
target populations, 321
T-cell, 39, 219
teaching, 50, 155, 198, 201, 202, 203, 221, 292, 296, 329
teaching strategies, 203
technical assistance, 249, 271, 312

technician, 325
technicians, 50, 83
technology, 31, 48, 143, 145, 194, 221, 312
temperature, 14, 221
temporal, 18
Tennessee, 285, 303, 305, 306, 308
terminally ill, 70
terminals, 224
terrorism, 165
Tetanus, 122
Texas, 171, 179, 186, 303, 305, 306, 308, 309, 338
textbooks, 101
textiles, 66, 67, 90
therapists, 50, 145
therapy, 20, 37, 39, 40, 79, 122, 123, 127, 135, 145, 164, 167, 185, 188, 189, 194, 219, 300, 335
third-generation cephalosporin, 175
threat, 2, 163
threatening, 2, 236
threats, 30
throat, 133, 287
thymus, 280
time, 4, 8, 11, 15, 19, 21, 23, 25, 29, 31, 34, 35, 40, 42, 49, 50, 51, 57, 58, 69, 71, 78, 81, 83, 84, 97, 100, 127, 135, 143, 144, 147, 198, 246, 258, 269, 280, 299, 304, 306, 307, 318, 322, 323, 324, 325, 326, 328, 339, 340
timing, 312
tinea corporis, 231
tissue, 24, 35, 41, 65, 73, 103, 105, 106, 118, 145, 186, 187, 190, 262, 287, 316
title, 282
T-lymphocytes, 167
tolerance, 222
total joint replacements, 316
toxic, 57, 158
toxin, 19, 22, 108, 133, 163, 166
toxins, 19
tracers, 244
trachea, 280
tracking, 43, 49, 162, 318, 320

traction, 267
training, 4, 20, 44, 48, 49, 50, 72, 75, 81, 83, 84, 143, 144, 145, 148, 149, 199, 201, 202, 217, 249, 256, 272, 291, 297, 298, 312, 317, 330, 331, 332, 333
training programs, 75, 84, 272
transfer, 12, 13, 22, 35, 93, 96, 137, 149, 166, 222
transfusion, 40, 103, 113, 119
transition, 1, 301
translation, 270
transplant, 2, 4, 6, 9, 83, 99, 103, 106, 139, 147, 151, 153, 161, 162, 187, 188, 189, 190, 219, 221, 225, 228, 231
transplant recipients, 151, 155, 189, 190, 228
transplantation, 40, 41, 105, 144, 188, 190, 206, 219, 225, 229
transport, 63, 66, 93, 94, 95, 98, 220, 340
trauma, 31, 177, 198, 199
travel, 13, 15, 25, 28, 30, 129, 130
trench mouth, 125
trend, 49, 60, 82, 176, 259
triage, 73, 83, 88, 97, 138, 148
trial, 147, 152, 167, 215, 217, 271
trichinosis, 41
tuberculosis, 9, 10, 12, 14, 15, 16, 35, 36, 37, 38, 43, 56, 57, 58, 59, 60, 62, 63, 64, 70, 73, 77, 79, 87, 96, 97, 98, 99, 100, 114, 123, 129, 130, 145, 148, 150, 153, 155, 156, 159, 160, 184, 186, 187, 197, 203, 206, 207, 208, 209, 212, 216, 218, 226, 227, 246
tularemia, 21, 22
twins, 178
typhus, 119, 124

U

U.S. Department of Agriculture, 329
ubiquitous, 17
ulcer, 106, 118, 226
umbilical cord, 68, 144
umbilical cord blood, 144
uncertainty, 16
uniform, 259, 265, 294, 352
unions, 303
United Kingdom, 23, 24
United States, 6, 16, 22, 23, 25, 26, 27, 28, 35, 37, 42, 69, 74, 136, 152, 163, 164, 166, 167, 171, 173, 174, 178, 183, 184, 186, 190, 193, 195, 208, 214, 215, 216, 222, 229, 231, 233, 234, 236, 242, 289, 291, 294, 300, 341, 342, 352
updating, 242, 252
upholstery, 80, 100, 147, 220
upper respiratory infection, 217
upper respiratory tract, 15, 74
urban areas, 289
urinary, 11, 35, 42, 44, 48, 124, 182, 236, 261, 289, 294, 298, 307, 342, 343, 347, 348
urinary tract, 42, 44, 48, 236, 261, 289, 294, 298, 307, 342
urinary tract infection, 42, 44, 48, 236, 261, 289, 294, 298, 307, 342
urine, 64, 86, 105, 128
US Department of Health and Human Services, 232
Utah, 336
UV light, 16

V

vaccination, 22, 32, 43, 49, 50, 68, 97, 124, 125, 135, 152, 166, 167, 201, 208, 215, 226, 227, 242, 245, 306, 307
vaccinations, 240, 251, 254
vaccine, 21, 22, 27, 43, 46, 68, 69, 78, 97, 98, 99, 103, 110, 112, 113, 114, 116, 120, 121, 124, 125, 133, 135, 167, 201, 202, 215, 216, 226, 227, 246
vacuum, 140
validation, 255, 285, 304, 309, 310, 312, 313, 327
validity, 148, 263
valley fever, 105
values, 170
vancomycin, 19, 20, 37, 107, 152, 153, 156, 163, 164, 175, 176, 197, 203, 204,

205, 206, 209, 210, 212, 213, 216, 219, 224, 225, 236, 261, 271, 289, 334
variability, 52, 55
variable, 14, 152
variables, 84
variation, 168, 292, 309, 336, 346
vascular surgery, 262
vector, 17, 40
vehicles, 17
vein, 336
velocity, 14
venipuncture, 72
ventilation, 14, 15, 16, 38, 42, 59, 77, 80, 82, 128, 137, 139, 142, 149, 220, 226
ventilators, 31, 65
Vermont, 303, 305, 306, 307, 308, 309
vesicle, 132
vesicular rickettsiosis, 119
vessels, 67
Vibrio cholerae, 108
videotape, 47, 198
viral gastroenteritis, 170
viral hemorrhagic fever, 21, 28, 106, 112, 113
viral hepatitis, 74
viral infection, 33, 39, 91, 100, 210, 219
viral vectors, 40
virology, 170, 171
virulence, 11
virus infection, 107, 116, 119, 152, 153, 156, 159, 172, 173, 175, 187, 189, 190, 196, 201, 206, 207, 219, 224, 225, 229
viruses, 2, 3, 11, 13, 15, 16, 18, 22, 27, 28, 29, 33, 34, 36, 39, 40, 58, 59, 60, 62, 67, 70, 74, 87, 100, 101, 107, 112, 126, 129, 130, 142, 144, 161, 166, 170, 171, 172, 184, 196, 211, 342
visible, 51, 66, 85, 128
vision, 55, 133, 196
voice, 47, 199
vomiting, 27, 28, 132, 133, 135, 160
voting, 242

W

war, 60, 217, 266
warrants, 259
water, 17, 20, 27, 28, 51, 65, 67, 85, 86, 90, 99, 102, 103, 108, 133, 139, 143, 144, 162, 188
weakness, 133, 134
wear, 57, 62, 70, 72, 74, 76, 77, 78, 80, 86, 87, 95, 97, 98, 137, 138, 149, 317
weight loss, 136
West Africa, 26
West Nile virus, 103, 189, 228
Western Hemisphere, 170
whitlow, 12, 155
WHO, 7, 135, 236, 238, 250, 252, 253, 281, 284
whooping cough, 116
windows, 80, 103, 113, 139
winter, 26
Wisconsin, 181
women, 99, 120, 125, 153
work environment, 42, 46, 48, 148
workers, 6, 26, 36, 46, 47, 56, 75, 83, 125, 136, 148, 152, 158, 161, 165, 169, 170, 184, 185, 197, 198, 199, 201, 202, 203, 204, 205, 206, 208, 211, 215, 225, 226, 231, 239, 240, 242, 244, 251, 254, 256, 285, 298, 307, 317, 335
workflow, 292, 297, 320, 321
workforce, 46
working groups, 323
workload, 194
workplace, 143, 148, 197, 207, 216, 248
workspace, 74
World Health Organization, 7, 24, 236, 238, 281
World Health Organization (WHO), 24
wound healing, 35
wound infection, 31, 32, 175, 176, 177, 204, 212, 228, 289
wrists, 53

X

xenotransplantation, 41, 190

Y

yellow fever, 103
young adults, 217

Z

zoonotic, 41
zoonotic infections, 41